PSEUDOPHAKOS

PSEUDOPHAKOS

NORMAN S. JAFFE, M.D.

Clinical Professor of Ophthalmology,
Bascom Palmer Eye Institute,
University of Miami School of Medicine;
Chairman, Department of Ophthalmology,
St. Francis Hospital, Miami Beach, Florida

MILES A. GALIN, M.D.

Professor of Ophthalmology and
Director of Ophthalmic Research,
New York Medical College,
New York, New York

HENRY HIRSCHMAN, M.D.

Chief of Ophthalmology, Pacific Hospital,
Long Beach, California

HENRY M. CLAYMAN, M.D.

Clinical Assistant Professor of Ophthalmology,
Bascom Palmer Eye Institute,
University of Miami School of Medicine;
Clinical Professor of Health Sciences,
Miami-Dade Community College,
Miami, Florida

with 257 *illustrations*

The C. V. Mosby Company

Saint Louis 1978

Printed in the United States of America

The C. V. Mosby Company
11830 Westline Industrial Drive, St. Louis, Missouri 63141

Library of Congress Cataloging in Publication Data

Main entry under title:

Pseudophakos.

Includes index.
1. Intraocular lenses. I. Jaffe, Norman S.
[DNLM: 1. Cataract extraction. 2. Lenses.
3. Prosthesis. 4. Lens, Crystalline. WW354 P974]
RE988.P75 617.7'52 77-27307
ISBN 0-8016-2401-0

CB/CB/B 9 8 7 6 5 4 3 2 1

FOREWORD

Revolutionary ideas are shocking. Rarely was the ophthalmological profession shocked more than by the idea of replacing a cataractous crystalline with a clear artificial lens. Initially the idea aroused such an overwhelming interest among leading ophthalmologists all over the world that the subsequent setbacks were deeply disappointing and difficult to accept.

Together with a few others I was privileged to continue work in this fascinating field, despite the fact that this was not readily and not everywhere understood. The four authors of this book, however, did understand, and by their now longstanding and large experience they have contributed enormously to our present knowledge about the use and the usefulness of artificial intraocular lenses. The pseudophakos has now attained a definite place in the treatment of aphakia. Patients wearing a pseudophakos successfully are among the ophthalmologist's happiest patients. Surgical techniques develop slowly. It is felt that the ultimate surgical technique is still far away. Yet it is to be appreciated that the authors of this book have stayed with lens designs and surgical techniques that have proven valid for a long time. It can only be hoped that this attitude may be an example for the reader and the beginner in the field. For writing this book and for their continuing efforts to give instruction to their colleagues, as well as for their careful approach, the authors deserve our admiration and gratitude. I wish *Pseudophakos* a wide distribution to the benefit of the many patients in the world suffering from cataract.

Cornelius D. Binkhorst

PREFACE

Intraocular lens implant surgery has survived its early disastrous history. The scene of this turbulence was mainly European. It was not until 1967 that Americans began performing implant surgery in appreciable numbers. By this time most of the serious drawbacks of early implants had been eliminated. Nevertheless, very few innovations in ophthalmology have caused as much debate as lens implant surgery. Most American ophthalmologists have exercised extreme caution in undertaking implant surgery because of a knowledge of the earlier experience of implant surgeons, the medicolegal climate in the United States, and the system of federal surveillance of medical devices and medical practice.

Implant surgery is not an American innovation, but certainly the United States has become the central stage for this surgery. While it is recognized that cataract extraction has achieved an extremely high rate of success, surgeons have constantly sought better methods for the optical correction of aphakia. No one doubts that the quality of vision obtained with a pseudophakos in situ more closely resembles that of the phakic eye than any other known method. However, since the surgery is more complex than a routine cataract extraction, it is expected that the rate of complications would be somewhat higher. With refinements in techniques and the availability of higher quality implants, the rate of complication has significantly declined.

In writing this book, we concede that the technique of lens implant surgery is still controversial and its progress extremely dynamic; therefore much of the material may be obsolete by the time it appears in print. Also, it is impossible to cover every detail of surgical technique or to describe experience with every implant. However, our combined experience has been considerable, to date comprising more than 6000 intraocular lens implantations.

Intraocular implant lens surgery has a considerable scientific basis, and this is emphasized particularly in the introduction and in the chapters on theory of pseudophakos, the molecular basis of implant materials, sterilization techniques, and the preoperative calculation of intraocular lens power. There are also some controversial areas, such as the role of regulatory agencies in the use of intraocular lenses, implants in pediatric patients, and especially, the indications and contraindications for intraocular implant lens surgery. There is increasing clamor in the United States for a reasonable set of guidelines for intraocular implant lens surgery. It is hoped that this book will help set the tone for these guidelines. There are also new directions for implant surgery, and this is particularly emphasized in the chapter on the Choyce implant.

We realize that the surgical principles presented are somewhat biased in that they reflect our own personal opinions; however, we believe that these principles provide a framework for intraocular implant lens surgery as it is practiced today. The emphasis on complications is apparent and applies to all implants currently available.

We dedicate this book to C. D. Binkhorst of the Netherlands, who is the acknowledged father of modern implant surgery. Nothing epitomizes the greatness of this man better than the statement made about him when he received the Snellen Award in Ophthalmology in 1974: "His skill is only exceeded by his integrity."

Norman S. Jaffe
Miles A. Galin
Henry Hirschman
Henry M. Clayman

CONTENTS

CHAPTER 1

Introduction

There is no more exciting field of work than that involving alloplastic (man-made) materials. The uses of metals and plastics for standard procedures in medicine and surgery are increasing rapidly, and research is reaching out into hitherto untried fields. To those of us who are involved closely with it, it is surely the most rewarding area in which to work.

For centuries humankind has longed to remove nonfunctioning portions of the body and replace them with new ones so as to prolong life and promote good health. As the knowledge and experience of the surgeon has grown, homotransplants and heterotransplants have been tried with varying degrees of success.

Use of these tissues and organs is often complicated by the immune rejection mechanism and has been plagued and will continue to be plagued by other tremendous problems, including difficulties in sterilization and storage of these parts. Even when we have overcome the formidable technical problems involved in organ transplantation from human or other living creatures, there will still remain knotty moral and legal problems. The fact that our population is rapidly aging will be of little help to the solution of this problem. Demand for homograft replacements will far outnumber the supply. It is for these reasons that the development of artificial implants has the impetus to forge ahead.

But replacement of parts of the human body with artificial parts is a truly challenging task. This is a technologic venture requiring the utmost from materials and those who will be making the actual repairs. The human body presents an amazingly hostile environment. Body fluids are both corrosive and electrically conducting, and the spare part must be called upon to function continuously—hopefully without requiring any repair during the lifetime of the individual. The only fortunate factor in this environment is that the temperature remains constant and does not subject the spare part to extremes.

A survey of the field of alloplastic replacement reveals that achievements have been remarkable. In the light of history, even replacement of such a relatively simple structure as an artery would be a tremendous achievement, but when considering the artificial kidney, lung, and heart, as well as cardiac pacers and other heart assist devices, one can be sure that we have come a long way. Thousands of patients are now alive and productive because they have had access to the results of earlier research work.

Historically, sutures were the earliest implanted materials. These were not synthetic materials, but were artificial in the sense that they were not substances occurring naturally in the human body. The Romans used direct suturing of wounds for their gladiators.

The first restorative surgery utilizing alloplastic materials appears to have been a skull repair in 1890 by Fränkel. Although polystyrene and certain vinyls were encountered in the laboratory as early as 1828, their potential in all areas was not developed until perhaps a century later, and surgery lagged even further behind. During the past 30 years a wide spectrum of synthetic materials has become commercially available as chemists and manufacturers begin to see their tremendous potential. They vary from rubbery to hard, and their properties cover a wide range of physical characteristics. These materials were originally developed strictly for industrial purposes. Only the barest beginning has been made in developing materials primarily for biomedical uses.

Enterprising surgeons, seeing the wide vistas opening up before them by the appearance of these new materials, have seized upon them and, in collaboration with engineers, are bringing about a revolution in surgery. Some of the most dramatic achievements in that field have occurred in the past several decades and most particularly in the past 10 years.

Silver and gold have long been used for intimate association with body parts. More recently such metals as titanium, which combines strength and lightness with an admirable resistance to corrosion, have come upon the scene. Titanium, tantalum, certain stainless steels, and chromium-cobalt alloys have established themselves as less expensive alternatives. But it was the appearance of the new and versatile plastics that gave a tremendous boost to the development of the new field of biomedical engineering. Certain of these materials are of low biologic reactivity so that they can be implanted today not only for simple reinforcements or for tissue augmentation but also for replacement of a functioning part. The intracameral lens is a case in point.

Because the structures of the eye are so small and delicate, one would not expect alloplastic materials to be of value in ophthalmology. But the eye surgeon, aware of the great needs in his specialty, was among the first to recognize the potential of such synthetic materials. Some of the oldest replacement implants were in this field. Experimentation with replacement materials has been attempted in almost every condition calling for eye surgery. A great deal of such work is as yet in the experimental stages, but use of synthetic materials has been standard practice in certain procedures for years.

One has only to look at the medical literature to see the extent to which artificial materials are being used in reconstructive surgery. Literally thousands of papers have been published in this area, and it is gratifying to note how many successful uses there are in standard procedures and how many experimental projects are being undertaken. The hydrocephalus drain, the arteriovenous shunt, and the cardiac pacemaker are three examples of standard uses for alloplastic materials in the body. These have been placed in thousands of patients over the past 10 years with surprisingly uniform acceptance by the body.

As stated above, eye surgeons were among the first to adopt the use of these artificial materials in the body. The first alloplastic material to be used in ophthalmology was in the early 1940s, followed shortly by the use of various materials in retinal detachment surgery. Since that time the use of synthetics has been tried in every phase of ophthalmology. A definitive review of the use of synthetics in ophthalmology in 1955 contained 73 references. This list has greatly increased, particularly in the past decade.

Synthetic materials are now being universally used in the more complex cases of retinal detachment. They have long been used in replacement of the eye contents after evisceration and as a replacement for the eye following enucleation. Intraocular lenses have been made of a number of materials and in many designs, and their development is continuing apace. Synthetics have been used to make artificial corneas, corneal endothelia and epithelia as water-impervious barriers within the cornea itself to prevent edema, and sheets of synthetic material have been used to prevent adhesions of various parts of the eye following surgery.

Alloplastic materials are being used

widely to replace body defects in and around the eye and to correct enophthalmos. A number of procedures have been described to maintain the integrity of a nasolacrimal duct that was occluded before operation. Some experimental work with alloplastic materials has been carried on to place glaucoma drains, for refilling the cataractous lens following removal of its contents, to replace portions of the extraocular muscle, to replace the vitreous gel following retinal detachment, and to serve as a transparent bandage over a corneal blowout. Synthetic adhesives are beginning to be developed, and these may be of untold value in ophthalmic surgery in the future.

The increasing use of implants in ophthalmology is only a small chapter in the emergence of biomedical engineering as a subject of enormous importance and potential. It cannot be considered solely a triumph of innovative surgery but rather the interdisciplinary effort of clinicians, bioengineers, and medical scientists.

The ophthalmic surgeon who derives satisfaction from the successful implantation of an intraocular lens must not lose sight of the fact that he is indebted to many—to the wisdom and skill of those imaginative surgeons who have foreseen and developed the techniques of implantation and to the engineers and scientists who have produced and tested the hardware.

This book is not intended as a treatise on the biochemistry of intraocular implant materials. The authors are basically clinicians. We can only hope to present a reasonable scientific background for a comprehensive presentation of the clinical aspects of intraocular lens implantation. There always exists a natural fear in an innovative field that the rapid proliferation of implant materials and techniques may be based upon inadequate scientific foundation. This has been partly offset by the successes achieved in so many patients. However, the interdisciplinary approach must be increasingly emphasized if the safety and efficacy of implants is to be established beyond doubt.

There is a natural tendency for the surgeon to separate the surgery from the science. The validity of the surgical indications for an implant are his to assess. He is responsible for the selection of a suitable implant, its implantation into the body, and the postoperative management of the patient. The complexities of such a task are enormous. Having been charged with the ultimate decision as to whether the operation will benefit the patient, it is not surprising that the surgeon tends to minimize the interdisciplinary approach. He must not lose sight of the considerable scientific basis for the use of implants. The talented implant surgeon employs this science as the framework for the more practical clinical aspects of his surgery. In the end, he is solely responsible for the quality of the implant design, its safety and efficacy, the choice of materials, his surgical skill, and the value of the whole procedure to the patient. Therefore he will benefit by making the surgical process of implanting a device into a patient a cooperative effort involving the surgeon, the biomedical engineer, and the medical scientist. It is hoped that this book, among other things, will stimulate the implant surgeon to reacquaint himself with the chemistry of polymers and metals so that he may be better equipped to evaluate the safety of these materials that are permanently implanted within the eye.

The ophthalmic implant surgeon should understand the relationship between intraocular implants and surgical implants. A surgical implant is an object made from nonliving material that is inserted into the human body, where it is intended to remain for a significant period of time in order to perform a specific function. While this may serve as a practical definition, it is replete with obvious ambiguities. If an implant is an object, it suggests prefabrication to a desired shape. Thus soft tissue substitutes such as silicone would not fit this definition, yet they are considered to be implants. The expression "nonliving material" eliminates transplanted material from living and nonliving donors. Insertion into the human body implies complete wound enclosure and includes partial insertion. For example, an intraocular lens satisfies the requirement of complete wound enclosure, whereas a keratoprosthesis, which is partly inside and partly outside the eye, does not. However, a keratoprosthesis is indeed a bona fide implant. In ophthalmology we are less concerned with the definition of significant period of time than are other surgical specialties. The intraocular lens is intended to remain in situ indefinitely, yet a device such as a drain or catheter may remain in the body for a short period of time. The term "function" is also ambiguous. What type of function do we mean? Is it the function of an original living organ, such as the substitution of an intraocular lens for the cataractous crystalline lens? What of shaped implants that serve to fill a space or therapeutic implants such as controlled-release drugs?

It should be clear that there is great difficulty in formulating an exact definition of a surgical implant. Rather than engaging in pursuit of such a definition, it would be more useful in the context of this book to consider only those areas of a practical definition that apply to intraocular lenses. It is apparent that we must establish logical boundaries, arbitrary though they may be. We must emphasize certain details. The object, as a prefabricated material, is vital to our discussion. In addition, our concern is with synthetic, man-made, or alloplastic materials rather than fresh or reconstituted tissues. The implant considered in this book is one which is completely enclosed within the eye. We are also vitally concerned with the long-term interaction between the implant and the tissues and fluids of the eye. We will become intimately involved with the three basic properties of materials: mechanical, physical, and chemical —for example, the mechanical function of the haptic supports of the lens implant, the physical property of transparency of polymethylmethacrylate for optical purposes, and the chemical properties, as manifested by the reactions exhibited between it and the environment of the eye.

As will be seen later, intraocular lens implants involve the use of polymer-based materials as well as metals. There has been relatively little increase in the availability of new metals for implant use in recent years. Stainless steel, Vitallium, and tantalum were in use for many years, but the only new metallic materials to be introduced since 1950, aside from a modification of the cobalt-based alloys to give a more ductile and stronger alternative to Vitallium, are titanium and, later, some alloys of this element. This has not been the case with plastics. The initial industrial development of today's major thermoplastics occurred between 1930 and 1940. In this period, just before World War II, polyethylene was manufactured on a commercial scale. It was an excellent electrical insulator and was used as a submarine cable insulator. At the same time, Imperial Chemical Industries of England began to market Perspex, which is polymethylmethacrylate. They found that a rigid transparent thermoplastics material could be produced at a commercially feasible cost. It became invaluable during the war for aircraft glazing. Nylon was developed in the United States by W. H. Carothers of DuPont as a fiber in the mid-1930s. These materials were not developed for biomedical use; therefore surgeons had to rely on commercial grades of plastics.

As the uses of synthetic materials multiply and the need for them becomes even more apparent, there will have to be more teamwork in their development and use than there has been previously. More and more we will depend upon extremely carefully controlled synthesis and purification of materials, on rigid design criteria, and on attention to the finest details in implantation. As new materials become available, they will have to be carefully studied. We must not only determine the immediate value of a particular one but also determine what chemical configurations elicit the least tissue response in combination with the most-needed characteristics. This will permit greater strides in tailor making surgical repair materials.

To this point the interdisciplinary approach has made available materials used in the manufacture of intraocular implant lenses. The same approach has been responsible for the outstanding progress in refinements of surgical techniques in cataract surgery. Increasing sophistication has been the hallmark of this progress. The contributions of surgeons, biomedical engineers, and medical scientists during the past 30 years are responsible for the current high level of perfection of the cataract operation. The successes being achieved in implant surgery today are directly attributable to this progress. For without precision in cataract surgery, what can implant surgery hope to accomplish?

The popularization of surgery on the soft eye has been the single most important advance in cataract surgery during the past quarter of a century. Digital pressure was a contribution made solely by surgeons. Safe and efficacious hyperosmotic agents administered by the oral or parenteral route are an example of the interdisciplinary approach.

The availability of alpha-chymotrypsin has made the intracapsular cataract extraction a safer procedure, particularly in patients under 60 years of age. Improved sutures and needles and better instruments have made the incision and closure of the cataract incision more precise. Postoperative abnormalities of anterior chamber depth are therefore becoming increasingly rare. This is a crucial prerequisite for safe implant surgery.

The technique of the actual cataract extraction itself has also been a part of this increasing sophistication. The unplanned extracapsular cataract extraction has virtually disappeared as a result of cryoextraction replacing the antiquated capsule forceps and erysiphake. The planned extracapsular cataract extraction is rapidly becoming a refined technique as a result of the development of phacoemulsification and its irrigation and aspiration features. Although the genesis of these developments emanated from clinicians, they would not have been possible without the cooperative effort of biomedical engineers and medical scientists.

Finally, the advent of microsurgical cataract surgery has made it possible to perform more precise surgery and to better manage postoperative complications. The microscope has been a blessing for neophyte surgeons. It has enabled them to perform procedures with a precision that older surgeons required many years to master. This is not to say that intracapsular cataract surgery cannot be well performed with surgical loupes, but who can deny that the microscope is a vital requirement for phacoemulsification and other extracapsular techniques. The effective preservation of the posterior lens capsule, precise capsulotomies, discissions, and trans pars plana membrane excisions are best performed with the microscope.

In summary, it is evident that the implant materials and the surgical techniques involved in their implantation have not been solely a triumph of innovative surgery but rather the interdisciplinary effort of clinicians, bioengineers, and medical scientists. This approach should assure the future progress of implant surgery.

CHAPTER 2

Molecular basis of implant materials

BASIC STRUCTURE

Polymers and metals

Carbon is capable of forming covalent bonds (electron sharing) with itself and other elements. The carbon atom has four valence electrons. When four hydrogen atoms are covalently bound in a tetrahedral manner to one carbon atom, methane (CH_4) is formed (Fig. 2-1). Ethane (C_2H_6) consists of two carbon atoms sharing an electron with each other and each also having three covalent bonds with hydrogen atoms. When the molecules are small, the intermolecular forces are weak, and the resulting substances exist as gases or liquids. As the number of atoms per molecule increases, there is a greater tendency to form solids. With very large molecules, electrostatic bonding (Van der Waals bonds) holds the molecules together, but, in addition, the intermolecular force is enormously increased by a physical entangling of the molecules. This results in substances in which the molecules may consist of many thousands of carbon atoms, each with their attendant hydrogen or other atoms. These substances are known as organic polymers. Generally, the greater the molecular weight, the higher the melting point and the greater the tendency to exist as a solid.

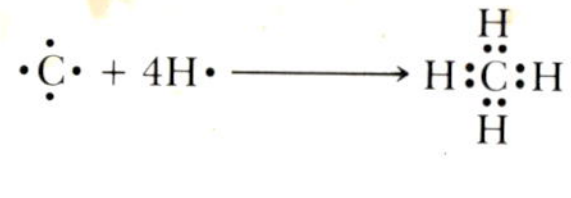

Fig. 2-1. Covalent bond is formed by sharing of one or more pairs of electrons between two atoms. An example is formation of methane.

The metallic bond differs from that seen with polymers. It is not covalent and is not spatially directional. Metallic atoms have only a small number of valence electrons. They therefore find it easier to lose rather than gain electrons to achieve a stable configuration. This is done by each atom's releasing its valence electrons and forming a "cloud" of free electrons. The electrically unbalanced structure that remains is called an ion, with a positive charge resulting from an excess of protons. The substance exists as a collection of positive ions surrounded by a cloud of free, negatively charged electrons. These substances are called metals, and the general electrostatic bond that exists between the ions and the electrons, and which therefore holds the ions together, is known as the metallic bond. Since bonding in metals is not directional, there are no constraints on the positions the atoms adopt with respect to each other. To achieve a minimum energy structure, metallic atoms are placed, layer on layer, in an ordered array. As a result of this structural order, these solids are said to be crystalline. It is the nature of this crystallinity that is important in determining the properties of the substance.

Returning to polymer-based materials, we have seen that carbon is able to produce polymers by combining with hydrogen and other atoms to form large molecules. Silicon is another element similarly capable (silicone rubber and silicone fluids). A monomer is defined as the small molecule that comprises the repeated structural unit in the large molecules.

The simplest organic polymer is polyethylene, whose structure is

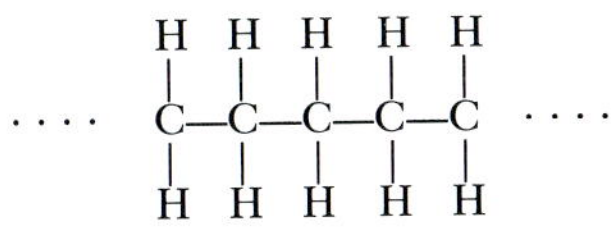

and is based on the ethylene monomer

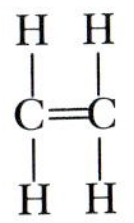

Techniques of polymer production

There are basically three ways by which polymers may be produced synthetically from simple starting materials. These techniques are referred to as addition polymerization, condensation polymerization, and rearrangement polymerization.

Addition polymerization. In addition polymerization a simple, low molecular weight molecule (monomer) that possesses a double bond is induced to break the double bond, and the resulting free valances are able to join up to other similar molecules (Fig. 2-2). In these cases the monomer is converted to a polymer, and no side products are formed.

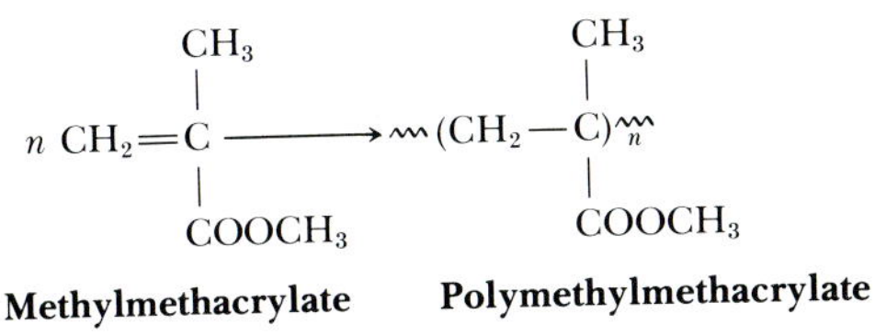

Fig. 2-2. In addition polymerization a simple, low molecular weight molecule (monomer) that possesses a double bond is induced to break the double bond, and the resulting free valences are able to join up to other similar molecules. The conversion of methylmethacrylate to polymethylmethacrylate is demonstrated.

$$nCH_2 = CH_2 \rightarrow -(CH_2-CH_2)_n-$$

Ethylene **Polyethylene**

Since there is only one type of monomer involved in the structure of polyethylene, it is known as a homopolymer. Since it is physically formed by the repeated addition of one monomer to another, it also is known as an addition polymer.

Polymethylmethacrylate (PMMA) is another addition polymer formed by the breaking of the double bond of methylmethacrylate.

In these examples the polymerization, as indicated, takes place by the opening of a carbon = carbon double bond. Other kinds of double and triple bonds are opened in the production of different addition polymers.

Condensation polymerization. A condensation polymer is made by a specific reaction between different substances. It differs from addition polymerization in that some small molecule is split out during the reaction. Furthermore, it is not essential that the monomer should contain a double bond. An example of condensation polymerization is the formation of the polyamide nylon 66 by the reaction of hexamethylenediamine and adipic acid. The reaction not only produces nylon 66, but also a by-product (water, in this case, Fig. 2-3).

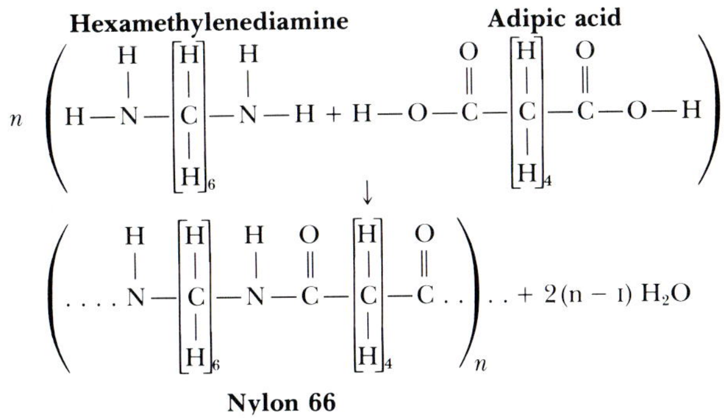

Fig. 2-3. Condensation polymerization involves a specific reaction between different substances. An example is formation of nylon 66 by the reaction between hexamethylenediamine and adipic acid. The reaction also produces a by-product, water in this case.

(c) 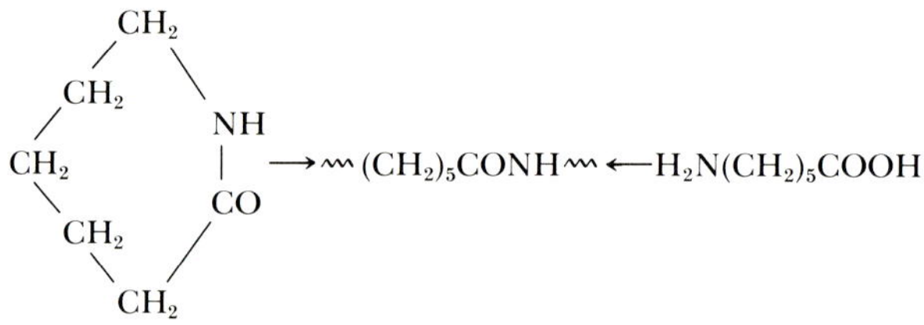

Fig. 2-4. Ring-opening polymerization. An example is the polymerization of ϵ-caprolactam (nylon 6).

Rearrangement polymerization. This approach to synthetic polymers is of somewhat less commercial importance. There is in fact no universally accepted description for the route, but the terms rearrangement polymerization and polyaddition are commonly used. In many respects this process is intermediate between addition and condensation polymerization. As with the former technique, there is no molecule split out, but the kinetics are akin to those of the latter. One particular form of rearrangement polymerization, of interest to ophthalmologists, is ring-opening polymerization. An example is the polymerization of ϵ-caprolactam (nylon 6) (Fig. 2-4).

An interesting feature of this example is that the polymer formed may also be produced by condensation polymerization.

Thermoplastics

Polymers such as polyethylene, PMMA, and polyamides are known as thermoplastics. They are characterized by their ability to become viscous fluids at elevated temperatures. This is in contrast to the other major class of polymers known as thermosetting resins, where there is no viscous state prior to the solid decomposing. Note that, in the examples given so far, the product of polymerization has been a long-chain molecule, a linear polymer. With such materials it should be possible for the molecules to slide past each other under pressure above a certain temperature such that the molecules have enough energy to overcome the intermolecular attractions. More simply stated, the material is capable of flow above a certain temperature, that is, it becomes plastic, whereas below this temperature it is to all intents and purposes a solid. This is characteristic of thermoplastic materials, the most important class of plastics material commercially available.

Transition temperatures and crystallinity. As stated above, various structural changes occur in thermoplastics on raising or lowering the temperature, and the properties displayed at room temperature are controlled by the relationship between room temperature and the transition temperatures. PMMA is an example of a polymer that exists at room temperatures below all the transition temperatures. This accounts for its rigidity. Polyethylene, on the other hand, exists above the transition region and is therefore relatively soft and flexible. Amorphous polymers show different property changes with variations in temperature than do crystalline polymers (see below). Thus a specific linear amorphous polymer such as PMMA can exist in a number of states according to the temperature and the average molecular weight of the polymer. At low molecular weights the polymer will be solid below some given temperature, while above that temperature it will be liquid. The melting point for such polymers will be quite sharp and is the temperature above which the molecules have sufficient energy to move independently of each other; that is, they are capable of viscous flow. Conversely, below this temperature the molecules have insufficient energy for flow and the mass behaves as a rigid solid. At high molecular weights, such a clearly defined melting point no longer occurs, and a rubbery intermediate zone is often observed. In this case, two transition temperatures may be observed, a rigid solid-rubber transition usually known as the glass transition temperature and, secondly, a generally very indefinite rubber-liquid transition sometimes referred to as the flow temperature. Amorphous polymers are transparent, and thus the materials are glasslike, and the state is sometimes referred to as the glassy state.

To demonstrate changes of orientation in linear amorphous polymers, if a sample of such a polymer is heated to a temperature above its glass transition point and then subjected to a tensile stress, the molecules will tend to align themselves in the general direction of the stress. If the mass is then cooled below its transition temperature while the molecule is still under stress, the molecules will become frozen while in an oriented state. PMMA, however, will revert completely to the original flat sheet from which it is prepared if it is heated above its glass transition temperature.

If a polymer molecule has a sufficiently regular structure, it may be capable of some degree of crystallization. Since the methyl and the methacrylate groups on alternate carbon atoms are relatively large in the case of PMMA, crystallization is inhibited and the polymer therefore exists in wholly amorphous form. It thus can be easily prepared in a clear form suitable for intraocular lenses. There are substantial differences between the crystallization of simple molecules such as water and copper sulfate and of polymers such as polyethylene and polyamides (nylons). The essential difference between the traditional concept of a crystal structure and crystalline polymers is that the former is a single crystal while the polymer is polycrystalline. By a single crystal is meant a crystalline particle grown without interruption from a single nucleus and relatively free from defects. The term polycrystallinity refers to a state in which clusters of single crystals are involved, developed from the more or less simultaneous growth of many nuclei. The resulting conglomerate may possess no readily discernible symmetry. There is a growing school of thought that polymer molecules fold upon themselves at intervals of about 10 nm to form lamellae that appear to be fundamental structures in a crystalline polymer. Crystallization spreads by the growth of individual lamellae as polymer molecules align themselves into position and start to fold.

It was stated earlier that, with thermoplastic materials, it should be possible for the molecules to slide past each other under pressure above a certain temperature such that the molecules have enough energy to overcome the intermolecular attractions. Thus they are capable of flow above this temperature. However, in a highly crystalline polymer there is little scope for segmental motion, since most of the segments of the polymer are involved in a lattice formation in which they have low mobility. These polymers are comparatively rigid in the mass, compared to amorphous polymers, and there is little difference in properties immediately above and below the glass transition temperature. In fact, the glass temperature zone may be difficult to find.

Changes in orientation of linear amorphous polymers were previously mentioned. However, if a crystalline polymer, such as nylon 66, is stretched at some temperature well below its melting point but above its transition temperature (for example, room temperature), additional crystallization will be induced and the crystalline structure will be aligned in the direction of extension. This results in oriented crystalline filaments or fibers that are much stronger than the unoriented product. This is the basis of the "cold-drawing" process of the synthetic fiber industry. Polyethylene terephthalate (Dacron) with a transition temperature of 67° C has to be cold-drawn at some higher temperature. Synthetic surgical sutures are manufactured from crystalline polymers.

Optical properties. The most important property of PMMA in relation to its use as an intraocular lens is its optical property. Most materials are opaque, including the metals and most polymers. Relatively few permit light to pass through them to any extent except the glasses and an occasional polymer.

Light incident on a solid may be affected in a number of ways. A certain amount of light will be absorbed by the material, a further amount will be scattered, and the remainder will be transmitted through the material. The transparency of a material describes the amount of light that is transmitted directly through the material. It may be expressed as the direct transmission factor, which is the ratio of the light flux transmitted through the material to the incident light flux. Thus, transparent materials have a high transmission factor, while opaque materials have a low value. The transmission factor, besides being dependent on the material in question, is a function of the wavelength of the light and the geometry and thickness of the specimen. In addition to transmission, light may be absorbed. This depends primarily on the molecular structure of the material. Light may also be scattered by a material. Scattering depends on the nature of the molecule and structural imperfections.

In order to achieve a product with a high clarity, it is important that the refractive index is constant throughout the sample in the line of direction between the object in view and the eye. The presence of interfaces between regions of different refractive index will cause scatter of the light rays. Amorphous polymers free from fillers or other impurities are transparent unless chemical groups are present that absorb visible light radiation. Generally, the greater the crystallinity of the polymer, the greater the light-scattering coefficient. However, crystalline polymers may or may not be transparent, depending on a number of factors. Where the crystalline structures, such as spherulites, are smaller than the wavelength of light, they do not interfere with the passage of light and the polymer is transparent. Where the structures formed are greater in diameter than the wavelength of light, the light waves will be scattered, if the crystal structures have a different refractive index than that of the amorphous regions of the polymer material.

High density polyethylene and nylon 66 are among the most highly crystalline polymers and are therefore essentially opaque. PMMA is amorphous and therefore transparent. It is the most suitable plastic material for optical applications. It has a low absorption coefficient and a minute scattering coefficient. Scattering by surface defects is eliminated by highly polishing its surface.

Plastics

The distinction between a polymer and a plastic should be understood. Although some polymers are used in a pure form for certain applications, most are used in a modified form. They usually require mixing with additives of one kind or another to yield useful end products. One accepted definition of a plastic is that end product substance which results from mixing a polymer with additives. The eighth edition of the *Condensed Chemical Dictionary* gives the following definition of a plastic: "A high polymer, usually synthetic, combined with other ingredients, such as curatives, fillers, reinforcing agents, colorants, plasticizers." To this ingredient list one might add antioxidants, stabilizers, antistatic agents, and lubricants. The term "plastic" does not specify one type of material; rather, it indicates a family of materials, since it encompasses a great number of diversified compounds. Thus it should be understood that almost every plastic that is used contains more than just the pure polymer and that it is the effect of the additive on the polymer that modifies its properties.

Additives

The alteration of the bulk properties of a polymer by the incorporation of additives is widely used in industry. Probably the most well-known commercial example of this occurs in rubber technology where variations in the choice of additives can produce such widely differing products as tires, rubber bands, battery boxes, latex foam upholstery, erasers, and tennis court surfaces.

Additives should have certain required features, unless by virtue of their function such requirements are excluded. The following is a list of these requirements:

1. They should be efficient in their function.
2. They should be stable under processing conditions.
3. They should be stable under service conditions.
4. They should not bleed or bloom.
5. They should be nontoxic and not impart taste or odor.
6. They should be cheap.
7. They should not adversely affect the properties of the polymer.

These requirements are self-explanatory, but the terms bleeding and blooming require discussion. Bleeding of an additive into an adjacent material occurs when the additive has a degree of solubility in the polymer and also in the adjacent liquid or solid material. Bleeding is much more extensive from polymers that are above their glass transmission temperature (and melting temperature, if crystalline) than from polymers below this temperature. Blooming is a separate phenomenon but is again associated with solubility. It occurs when an additive has totally dissolved in the polymer at the processing temperature but is only partially soluble at ambient temperature. As a result, some of the additive is thrown out of solution on cooling, and some of this may collect on the surface of the polymer mass.

Physically, additives may be divided into four groups: solids, rubbers, liquids, and gases, the last of these being employed for making cellular polymers. However, in terms of function, there are larger numbers of groups, some of which follow.

Fillers are usually solid additives incorporated into the polymer to modify its physical (usually mechanical) properties.

Plasticizers and softeners, when first used, primarily acted as spacers between the polymer molecules. Less energy was therefore required for molecular bond rotation, and polymers became capable of flow at temperatures below their decomposition temperature. It was subsequently found that plasticizers could serve two additional purposes: to lower the melt viscosity and to change physical properties of the product such as to increase softness and flexibility and decrease the cold flex temperature (a measure of the temperature below which the polymer compound loses its flexibility).

Lubricants and flow promoters are grouped into three categories. The first reduces the friction of moldings and other finished products when they are rubbed against adjacent materials which may or may not be of the same composition. Examples are graphite and molybdenum disulfide used in 1% to 2% quantities in nylons and other thermoplastics employed in gear and bearing applications. A second type is external lubricants that have a low compatibility with the polymer and, in addition, often possess polar groups to enhance their affinity to metals. The third group is comprised of low molecular weight materials that promote the flow of the polymer in the melt but which, unlike plasticizers, have little effect on the solid state properties. These have been called internal lubricants.

Antiaging additives. Most plastic materials deteriorate with the passage of time. The changes in the properties are due to structural modifications of which there are four main types:

1. Chain scission, resulting in a loss of strength and toughness
2. Cross-linking, which may lead to hardening, brittleness, and changes in solubility
3. Development of chromophoric groups, leading to color formation
4. Development of polar groups, such as carbonyl groups in polyolefins, causing a deterioration in electrical insulation and also changes in chemical reactivity

Such structural changes are a consequence of chemical reactions of which the most common are oxidation, ozone attack, dehydrochlorination, and ultraviolet attack.

Colorants. There are basically four methods used for coloring polymers: surface coating (for example, painting), surface dyeing, introduction of color-forming groups into the polymer molecules, and mass coloration.

Miscellaneous. Other additives include heat stabilizers, antioxidants, ultraviolet light absorbers, antiozonants, stabilizers against dechlorination, flame retarders, blowing agents, cross-linking agents, and photodegradants.

• • •

The most important constituents of all currently used intraocular lenses are polymethylmethacrylate, nylon, polypropylene, and metal (platinum-iridium and titanium). They will be described in order.

Polymethylmethacrylate (PMMA)

PMMA is, commercially, the most important member of a range of acrylic polymers that may be considered structurally as derivatives of acrylic acid. It forms the optical portion of all currently used intraocular lenses.

History. Historically, Röhm[1] reported on his studies of acrylic polymers for his doctoral thesis in 1901. The Röhm and Haas Co. in Darmstadt, Germany, commenced limited production of polymethylmethacrylate under the trade names Acryloid and Plexigum. These were soft, gummy products of interest as surface coatings, rather than as moldable plastics materials. About 1930, R. Hill[1] prepared PMMA and found it to be a rigid, transparent polymer, potentially useful as an aircraft glazing material. In 1932 J. W. C. Crawford[1] discovered a new route to the monomer using cheap and readily available chemicals: acetone, hydrocyanic acid, methanol, and sulfuric acid. His process is used today, with minor modifications, throughout the world. Sheet PMMA became prominent during World War II for aircraft glazing, as predicted by Hill in his early patents. Since then it has found other uses in many fields. Current examples of commercial sheet PMMA are Perspex (Imperial Chemical Industries, England), Oroglas (Rohm and Haas, United States), and Plexiglas (Röhm and Haas, Germany).

Preparation of monomer. As stated, the successful commercial utilization of PMMA is due largely to the process of producing the monomer from acetone, as developed by Crawford. Some details of the process as operated by the Rohm and Haas Co. of Philadelphia have been disclosed.

Acetone is first reacted with hydrogen cyanide to give acetone cyanohydrin (Fig. 2-5, *A*). The cyanohydrin is then treated with 98% sulfuric acid in a cooled hydrolysis kettle to yield methacrylamide sulfate (Fig. 2-5, *B*). The sulfate is not isolated from the reaction mixture, which passes into an esterification kettle and reacts continuously with methanol (Fig. 2-5, *C*). The esterified stream, which may contain inhibitors to prevent premature polymerization, is then passed to a stripping column, which separates the methylmethacrylate, methanol, and some water from the residue made up of sulfuric acid, ammonium bisulfate, and the

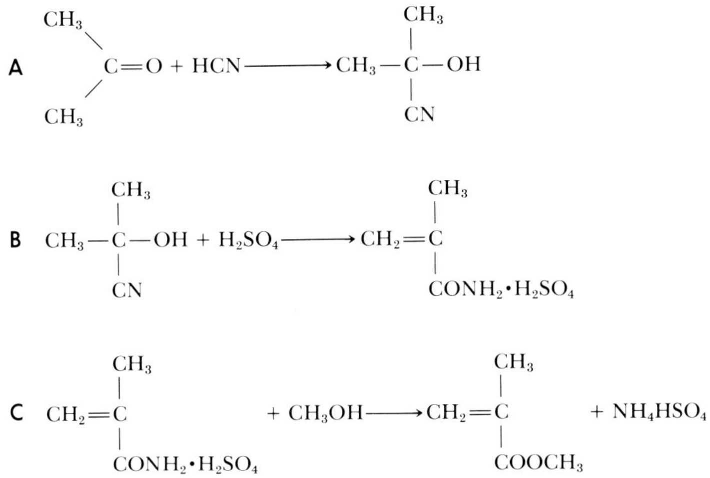

Fig. 2-5. A, Methylmethacrylate monomer is derived from acetone, which is first reacted with hydrogen cyanide to give acetone cyanohydrin. **B,** Acetone cyanohydrin is reacted with sulfuric acid to give methacrylamide sulfate. **C,** Methacrylamide sulfate is reacted with methanol to give methylmethacrylate.

remainder of the water. The methylmethacrylate is subsequently separated and purified by further distillation.

Polymerization. Methylmethacrylate will polymerize readily, and the effect may be observed with uninhibited samples of monomers during storage. Therefore in commercial practice the monomer is supplied with up to 0.1% of an inhibitor such as hydroquinone, which is removed before polymerization, either by distillation under reduced pressure or, in some cases, by washing with an alkaline solution.

Commercial polymerization involves free radical techniques using peroxides or azodiisobutyronitrile at temperatures up to 100° C. The presence of oxygen in the system will affect the rate of reaction and the nature of the products, owing to the formation of methacrylate peroxides in a side reaction. Therefore it is common practice to polymerize in the absence of oxygen, either by bulk polymerization in a full cell or chamber or by blanketing the monomer with an inert gas. It has been observed that in the polymerization of methylmethacrylate there is an acceleration in the rate of conversion after about 20% of the monomer has been converted. The average molecular weight of the polymer also increases during polymerization. This effect, known variously as the gel effect, Trommsdorff effect, or autoacceleration effect, is explained by the slowing down of the chain termination reaction during conversion. The reason for the drop in termination rate is that, as the reaction mixture becomes more viscous, the radical ends of the polymer chains find increased difficulty in diffusing toward each other, leading to the important mutual termination reaction. This autoacceleration effect appears most marked with polymers that are insoluble in their monomers. In these circumstances the radical end becomes entrapped in the polymer, and termination reactions become very difficult. It has been suggested that, in thermodynamic terms, methylmethacrylate is a relatively poor solvent for polymethylmethacrylate because it causes radicals to coil while in solution. The termination reaction is then determined by the rate at which the radical ends come to the surface of the coil and hence become available for mutual termination.

Since the average molecular weight of most bulk polymerized PMMA is too high to give a material that has adequate flow properties for injection molding and extrusion, a method has been devised to reduce the molecular weight of the polymer by mechanical scission. The technique is known as suspension polymerization. It can be carried out rapidly, usually in less than 1 hour.

Properties. Commercial PMMA, from which intraocular lenses are made, is a transparent material, and microscopic and x-ray analyses generally indicate that it is amorphous. Combining the facts of a glass transition temperature of 104° C with its amorphous nature, commercial PMMA is a hard, transparent plastics material in its normal conditions of use. Cast material (Perspex) is stated to have an average molecular weight of about 10^6. While the glass transition temperature is about 104° C, the molecular entanglements are so extensive that the material is incapable of flow below its decomposition temperature (approximately 170° C). There is thus a reasonably wide, rubbery range, and it is in this phase that such material is normally shaped. For injection molding and extrusion, much lower molecular weight materials are employed. Such polymers have a reasonable melt viscosity but marginally lower heat distortion temperatures and mechanical properties.

As just indicated, PMMA is a hard, rigid, transparent material. Commercial grades have extremely good weathering resistance compared with other thermoplastics. It is superior to untreated glass in terms of impact resistance, and although it cracks, any fragments formed are less sharp and jagged than those of glass and, normally, consequently less harmful. Although harder than most other thermoplastics, the scratch resistance does leave something to be desired. Shallow scratches may, however, be removed by polishing.

The optical properties of PMMA are particularly important. It absorbs very little light, but there is about 4% reflection at each polymer-air interface for normal incident light. Thus the light transmission of normal incident light through a parallel sheet of acrylic material free from blemishes is about 92%.

PMMA may be blended with a number of additives. Of these the most important are dyes and pigments, and these should be stable to both processing and service conditions. Further improvements in light stability may be achieved by addition of small quantities of ultraviolet absorbers.

The historical development of PMMA, based on its use as an aircraft glazing material and for applications in intraocular lens implant surgery, has not changed its usefulness as an aircraft glazing material. In aircraft it is used extensively on airplanes that fly at speeds less than Mach 10. They also form the familiar "bubble" body of many helicopters.

Although the above discussion may appear highly technical to many ophthalmic clinicians, the surgeon is reminded that PMMA forms the optical portion of the intraocular lens he permanently implants within the human eye. Therefore he should possess some background knowledge of the commercial product that is supplied to him by industry.

Polyamides

Polyamides are condensation products that contain recurring amide groups as integral parts of the main polymer chain. Polyamides are frequently referred to as nylons, a generic term that has been adopted by the U.S. Federal Trade Commission for designating fibers of the polyamide type. Its official definition is as follows: "Nylon: a manufactured fiber in which fiber-forming substances are any long-chain synthetic polyamide having recurring amide groups (−CONH−) as an integral part of the polymer chain." Polyamide fibers are used in the supporting structure of the optical portion of an intraocular lens and for sutures used to hinge the implant to the iris.

History. The early development of the nylons is mainly due to the work of W. H. Carothers[1] and his colleagues who first synthesized nylon 66 in 1935 after extensive and classic research into condensation polymerization. Commercial production of this polymer for subsequent conversion into fibers was commenced by the DuPont Co. in December 1939. In an attempt to circumvent the DuPont patents, German chemists investigated a wide range of synthetic fiber-forming polymers in the late 1930s. This work resulted in the successful introduction of nylon 6. Nylon 7 (Enanth) and nylon 9 (Pelargone) have been investigated as fibers in the Soviet Union. It is a tribute to the vision of the early developers of nylon 66 and nylon 6 that so many years later these two polyamides represent more than 98% of the total polyamide volume being converted to fibers.

Nomenclature. A simple method of nomenclature for polyamides is commonly employed, which designates the number of carbon atoms in the repeating units. For example, the polyamide made from ε-caprolactam, which contains 6 carbons, is known as nylon 6. If aminoundecenoic acid were employed, the monomer, which contains 11 carbon atoms, would form nylon 11. The reaction between the 6-carbon-atom hexamethylenediamine and the 6-carbon diacid (dicarboxylic or dibasic acid), adipic acid, produces nylon 66. If sebacic acid, a 10-carbon-atom diacid, were employed with hexamethylenediamine, the polymer would be called nylon 610. It is seen that the number of carbon atoms in the diamine is designated first and the number in the diacid is designated second.

Preparation of polyamides. Of the many possible methods for preparing linear polyamides, three are of commercial importance:

1. The reaction of a diamine with a dicarboxylic acid (Fig. 2-3)
2. Self-condensation of an ω-amino acid

$$\eta NH_2\ R\ COOH \rightarrow \text{—(—NHRCO)}\eta\text{—} + \eta H_2O$$

3. Opening of a lactam ring (Fig. 2-4)

Nylon 66 is manufactured by reacting equal amounts of hexamethylenediamine and adipic acid. (The favored starting point for the production of adipic acid is benzene.) A salt is first formed from the diamine and the adipic acid in a water and alcohol solution. An aqueous solution of the salt is then subjected to heat and pressure to cause dissociation followed by condensation to the polyamide. The pressure is reduced and condensation proceeds to a high molecular weight polymer. The molecular weight of the polymer is ordinarily controlled by the use of a chain terminator such as acetic acid.

Because it is easier to make and to purify, caprolactam is preferred to ω-aminocaproic acid for the manufacture of nylon 6. Commercial production is based on cyclohexanol, which may be produced by a number of routes from benzenes. The polymerization of ε-caprolactam is usually accomplished by heating the monomer to above 250° C in the presence of catalysts, such as water and phosphoric acid, and chain terminators, such as acetic acid.

Whatever method is chosen for polymerization of polyamides, it is important that there should be an equivalence in the number of amine and acid groups for polymers of the highest molecular weight to be obtained. In the case of the amino acids and lactams, this is ensured by the use of pure monomer, but when diamines and dibasic acids are used, it is necessary to form a salt to ensure such an equivalence.

Relation of structure and properties. Aliphatic polyamides such as nylons 66, 6, and 610 are linear polymers and thus thermoplastic. They contain —CONH— groups spaced out at regular intervals so that the polymers crystallize with a high intermolecular attraction. These polymer chains also have aliphatic chain segments that give a measure of flexibility in the amorphous region. Thus the combination of high interchain attraction in the crystalline zones and flexibility in the amorphous zones leads to polymers that are tough above their apparent glass transition temperatures. The strength of a polymer is due to the covalent interatomic bonds within the molecules, while the intermolecular bonds are really sources of weakness. In a fiber such as nylon the molecular chains are aligned so that the great majority are oriented axially, thus giving a great intrinsic strength to the fiber in this direction. Thus the strength of the fiber is no longer controlled by the weak intermolecular bonds. This is easier done with polymers that readily crystallize.

There are a number of structural variables that can considerably affect the properties of the aliphatic polyamides:

1. Distance between the repeating —CONH— group. In the case of nylon 11, this is approximately twice that of nylon 6. Thus nylon 11 has a lower interchain attraction, is softer, has a lower melting point, and lower water absorption.
2. Number of methylene groups in the intermediates. It has been observed that polymers from intermediates with an even number of methylene groups have higher melting points than similar polymers with an odd number of methylene groups. Thus nylon 66 has a higher melting point than either nylon 56 or 76.
3. Molecular weight. Specific types of nylon, for example, 66, are frequently available in forms differing in molecular weight. The main difference between such grades is in melt viscosity, the more viscous grades being more suitable for processing by extrusion techniques.
4. N-substitution. Replacement of the hydrogen atom in the —CONH— group by such groups as CH_3 and —CH_2OCH_3 will cause a reduction in the interchain attraction and a consequent decrease in softening point.
5. Copolymerization. This usually leads to less crystalline and frequently amorphous materials.

The properties of the nylons are considerably affected by the amount of crystallization. The greater the degree of crystallinity, the less the water absorption and hence the less the effect of humidity on the properties of the polymer.

All nylons are hygroscopic. However, they must be processed essentially dry, usually below 0.3% water, to prevent hydrolysis; that is, a reversal of the reaction by which they are formed. When molded parts are exposed to the atmosphere, they slowly absorb water until an equilibrium is reached. This is accompanied by changes in dimensions and properties that must be considered in critical designing. Water acts as a plasticizer and lowers the modules, yield stress, and hardness of nylon, but increases elongation and toughness. Polyamides are generally resistant to chemicals and solvents and are not normally attacked by exposure to pure water. The effects of moisture just described are due to the plasticizing action of water at high temperatures for prolonged periods of time; in this case some hydrolysis of the amide groups results in degradation of the nylon. Degradation of nylon in vivo has been observed by many investigators. This is of importance only when retention of tensile strength for long periods of time is necessary. The use of nylon sutures for fixation of an intraocular lens is dependent on long-term strength retention. Nylon is suspect in this regard. Degradation is enhanced by poor manufacturing processes. For example, manufacturers who do not sufficiently stretch and therefore orient and crystallize the molecules comprising the filament may produce a suture that is less resistant to hydrolysis than one that has been well oriented. Another possible source of potential weakness is the method of sterilization (irradiation or ethylene oxide), but this has not been well documented.

Additives. Additives used in nylon can be grouped as follows:

1. Heat stabilizers
2. Light stabilizers
3. Plasticizers
4. Lubricants
5. Reinforcing fillers
6. Pigments
7. Fungicides

With the possible exception of pigments, which may be dry-blended by the processor, additives are incorporated by the manufacturers, and only a limited amount of information about them is normally made available.

Uses of nylon. For the best mechanical properties, nylon 66 would be considered, but this material is probably the most difficult to process and has a high water absorption value. Nylon 6 is easier to process but has slightly inferior mechanical properties and an even higher water absorption. Nylon monofilaments have found application in surgical sutures, brush tufting, wigs, sports equipment, braiding, and outdoor upholstery. Nylon is used as the haptic supporting device of most intraocular lenses. Nylon sutures are also commonly used for implant fixation within the eye.

Polypropylene

Most currently popular iris-supported intraocular lenses employ some type of suture to prevent dislocation (for example, transiridectomy suture used with the Binkhorst iris-clip implant and the iris suture used with the Worst Medallion 2-loop implant). Nylon 6 or nylon 66 sutures have been the most popular. Polyamides have just been described. Polypropylene sutures will probably replace nylon, since there has been some concern over the loss of tensile strength inherent in the nylon sutures available today. A crucial requirement is the need for an iris-fixation suture for intraocular lens implantation that will remain in place and maintain its tensile strength indefinitely.

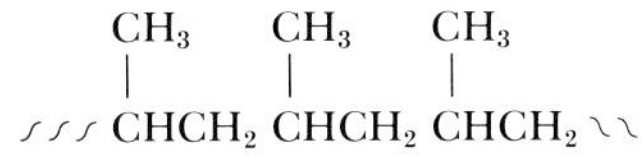

Fig. 2-6. Polypropylene (Prolene), the lightest major plastic, has no hydrolyzable linkages, unlike nylon.

Polypropylene (Prolene, Ethicon) sutures have been marketed for several years. The material was introduced primarily for cardiovascular surgery, but its application has extended to almost every specialty.

The structure of polypropylene is shown in Fig. 2-6. Since 1954 a major development in polymer chemistry has been a new technique leading to polymers with unusual structures. Polypropylene is produced in this way by coordination polymerization, which governs the orientation with which a monomer approaches the growing chain end. Quite often, coordination polymerization is carried out using a catalyst, usually a Ziegler catalyst. The latter are complexes formed by the interaction of alkyls of metals of groups I to III in the periodic table with halides and other derivatives of transition metals of groups IV to VIII. A typical coordination catalyst is a complex between an aluminum alkyl and a titanium halide.

In principle the catalyst system used governs the way in which a monomer and a growing chain approach each other, and because of this it is possible to produce stereoregular polymers. One way in which such stereospecificity occurs is by the growing polymer molecule forming a complex with the catalyst, which is also complexed with a monomer molecule. In this way, growing polymers and monomers are brought together in a highly specific fashion. The product of reaction of the growing polymer molecule and the monomer molecule is a further growing molecule that will then again complex itself with the catalyst, and the cycle may be repeated.

There are three possible molecular arrangements of crystalline polypropylene, the atactic, syndiotactic, and isotactic forms, the differences lying in the position of the CH_3 groups of the molecular chains. Using Ziegler catalysts, essentially isotactic polypropylene can be produced, which is, therefore, highly crystalline. The isotactic form is the most regular, since the methyl groups are all on one side of the molecule.

Polypropylene is the lightest major plastic with a density of 0.905. Its high crystallinity imparts to it high tensile strength. It is highly resistant to environmental stress. It is, unlike nylon, a polymer with no hydrolyzable linkages and has been shown to be stable indefinitely in vivo. Obviously this is a major advantage for intraocular sutures. This property made it particularly useful for sutures in areas such as cardiovascular device fixation and bypass surgery where long-term stability is essential.

The physical properties of 9-0 and 10-0 nylon and polypropylene sutures are similar except for one major difference. Polypropylene can be stretched to a much greater length (without breaking) than nylon. Tissue reaction to this suture has been shown to be less than that of any other suture and equivalent to that of stainless steel. The biologic stability of polypropylene sutures and its low tissue reaction appears to make it ideal for the transiridectomy or iris suture in intraocular implant lens surgery. To avoid the disadvantages discussed with the degradation of nylon, some manufacturers are supplying intraocular lenses with polypropylene haptic loops. Its clinical value is now being evaluated.

Platinum metals

The supporting element of some of the recently introduced intraocular lenses consists of platinum or platinum-iridium. These materials belong to a group of elements known as the platinum metals. Others in this group are ruthenium, rhodium, palladium, and osmium. They are characterized by their rarity, high density, and mobility. They have been useful in the electrical and chemical industries due to their ability to resist many forms of environmental attack and therefore to retain their function under critical conditions. They are not useful as implant materials in situations involving significant stresses because of their poor mechanical properties. Their main use is as electrodes, with the alloy platinum-iridium being particularly useful. The iridium is added to the platinum to give it greater rigidity. The great advantage here lies in the fact that these materials are resistant to oxidation; the subsequent absence of surface film formation assures a low contact resistance. All these metals except osmium can be cast, hot-forged, and worked fairly readily. Deep-drawing of wire is particularly easy. Platinum and platinum-iridium wire loops have been used to attach an intraocular lens to the posterior capsule of the crystalline lens. They have been substituted for nylon loops in some intraocular implants.

Titanium

Titanium has recently gained popularity as a material for the loops of some intraocular lenses. It is the most recently introduced of the main metallic implant materials used in other parts of the body. It is conventionally used in the pure, or at least commercially pure, form. There are available a range of commercially pure grades, depending on the exact amount of impurities. The principal impurities are oxygen (0.5%) and iron (0.2%). The variation in the amount of impurities results in a variation in the mechanical properties displayed and is therefore of great importance. The higher the impurity content, the stronger but less ductile the metal. Resistance to stress, which is important in orthopedic implants, is not crucial in intraocular lenses.

The two most important properties of titanium are its low specific gravity and its excellent corrosion resistance. Since the weight of an intraocular lens supported by the iris must be extremely low, the lightness of titanium (specific gravity of 4.5, compared to a value of 7.9 for stainless steel) is ideal. Titanium is intrinsically very reactive, and the thin tenacious film of the oxide that forms on the surface protects the metal from a wide range of corrosive media. Titanium is particularly resistant to attack in saline solutions, which are normally considered hostile media.

REACTIONS AFTER IMPLANTING

Such a wide range of mechanical properties is being offered by modern materials that more and more of them will be drawn into use as possible implants. It is not enough, of course, that such a material have correct mechanical properties. At least as important is its reaction when in contact with the tissues.

The term "tissue compatibility" involves the interaction between host and implant. This embraces two sides of the same coin. On one side is the effect of the tissues and body fluids on the implant. On the other side is the effect of the implant on the tissues. Both of these must be given equal consideration.

Reaction of tissues to implanted materials

The effects of an implant on the tissues may be either local or systemic or both. Results may be immediate or may be delayed. The implant may cause a toxic or an allergic reaction, may provoke a foreign body reaction in which the body attempts to involve it with giant cells and fibrous tissue, or may introduce microorganisms and produce an infection.

The foreign material may contain extractable substances that are truly toxic. These, if present, frequently cause local cell death or a local inflammatory reaction as they leach out, but they can produce in addition more generalized toxic symptoms. Among the possible local effects of the foreign material on the tissues are acute inflammatory responses accompanied by cell and tissue death or injury, exudate formation, vascular responses such as redness, or long-term effects such as excessive hyperplasia.

The amount of tissue injury and cell necrosis depends on the nature of the irritant. Certain materials elicit minimal response. Those that bring about an inflammatory response with cell necrosis may cause release and degradation of the materials normally contained in cells. These degradation substances in turn may produce either local or systemic effects.

Any synthetic implant from which potential toxins leach out, either because of faulty fabrication or after breakdown, could lead at any time to immunologic or allergic reaction, inflammation, and rejection.

A prime consideration in the choice of materials utilized for certain types of implant is the amount of encapsulation the material will evoke. It has been noted in arterial prosthetic surgery that different materials evoke different thicknesses of capsule. Little[2] states that while certain hard plastics may initiate only a slight fibroblastic reaction two to four cells deep, a similarly inert material with a soft surface might under similar circumstances have only a single layer of cells encapsulating it. Work is being done now to determine how much proliferation is caused by various materials so as to be able to pinpoint those that evoke the thinnest and most permeable connective tissue capsules.

Certain synthetics or their breakdown products are capable of being transferred and excreted by the body. This could lead to secondary effects in the liver and kidneys, to hypertension, or to deposition in scattered internal organs. In the eye there is always the concern that leaching from the implant or products from the biodegradation of the foreign material, or actual physical contact of the implant with the cornea, may cause corneal opacification. In such case, no matter how successful the lens implant in itself may be, it is useless to the patient.

Less well understood are the reactions of the tissues to physical stimuli. Pressure may result in tissue death and necrotic changes. Many physical reactions to implants are caused by the condition of their surfaces. A soft or rubbery surface might be expected to have little or no physical effect on the surrounding tissues and is therefore considered more desirable than hard ones. Most satisfactory of these rubberlike materials are the silicones. Natural rubber may be satisfactory for some time, but later the surfaces oxidize and become hard and abrasive.

A material that has been cut or machined and then viewed under the electron microscope shows the irregularities in the surface as sharp ridges or spikes; if hard, these may result in cell abrasion. Particles of fillers and pigments, or polymer granules exposed after leaching out of the plasticizer, can also cause this effect.

Actual migration of the implant through the tissues can be caused by uneven pressure on a material that has a sharp edge. This can frequently result in the ejection of the foreign material through the skin. In the eye, physical contact of the implant with the cornea may lead to opacification of the cornea. This may not be for toxic reasons inherent in the foreign material itself, but rather may be a result of physiologic aberrations caused by blockage of the normal flow of necessary materials.

One cannot predict simply by studying the chemical or physical makeup of a substance whether it will be compatible with the body. Each material considered for a specific application must be tested empirically and, if possible, under conditions of intended use in laboratory animals; then, if satisfactory results are obtained, it can be utilized for placement in humans.

Carcinogenesis

Implantation of various materials in mice, rats, and hamsters has been found to increase the rate of tumor formation. So many different kinds of materials have been found to increase the incidence of rodent tumors that certain investigators have reached the conclusion that *any* implanted substance has the ability to do this in specially-bred, cancer-prone mice.

Such published data are difficult to reconcile with the observation that no proven case of induced malignancy is known to have resulted in humans from permanent implantation of an artificial material. Harris[3] made an 11-year survey of 10,000 implants, including Ivalon, Etheron, polyethylene, Surgifoam, and polyurethane, that had been used for augmentation mammaplasties; not one substantiated case of malignancy was reported in the entire series. Hoopes, Edgerton, and Shelley[4] stated that since the usual incidence of breast cancer in women is 5½% and since 40,000 women have undergone augmentation mammaplasties, at least 2,000 should develop the disease. Surprisingly, only six such cases have been found; in none was the cancer in direct proximity to the implant. They concluded that "there is no current evidence to suggest that prosthetic material enhances the opportunity to develop mammary cancer in humans."

There are obvious and unexplained differences in tumor induction between rodents and higher species. Where cancerous change is concerned, it appears to be impossible to draw conclusions that are applicable to humans from results observed in rodents. Nevertheless it is always necessary to keep possible carcinogenicity in mind and weigh it carefully against the advantages of the implant.

DETERIORATION OF IMPLANT MATERIALS

Having considered the properties of implant materials, the crucial aspect of their long-term behavior is now examined. This is essentially a description of how the structure and the various properties of the material change with time. Resistance to deterioration is an essential requirement of all implants, but especially intraocular lenses. Not only may the environment in which the implant is placed alter the structure and properties of the implant material, and therefore the function of the implant, but, as previously discussed, the by-products of these changes may have a harmful effect on the tissues of the environment. Thus we shall consider both plastic and metallic deterioration.

Deterioration of a plastic is generally known as degradation. This usually involves a change in the molecular structure of the polymer that is brought about by the catalytic effect of various features of the environment such as heat, ultraviolet light, and ionizing radiations. The length of the molecules may change; some of the side groups attached to the basic chains may be released and others added; the relationship between one molecule and its neighbors may be altered, either increasing or decreasing the cross-linking, and so on. These are usually slow changes. It is known that molecular chain shortening results in a decrease of material strength. An increase in the degree of cross-linking makes the material more brittle. Changes in the nature of the side groups affects the physical properties of the material, such as conductivity, opacity, and color. Release of the by-products of polymer degradation into the surrounding tissues has not yet been studied in detail.

The five main degradation effects of polymers are

1. Random chain scission
2. Depolymerization
3. Cross-linking
4. Bond changes
5. Side group changes

Random chain scission involves the breaking of the molecular chain at random points, leaving fragments that are large in comparison with the monomer unit.

Depolymerization resembles chain scission in that it involves the breaking of bonds on the basic carbon chain. However, in this case the points of initial attack are at chain ends or at specific weak links in the chain, and once initiated, the attack propagates along the chain either until it is entirely converted to the monomer or until some secondary process interferes with its progress. The thermal degradation of PMMA provides a good example, over 90% of the original monomer being reclaimed. When methylmethacrylate is polymerized, the molecular chain has to terminate in some manner, and this is commonly achieved by what is called disproportionation of radicals.

Two chains, each with an unsaturated bond at the end, may react, terminating one chain by the addition of a hydrogen atom to satisfy that bond and the other chain by the loss of the hydrogen atom and the formation of a double carbon bond (Fig. 2-7, *A* and *B*). It is at chain ends such as these that the depolymerization process starts, for the bond joining an unsaturated radical on the end of the chain (that is, a radical having a double bond between the carbon atoms) to the remainder of the chain is relatively weak and susceptible to environmental attack. In this case the monomer methylmethacrylate is produced (Fig. 2-7, *C*). Since the new chain also terminates with an unsaturated radical, the process will become autocatalytic. This is sometimes called an "unzipping" reaction, for obvious reasons. It is possible, as in the case of PMMA, for large amounts of monomer to be produced in this way. The amount of monomer produced by degrading agencies varies in different polymers, the

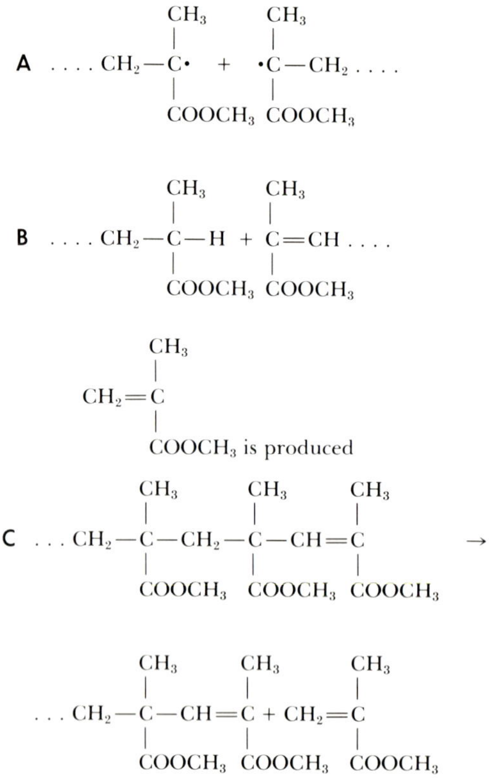

Fig. 2-7. A, Disproportionation of radicals. Two chains, each with unsaturated bond at end (denoted •), react. **B,** One chain is terminated by addition of hydrogen atom to satisfy that bond, and other chain by loss of hydrogen atom and formation of double carbon bond. **C,** Depolymerization of polymethylmethacrylate. This is commonly known as an "unzipping" reaction.

principal factor being the structure of the polymer.

Cross-linking is most likely to occur under the influence of ultraviolet and ionizing radiations. In the case of polyethylene, degradation occurs on exposure to sunlight. This results in ionization of some of the hydrogen atoms. If the electron can escape, a secondary process of the liberation of a hydrogen atom and the formation of a free radical may follow because of inherent instability of the ionized structure.

Changes in the nature of bonds between carbon atoms on the basic molecular chain may occur without any kind of chain scission or cross-linking. The thermal degradation of polyvinyl chloride illustrates this point, undergoing a process known as dehydrohalogenation. The polymer changes fairly quickly from colorless to pale brown and finally becomes black, with hydrogen chloride (HCl) liberated from the polymer.

Side group changes may also occur, often without radically altering the molecular weight of the material. Hydrolysis (reaction with water) often involves these side chains. Polyvinyl acetate, for instance, is converted to polyvinyl alcohol by the catalytic action of water. Since polyvinyl acetate is insoluble in water and polyvinyl alcohol is water soluble, such reactions have great implications.

EFFECTS OF STERILIZING AGENTS ON MEDICAL PLASTICS

Effective sterilization of medical implants may adversely affect the plastic itself. Plester[5] reviewed the various methods available. However, there are very few plastics that can be safely sterilized by all methods, and there are no methods that can be used for all plastics. The usual sterilization techniques include dry heat, moist heat, radiation, and chemical sterilants.

Dry heat involves temperatures ranging from 160° to 190° C, the recommended exposure decreasing with increasing temperature. This process is unsuitable for many plastics, as these temperatures cause the materials to soften or deform. Polyethylene falls into this category. Even if the softening point is not reached, oxidation may become a problem, such as with nylon 66. The only commonly used medical plastics that can be dry-heat sterilized are polytetrafluoroethylene (PTFE) and silicone rubber, both noted for their thermal stability.

The temperatures involved in steam sterilization are lower, ranging from 121° to 134° C, and hence oxidative degradation is not a problem. There are still some plastics that will soften at these temperatures. Any form of heat sterilization may cause distortion of materials.

Radiation is a favored alternative to heat sterilization. Gamma-ray radiation obtained from the radioactive cobalt-60 isotope, or possibly electrons produced by high-voltage accelerators, are commonly employed, these two methods having roughly similar effects. Although all plastics are affected to some extent by radiation, there are many where the accepted dose level of about 2.5 Mrad is below the level where any significant changes are produced. Nylon, polyethylene terephthalate (Dacron), polyethylene, polyvinyl chloride, and polystyrene can all be safely sterilized by irradiation. Nylon 6 and nylon 66 tend to harden at high doses. PMMA may turn brown, become brittle, and crack.

Chemical sterilization is often used, especially with gases such as ethylene oxide. Sodium hydroxide is another popular chemical sterilant. The major problems associated with chemical sterilants concern the dose levels to produce efficient sterilization and the removal of all traces of the chemicals prior to implantation to avoid any tissue reactions. The Ridley caustic soda method is discussed later.

The effects of the external environment and sterilants on polymers are much easier to assess than the effects of the body environment. In fact, very little is known about the degeneration of plastics after implantation. None of the usual degrading agencies are active within the body. Implants are not exposed to damaging temperatures or most of the effects of ultraviolet or gamma radiation. There is no atmospheric oxygen or ozone, thus precluding attack by these radiations. It is conceivable, although unlikely, that an intraocular lens may be affected by ultraviolet radiation. The list of possible causes of plastic degeneration is small and includes hydrolysis, reactions with the oxidizing media of the body, reactions with free radicals in the body, enzyme-catalyzed degradation, and possibly, in case of infection, microbial degradation. Obviously the intraocular environment should be a poor supporter of these degradation agencies. The most important damaging effects on plastic implants are due to hydrolysis.

PMMA has thus far shown no degradation in vivo. However, nylon is often used as supporting structures for the optical portion of an intraocular lens. Nylon fell into disrepute as an implantable polymer because it has shown rapid degradation with ultimate loss of tensile strength. In some cases it has provoked intolerable tissue reactions. This must prove confusing to the ophthalmic surgeon who has considered nylon to be a very inert material evoking little, if any, inflammatory response. This may be due to the availability of several different types of nylon, depending on the exact monomers involved in the construction of the molecules. Also, nylon has exhibited great strength when used in its fibrous form, as in ophthalmic surgery. Nylon also probably reacts differently in other parts of the body. The main drawbacks of nylon are due to its hydrophilic and hydrolyzable nature. Nylons readily absorb water and thus lose tensile strength. It has also been suggested that proteolytic enzymes might aid in hydrolysis by attacking the amide group of the nylon polymer. Dacron (polyethylene terephthalate) has been shown to be more resistant to degradation than nylon, but this superiority is not conclusive.

Deterioration of metallic implants is quite different from polymeric degradation. The destruction of metallic structures by the action of the surrounding medium is defined as corrosion. While this is obviously of paramount importance in orthopedic implants, it is probably of little significance in eye surgery. Therefore it has received scant attention. Platinum, platinum-iridium, and titanium are now being used as supports for some intraocular lenses. Other metallic materials are likely to follow. Although the majority of corrosion processes involve solutions and are electrochemical in nature, the most important reactions involving metals and their environment are metal-gas reactions and specifically metal-oxygen reactions. Most metals oxidize in contact with air. Of all the metals, titanium is probably the most corrosion resistant.

In order for a metal to be corrosion resistant it must, upon initial exposure to the atmosphere, form a thin, uniform oxide layer that remains continuous with and adherent to the metal. For this to happen the oxide film must be self-limiting; that is, it must grow to a size sufficient to afford protection and then cease to grow. Another crucial requirement is that the oxide film must be coherent with the underlying metal. Oxygen ions are not normally the same size as metal ions, and the interatomic spacing in the oxide lattice is generally different from that in the metal. If the differences in the atomic structures of oxide and metal are very great (manifest, for example, by their densities), then the strain in the oxide lattice necessary to accommodate the change may be large enough to disrupt the film-metal interface. This results in cracks in the oxide film, which may leave the underlying metal exposed to attack.

IDEAL IMPLANT MATERIAL

For obvious reasons, autogenous tissues are preferable to synthetic materials for implantation. But it is also obvious that there are many situations in which synthetic materials must be used. The autogenous tissue may not be available, or in some cases the synthetic material may actually be preferable to the autogenous tissue for one reason or another.

Most alloplastic materials are unlimited in their availability. Their use obviates an additional operative procedure to obtain the necessary autograft material. This secondary procedure usually requires a general anesthetic, prolongs the operation, leaves scars, and causes the patient to have postoperative pain and perhaps later sequellae such as undesirable adhesions. One must also consider that autogenous grafts are sometimes absorbed and sometimes develop such alterations that they fail to perform their function properly.

Seales[6] has set forth eight criteria that any proposed implant material must fulfill. The material must be

1. Chemically inert
2. Not physically modified by contact with tissues
3. Acceptable to the body with no inflammation or foreign body reaction
4. Noncarcinogenic
5. Nonallergenic
6. Capable of fabrication to desired form
7. Capable of resisting mechanical strains
8. Readily sterilizable

To the above requirements should be added the ability to be safely and easily removed. The ophthalmologist, who has a vested interest in replacement of the lens, would in addition to these insist upon a low specific gravity, optimum refractive qualities, color stability, nonclouding, and ability to stimulate only the most minimal amount of capsule formation around it.

It is a generally accepted statement that an implant should arouse little or no tissue reaction. But in certain situations such lack of response is not desirable. Solid implants thus will tend to become free-floating, with a cystlike sac formed about the mass. Early mild reaction may be of little later consequence and in fact may be of value. In many prostheses widely used at present, Dacron cloth is permanently attached on the outside. Here the reactivity of the Dacron is of value, since it stimulates the proliferation of tissues that ramify through the cloth, making for later firm fixation of the implant.

The requirement that every implant must remain permanently unchanged in the tissues likewise does not hold good for every situation. As examples, consider tissue adhesives and sutures; here controlled biodegradability may be desirable.

Although the safety and efficacy of intraocular implants have increased enormously, it is apparent that the ideal intraocular implant lens has not yet been achieved. There has been universal acceptance of PMMA as the constituent of the optical portion of the implant. Yet it is possible that other materials in the future might be more desirable. A theoretical example is lightweight glass capable of spectral transmission so that the "blue vision" of aphakia is eliminated. There have been many changes in the materials used for the haptic portion of some of the commonly used iris-supported and capsule-supported intraocular lenses. Examples are nylon, polypropylene, PMMA, platinum-iridium, and titanium.

As stated in Chapter One, the ideal intraocular implant lens can only be approached through the interdisciplinary effort of clinicians, bioengineers, and medical scientists.

REFERENCES

1. Brydson, J. A.: Plastics materials, London, 1975, Newnes-Butterworths, pp. 328, 392.
2. Little, K.: The interaction of plastics and tissues, Biochem. Eng., p. 404, 1968.
3. Harris, H.: Survey of breast implants from the point of view of carcinogenesis, Plast. Reconstr. Surg. **28**:81, 1961.
4. Hoopes, J., Edgerton, M., Jr., and Shelley, W.: Use of the organic synthetics for augmentation mammaplasty and their relation to breast cancer. Presented at annual meeting of American Society for Plastic and Reconstructive Surgery, Las Vegas, October 6, 1966.
5. Plester, D. W.: The effects of sterilizing processes on plastics, Biomed. Eng. **5**:443, 1970.
6. Seales, J.: Discussion on metals and synthetic materials in relation to soft tissues: tissue reaction to synthetic materials, Proc. R. Soc. Med. **46**:647, 1953.

CHAPTER 3

Theory of pseudophakos

COMPARISON OF CURRENT METHODS OF OPTICAL CORRECTION OF APHAKIA

In view of the fact that a spectacle lens and a contact lens are safe appliances since they can be removed or replaced if defective, what accounts for the current popularity of intraocular lenses? This is easily explained by examining the three available methods of optical correction of aphakia: (1) spectacle lens in front of the eye, (2) contact lens on the eye, and (3) intraocular lens inside the eye.

Spectacle lenses

Spectacle lenses were better accepted 30 years ago than today for two reasons. First, no other method of optical correction was available. Second, cataract surgery was rarely performed before the cataract was mature or nearly so in one eye and vision markedly reduced in the second eye. Therefore the improvement in vision appeared dramatic to the patient, and this made his psychologic adjustment to aphakia easier. With the advent of the intracapsular cataract extraction and its subsequent sophistication, cataract extraction is now often performed earlier. In addition, surgery is being performed on older patients who adapt to the handicaps of spectacle lenses with less facility.

Woods[1] outlined the disadvantages of spectacle lenses in aphakia after having personally undergone cataract extraction in both eyes:

1. The image size is magnified by about 25%. When the aphakic patient first receives his aphakic spectacles, he is immediately astounded by the increase in the size of familiar objects. If he is aphakic in one eye only and still has some fair residual vision in the second eye, the attempt at binocular vision produces a superimposed diplopia. Useful binocular vision is impossible until the second eye is operated on. However, even if binocularity is restored by surgery on the second eye, the magnification of familiar objects causes false spatial orientation. This results in a series of minor domestic tragedies such as overturned tumblers, spilling of ink, and broken flower vases.

2. Spherical aberration. The aphakic patient suddenly finds himself in a parabolic world. Ocular movements cause this parabolic world to squirm like a writhing snake. Straight lines are transformed into curves. A pincushion distortion occurs.

3. Poor coordination of manual movements. The new visual imagery causes incessant clumsiness with simple tasks, such as sharpening a pencil, carving a turkey, or placing a key in a lock.

Fortunately the newly created aphakic patient can be assured that his three most obvious difficulties—false orientation, spherical aberration, and lack of coordination—can ultimately be partly overcome with time, practice, and good aspheric spectacles. There are two other problems that are so difficult to overcome they must be endured. These follow.

4. Restricted peripheral field (Figs. 3-1 and 3-2). The visual field of the normal, uncorrected aphakic eye does not differ

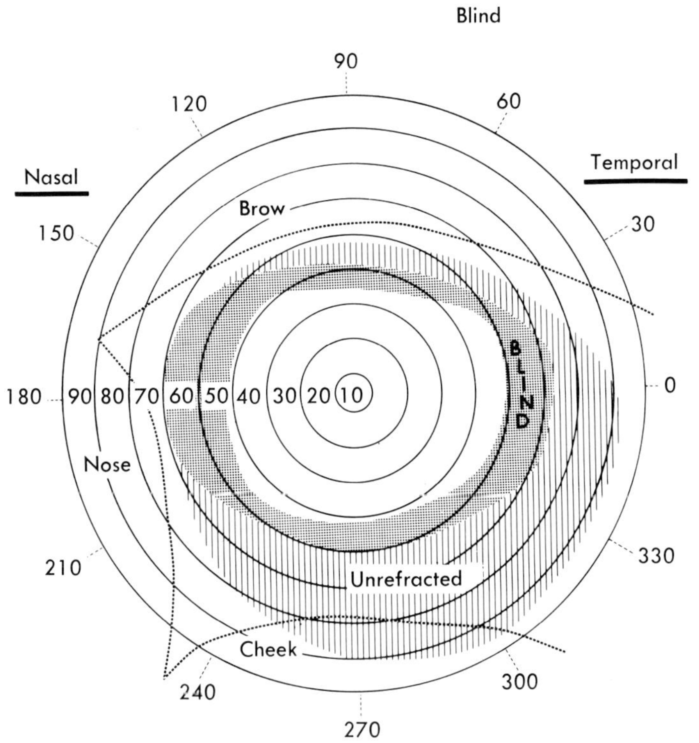

Fig. 3-1. Effect of aphakia spectacle lens on visual field. (From Dabezies, O. H., Jr.: Contact and Intraocular Lens J. **2**:8-13, 1976.)

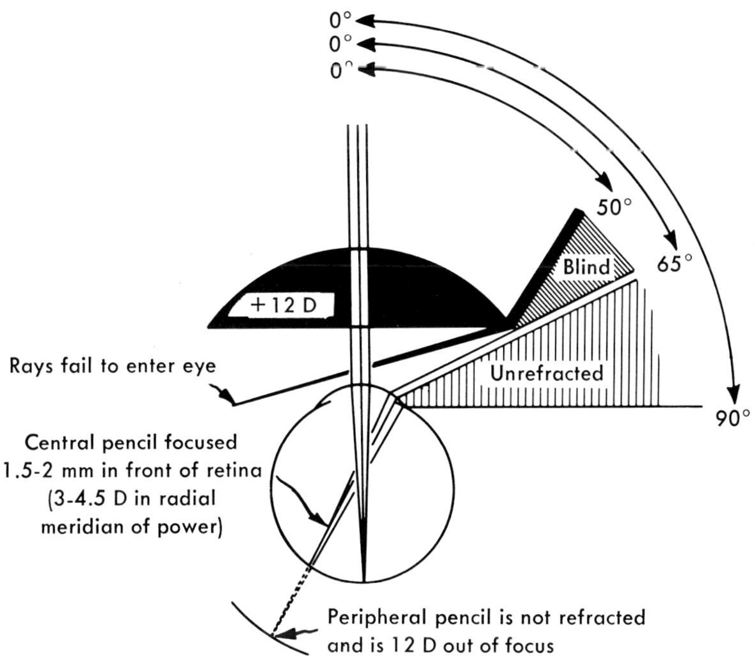

Fig. 3-2. Spectacle lens–corrected aphakia. Refraction of peripheral rays by high-plus nonapheric spectacle lens creates ring scotoma from 50° to 65°. (From Dabezies, O. H., Jr.: Contact and Intraocular Lens J. **2**:8-13, 1976.)

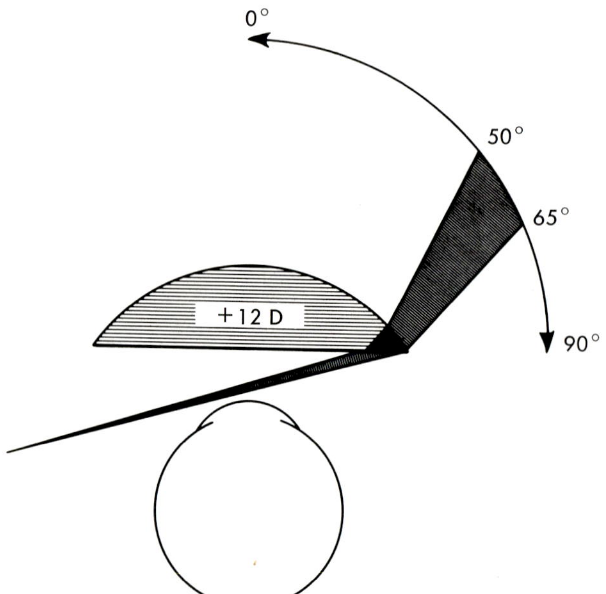

Fig. 3-3. Peripheral prismatic effect of high-plus lens. Rays from 50° to 65° fail to pass into eye. (From Dabezies, O. H., Jr.: Contact and Intraocular Lens J. **2**:8-13, 1976.)

from that of the normal phakic eye if appropriately larger test objects are used. The peripheral restriction of the visual field results from the use of aphakic spectacles. There are three causes for this reduction in field:

a. Small size of aphakic lenticular spectacle
b. Ring scotoma
c. Unrefracted field of vision outside spectacle lens

The usual small size of the average aphakic lenticular spectacle moves the ring scotoma more centrally and leaves a greater amount of unrefracted visual field outside the spectacle lens.

The ring scotoma takes the general shape of the spectacle lens, is about 12° to 15° wide, and surrounds the refracted visual field. As pointed out by Dabezies,[2] the edge of an aphakic spectacle can be considered to be a base in a prism that bends light rays toward its base. Because of the considerable prismatic effect at the periphery of the spectacle lens, a ray in the area of 50° to 65° from central fixation strikes the periphery of the lens, is bent 13° to the base, fails to pass into the eye, and therefore is not seen (Fig. 3-3). This "blind" area completely circumscribes the restricted field of the aphakic eye. Dabezies[2] reminds us that this blind area is not a true scotoma of the eye, but rather an optically produced defect in the visual field due to the prismatic effect at the periphery of the lens.

The ring scotoma is not stationary. Its movements are initiated by movements of the eye. It is well known by all aphakic patients wearing spectacles that, in ordinary group conversation, faces pop in and out of the blind area with the annoying insolence of a jack-in-the-box. Thus objects observed in the unrefracted visual field (peripheral) may disappear if the gaze is moved toward them, since they move into the blind area. Welsh[3] referred to this as the roving ring scotoma, which is descriptive enough to be popularly accepted in spite of Linksz's[4] observation that "it is obviously the eye rather than the scotoma which does the moving."

A

B

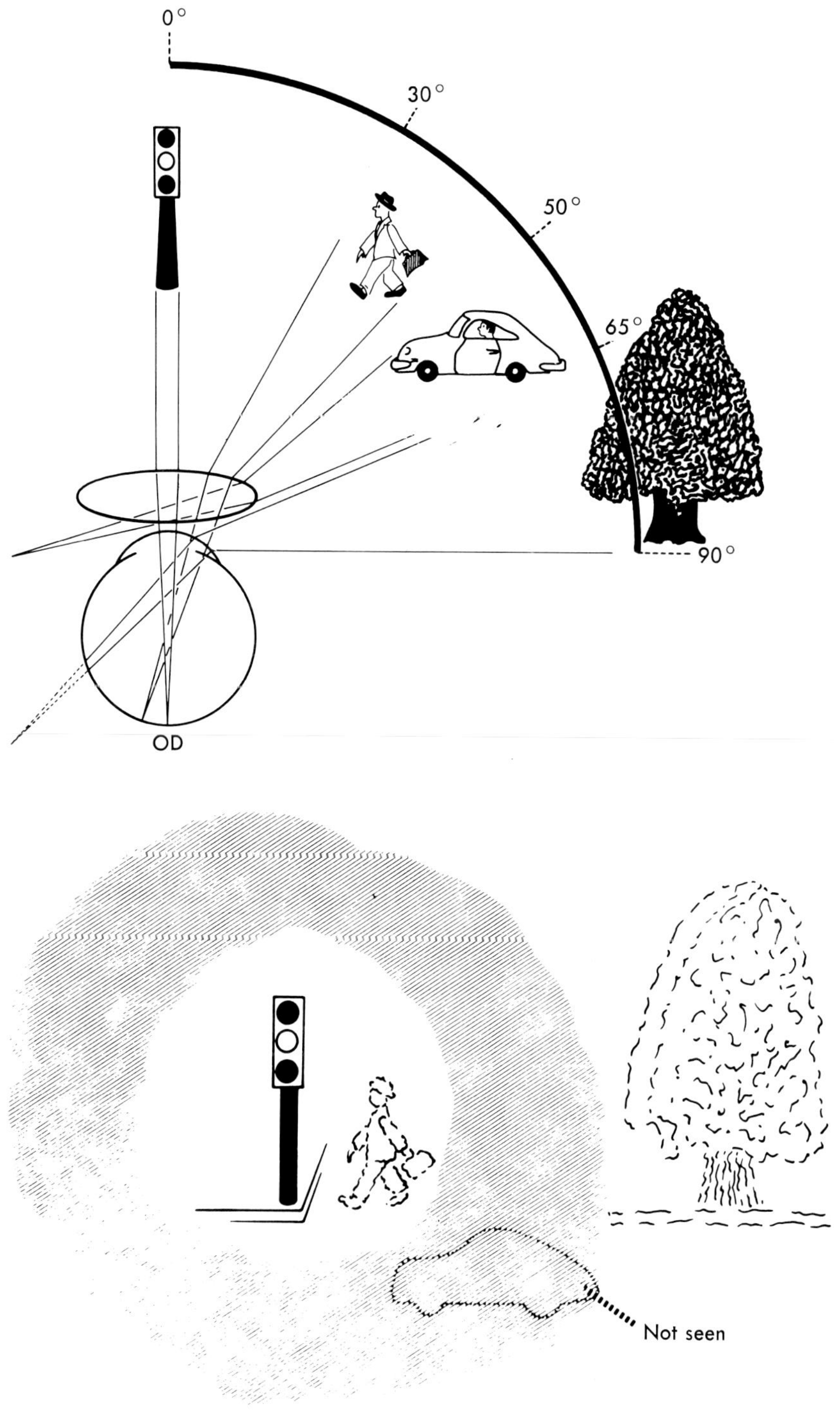

Fig. 3-4. A, Aphakia spectacle lens–corrected vision in straight-ahead gaze. Rays 50° to 65° fail to enter eye. Rays 65° to 90° are unrefracted by spectacle glass. **B,** View as seen by patient. Ring scotoma (optically blind area). (From Dabezies, O. H., Jr.: Contact and Intraocular Lens J. **2:**8-13, 1976.)

A

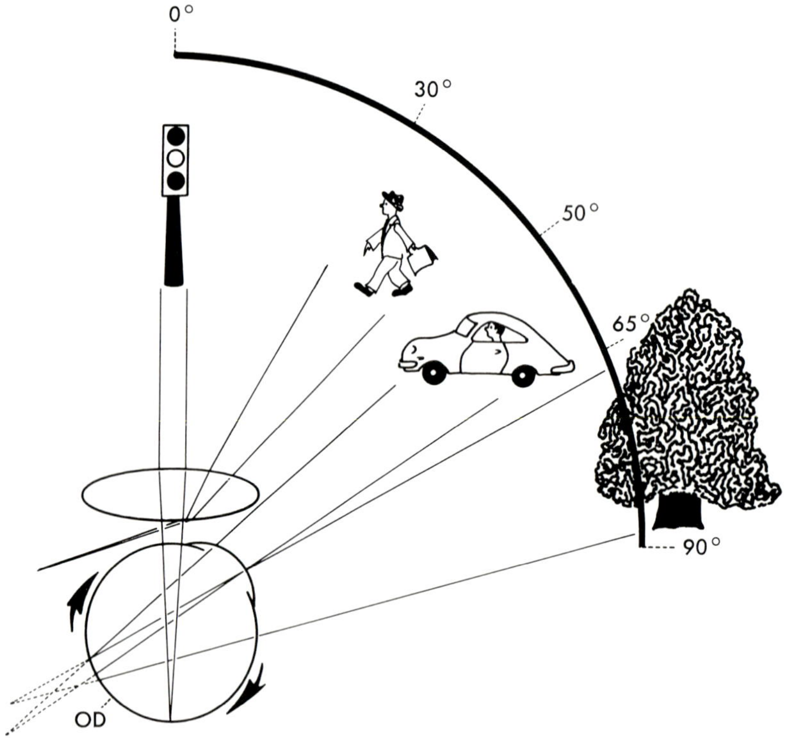

B

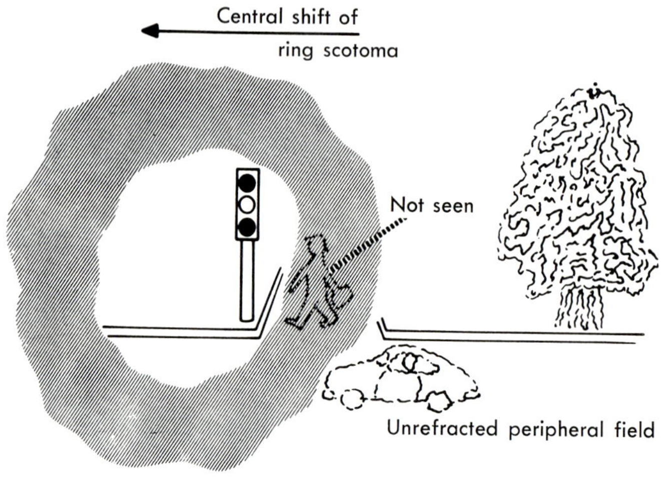

Fig. 3-5. A, Aphakia spectacle lens–corrected vision when gaze directed laterally. Rays 30° to 50° fail to enter eye. Rays 50° to 90° are unrefracted, as they fail to enter spectacle glass. **B,** View as seen by patient. Due to central shift of ring scotoma, person disappears. When gaze returns centrally, person reappears (jack-in-the-box phenomenon). (From Dabezies, O. H., Jr.: Contact and Intraocular Lens J. **2**:8-13, 1976.)

To illustrate the jack-in-the-box phenomenon, consider a patient wearing aphakic spectacles gazing directly ahead through the center of his lens (Fig. 3-4). The center of the refractive field of view corresponds to the optical axis of the spectacle lens. The ring scotoma extends from 50° to 65° of the visual field. If the eye rotates temporally (Fig. 3-5) (the head is not rotated), and fixates on an object 30° from the original optical axis, the eye is now gazing through the midperiphery of the spectacle lens. Objects formerly located at 30° to 50° in the original, straight-ahead field are deflected by the prismatic effect of the spectacle lens (base in effect) so that they no longer enter the eye. The blind area (ring scotoma) has moved centrally and lies 30° lateral to the new optic axis. At the same time, objects formerly hidden inside the ring scotoma now appear. In summary, in the straight-ahead position the blind area begins approximately 50° from the optical axis. When the patient shifts his gaze 30° laterally, the blind area now begins 30° from the optical axis. This shifting centralward of the blind area causes the jack-in-the-box phenomenon.

The other major cause of the complaint of poor side vision is the fact that the visual field, extending from the temporal 65° to the most peripheral portion of the visual field at 85°, is unrefracted, since light rays from this area are too far peripheral (temporal to the spectacle frame) to enter the spectacle lens. However, the unrefracted rays do pass into the eye. The resultant peripheral vision that surrounds the ring scotoma is very blurred but is nevertheless helpful to the patient in establishing overall space orientation.

The plight of the spectacle-corrected aphakic patient was humorously described in a paper entitled "Cadillacs, Volkswagens, and Aphakic Corrections."[5] The author, a bilaterally aphakic ophthalmologist, made the following observations regarding the ring scotoma. With 3 mm pupils, wearing 45 mm aspheric lenses at a vertex distance of 12 mm and a spectacle lens power of OD +10.00 +0.75 × 20° = 20/10, OS +8.50 +1.00 × 160° = 20/10, the scotoma measured 15°, using a 1° test object at 330 mm. The position of the scotoma was between 40° and 55°. Experimenting in his parking lot, he found that this scotoma obscured a Cadillac at 45 ft (13.5 m) and a Volkswagen at 40 ft (12 m). A person was completely obscured at 4 ft (1.2 m).

A means of simulating the plight of aphakic patients was suggested.[6] A −14 D contact lens is placed on the cornea and a +12 D spectacle is worn in front of the eye. This will convince any ophthalmologist that the adjustment to aphakic spectacles is not a minor problem.

5. Continual adjustment of aphakic spectacles. The glasses must be accurately centered and adjusted. Since the optically active aphakic patient uses only the optical center of his lens, any maladjustment of the pupillary distance introduces at once a prismatic error that greatly reduces visual efficiency. Similarly, a fraction of a millimeter in the vertical adjustment produces a similar error. In addition, small variations in vertex distance introduce relatively large errors of refraction. As any optician will attest, the spectacle-corrected aphakic occupies much of his valuable time with incessant requests for spectacle adjustments.

Contact lenses

Contact lenses, for the patient who can wear them, are far less visually disabling than aphakic spectacles. Linksz[4] cited the following:

1. No significant magnification (only about 7%)
2. No appreciable spherical aberration, no pincushion distortion
3. No ring scotoma, no jack-in-the-box phenomenon or roving ring scotoma, and therefore full peripheral vision

There are other advantages. There is practically no false spatial orientation.

They are safer than intraocular lenses in that they can be discontinued with less difficulty. They are effective in some superficially scarred corneas that result in irregular astigmatism. They are more comfortable in eyes after cataract extraction, probably due to the reduced corneal sensitivity.

In general, they are more practical in the younger aphakic patients than the elderly. This is the main disadvantage. Most elderly patients do not possess the manual dexterity required to insert and remove them. To these may be added patients with infirmities such as rheumatoid arthritis, Parkinsonism, hemiplegia, and senility. Also, many elderly patients live alone in somewhat less than adequate hygienic conditions. Experience has shown that the majority of unilaterally aphakic elderly patients discard their contact lenses relatively soon, and the great majority are no longer using them after a few years.[7] The elderly bilaterally aphakic patient usually finds contact lenses even more difficult to manage, since they must use aphakic spectacles to initiate the process of insertion and sometimes the removal. However, they wear them more faithfully than the unilateral aphake, probably because the poor vision of two uncorrected aphakic eyes leads to better motivation. While a 60-year-old patient may satisfactorily manage contact lenses even with advancing age, the 70-year-old patient usually experiences frustration in his attempt to learn how to manage them.

Most ophthalmologists have found the contact lens correction of the unilaterally aphakic child resulting from trauma to be disappointing. Amblyopia and ocular deviation are rarely prevented. On the other hand, there is growing evidence that intraocular lenses may be far superior in this regard (see below).

Soft contact lenses may prove to be more applicable in the elderly patient if technologic sophistication increases so that the lenses may be worn for long periods of time. To date, this goal has not been reached.

Intraocular lenses

Intraocular lenses provide many advantages over both spectacle and contact lenses. The elimination of perceptual problems, as discussed with contact lenses, requires no repetition. In addition, image size disparity is reduced still further. A comparison[8] of 30 unilaterally aphakic adult patients wearing a contact lens with 30 unilaterally aphakic adult patients with an intraocular iris-clip implant showed an average retinal image size increase of 6.99% in the former group and 1.92% in the latter. The figure of 1.92% was later corrected to 0.20% minification.[9] The difference arose over computing the average of cases with magnification and of cases with minification. The AO Space Eikonometer was used for all measurements. An average visual acuity of the operated eye of 0.8 was found in both groups. The patients using contact lenses were considerably younger (49.6 years) than those with implants (67.7 years). Using the Wirt stereopsis test, the contact lens group recorded an average of 45.7% and the implant group 81.8%, in spite of the 18.1 years difference in their average ages.

Since the intraocular lens is intended to remain in situ permanently, it eliminates all the difficulties in inserting and removing contact lenses encountered by elderly patients and those with infirmities such as Parkinsonism and so on.

The use of an intraocular lens may be advantageous for those working in unusual environments (cattle ranchers, miners, and so on) and for those whose visual requirements for occupation must be fulfilled (pilots, army, navy, marines, and so on).

The potential for prevention of amblyopia in young children who suffer a traumatic cataract is high. Ophthalmologists have been frustrated in their attempts to prevent amblyopia in these children. At ages 2 to 7 years it is extremely difficult to employ a contact lens following removal of the traumatic cataract. Binkhorst and Gobin[10] fitted 10 of 22 unilaterally aphakic children with contact lenses and reported that suppression or diplopia developed in all cases. Van Balen[11] found that only 3 of 15 unilaterally aphakic children under the age of 14 could be treated adequately with a contact lens. A comprehensive report of the techniques and perspectives of lens implants in children, including an orthoptic analysis of all treated cases, was presented by Bierlaagh and co-workers.[12] They treated 29 patients less than 15 years of age who had unilateral pseudophakia after lens injury. The patients were divided into three groups according to the age at which injury occurred. They represented a consecutive series of cases of traumatic cataract treated by lens implant. The causes of the cataract were contusion of the eye as well as perforating injury with or without an intraocular foreign body. A few cases had very severely damaged anterior segments. During a follow-up period of 1 to 9 years, a complication was seen only once, and that in a severely damaged eye in which a band-shaped keratopathy developed as a result of the injury and repeated subsequent surgical interventions. All other eyes were doing well in spite of corneal scarring and other posttraumatic pathology as well as an occasional inevitable case of amblyopia. Twenty-three of the 29 eyes had 0.5 visual acuity or better and only 1 eye had less than 0.1 visual acuity. The summary of orthoptic evaluation of all patients revealed that in every age category the final result far exceeded that of any other known method of treating these difficult problems. This subject is discussed in greater detail in Chapter 11.

The disadvantages of an intraocular implant center about the surgery itself. The surgery requires adequate education in the proper selection of cases, the choice of surgical procedure, and the technique of the surgery itself. This is a formidable responsibility of the surgeon. It has not been statistically determined that implant surgery leads to more complications than routine cataract surgery. However, if this proves to be the case, it must then be determined if the previously mentioned disadvantages of other forms of optical correction of aphakia outweigh any greater risk involved in the implantation of an intraocular lens. It is apparent that implant surgeons and their patients are sufficiently happy with their surgical results that the procedure appears to be gaining in popularity. The specific disadvantages of operative and postoperative complications of implant surgery will be considered later.

ANISEIKONIA

The subject of aniseikonia appears to be a central theme in the various methods of the optical correction of aphakia. Much has been written on the limit of tolerance of image size disparity for comfortable binocular vision. Most authors consider 5% to 8% to be the limit.[13-18]

Patients wearing a spectacle lens are not usually disturbed by aniseikonia, since it is so great (22% to 35%) that binocular fusion in the monocularly aphakic patient is impossible. They use only one eye, either with aphakic spectacles or without, for all visual activities. Patients who use a contact lens on the aphakic eye do not possess the binocular visual efficiency of those with an intraocular lens. The degree of aniseikonia may exceed tolerable limits for some but apparently not for others.

If iseikonia is the aim in unilateral implantations, Binkhorst[19] attempts to equal the posterior focal length of the uncorrected pseudophakic eye to that of the uncorrected fellow eye. Thus the corneal power of the eye to be operated on (corrected with the spectacle correction of the fellow eye) and the axial length of the fellow eye are decisive. The latter has to be corrected due to the forward displacement of the second principal plane in the pseudophakic eye as compared with its position in the phakic eye. In the schematic phakic eye this displacement is −0.657 mm, corresponding with a −1.69 D anisometropia.

There are many formulas and convenient nomograms for the selection of a suitable power lens. This is discussed in greater detail in Chapter 6.

SUMMARY

The theory of pseudophakos is based on the disadvantages inherent in the spectacle and contact lens methods of correcting aphakia. There are advantages and disadvantages in all three methods. The surgeon is charged with the responsibility of deciding which is best for the patient. This decision can only be based on a thorough understanding of what confronts the patient whose eye will lose its crystalline lens.

REFERENCES

1. Woods, A. C.: The adjustment to aphakia, Am. J. Ophthalmol. **35**:118-122, 1952.
2. Dabezies, O. H., Jr.: Defects of vision through aphakic spectacle lenses, Contact Intraocular Lens J. **2**:8-20, 1976.
3. Welsh, R. C.: The roving ring scotoma with its Jack-in-the-box phenomenon of strong-plus (aphakic) spectacle lenses, Am. J. Ophthalmol. **51**:1277-1281, 1961.
4. Linksz, A.: Optical complications of aphakia. In Theodore, F. H., editor: Complications after cataract surgery, Boston, 1964, Little, Brown and Co., pp. 597-634.
5. McLemore, C.: Cadillacs, Volkswagens, and aphakic corrections, Arch. Ophthalmol. **70**: 734-735, 1963.
6. Welsh, R. C.: Experimental simulation of aphakia, Br. J. Ophthalmol. **49**:84-86, 1965.
7. Nordlohne, M. E.: The intraocular implant lens. Development and results with special reference to the Binkhorst lens, The Hague, 1975, Dr. W. Junk, N. V., Publishers, p. 5.
8. Girard, L. J., Friedman, C. D., Moore, C. D., Blau, R. I., Binkhorst, C. D., and Gobin, M. H. M. A.: Intraocular implants and contact lenses, Arch. Ophthalmol. **68**:762-775, 1962.
9. Binkhorst, C. D., and Gobin, M. H. M. A.: Injuries to the eye with lens opacity in young children, Ophthalmologica **148**:169-183, 1964.
10. Binkhorst, C. D., and Gobin, M. H. M. A.: Pseudophakia after lens injury in children, Ophthalmologica **154**:81-87, 1967.
11. van Balen, A. T. M.: Binkhorst's method of implantation of pseudophakoi in unilateral traumatic cataract, Ophthalmologica **165**:490-494, 1972.
12. Bierlaagh, J. J. M., Van der Wee, A., Kats, A., Leonard, P. A. M., and Binkhorst, C. D.: Technique and perspectives of lens implants (pseudophakia) in children, Proceedings of the Second International Orthoptic Congress, Amsterdam, May 1971, Amsterdam, 1971, Excerpta Medica.
13. Ogle, K. N., Burian, H. M., and Bannon, R. E.: On the correction of unilateral aphakia with contact lenses, Arch. Ophthalmol. **59**:639-652, 1958.
14. Linksz, A.: Aniseikonia: with notes on the Jackson-Lancaster controversy, Fifteenth Jackson Memorial Lecture, Trans. Am. Acad. Ophthalmol. Otolaryngol. **63**:117-140, 1959.
15. Choyce, D. P.: All-acrylic anterior-chamber implants in ophthalmic surgery, Lancet **2**:165-171, 1961.
16. Troutman, R. C.: Artiphakia and aniseikonia, Trans. Am. Ophthalmol. Soc. **60**:590-658, 1962.
17. Crone, R. A., and Leuridan, O. M. A.: Tolerance for aniseikonia. I. Diplopia thresholds in the vertical and horizontal meridians of the visual field, Albrecht von Graefes Arch. Klin. Ophthalmol. **188**:1-16, 1973.
18. Crone, R. A., and Leuridan, O. M. A.: Tolerance for aniseikonia. II. Determination based on the amplitude of cyclofusion, Albrecht von Graefes Arch. Klin. Ophthalmol. **188**:17-22, 1973.
19. Binkhorst, C. D.: The iridocapsular (two-loop) lens and the iris clip (four-loop) lens in pseudophakia, Trans. Am. Acad. Ophthalmol. Otolaryngol. **77**:589-617, 1973.

CHAPTER 4

History of pseudophakos

The history of intraocular lenses has always been exciting, often frustrating, but finally rewarding.

Although the current era of intraocular lenses dates back to 1949, the concept had occurred long before. It has been reported[1-3] that Casanova (1725–1798) referred in his memoirs to the Italian oculist Tadini, who discussed with him the idea of implanting an artificial lens after a cataract extraction in 1764–1765. Casanova is said to have passed this thought to the Dresden court ophthalmologist, Casaamata. Around 1795, Casaamata attempted to introduce a glass lens into an eye after a cataract operation, but the lens immediately slid posteriorly toward the fundus. More recently, Marchi[4] (1940) attempted without success to fixate quartz lenses with platinum wires in the anterior chamber of animals.

The modern history of intraocular lenses began with the contributions of Ridley, who was inspired by a comment made by a medical student who, while observing Ridley close the incision after an intracapsular cataract extraction, exclaimed that he had forgotten to replace the diseased lens with a new one.[5,6] During the Battle of Britain in World War II, many plastic canopies of Spitfire airplanes were shattered by enemy gunfire. This plastic material (polymethylmethacrylate) occasionally lodged inside the eyes of pilots. It was noted that there resulted little, if any, reaction to the plastic material, provided these fragments did not move about inside the eye. Thus in 1949 it occurred to Ridley that such a plastic substance might be used to replace the human lens. He observed[5,7,8] that "plastic compounds have been widely used in surgery, especially for filling gaps in bones, not only of the skull, but also in joint cavities where movement and the presence of synovial fluid resembles to some degree conditions inside the eye." Other materials were also considered in the manufacture of intraocular lenses. One of these was silicate glass.[9] However, its main disadvantage was its greater weight.

POSTERIOR CHAMBER LENSES

On November 29, 1949, Ridley implanted his first intraocular lens. He seemed convinced that "the proper place for an artificial lenticulus must surely be where nature intended the crystalline to be, viz. in the posterior chamber."[10] His first experiences were far from outstanding. His first model was a biconvex polymethylmethacrylate lens of about the same shape as the crystalline lens. The diameter, however, was 8.35 mm, approximately 1 mm smaller than the normal human lens, which was intended to facilitate insertion and avoid undue pressure on the ciliary body. Its weight in air was 112 mg. In his initial effort he implanted the lens in the posterior chamber of an eye of a 45-year-old female after an extracapsular cataract extraction. Due to an error in optical calculation, the patient became highly myopic (−18.00 sphere −6.00 cylinder × 120°), but corrected visual acuity was 20/60. His second attempt, on August 23, 1950, led to a similar

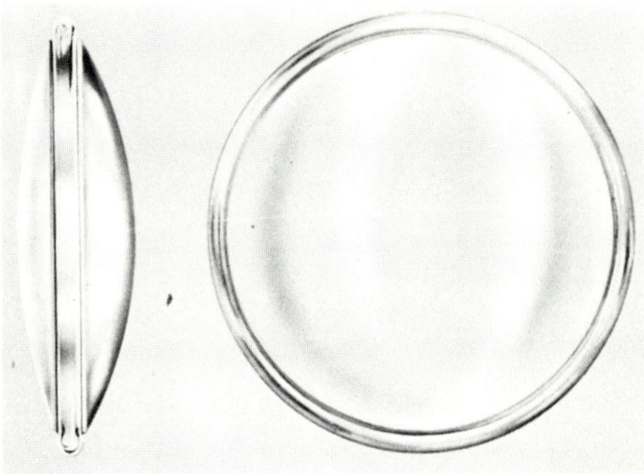

Fig. 4-1. Ridley posterior chamber lens. (From Jaffe, N. S.: Cataract surgery and its complications, ed. 2, St. Louis, 1976, The C. V. Mosby Co.)

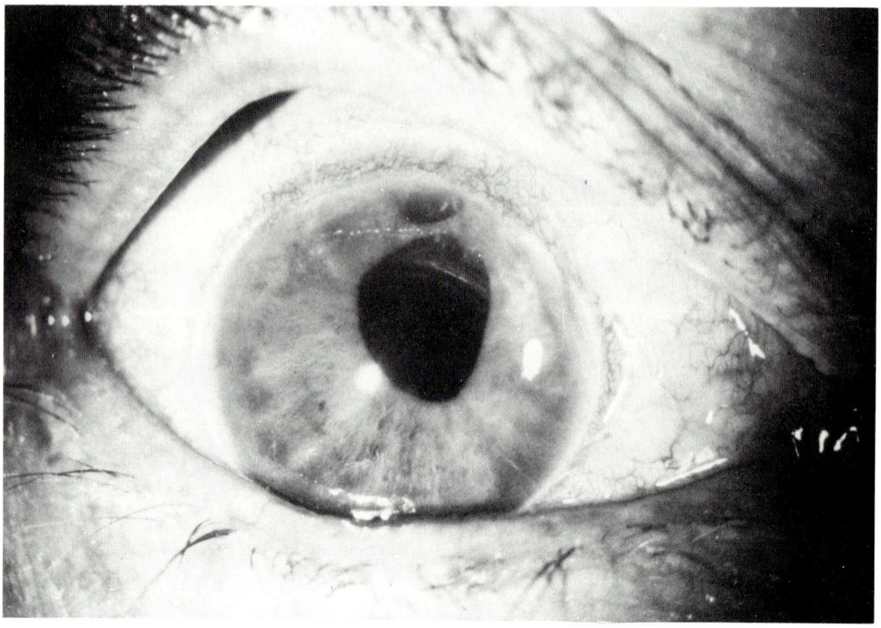

Fig. 4-2. Ridley posterior chamber lens in eye of 62-year-old patient 19 years after its implantation. Note upper edge of pseudophakos in pupillary area. Pupil is eccentric. Visual acuity with correction is 20/40. (From Jaffe, N. S.: Cataract surgery and its complications, ed. 2, St. Louis, 1976, The C. V. Mosby Co.)

result. The design of the lens was then changed (Fig. 4-1), but it could still only be used after an extracapsular lens extraction, and the operation had to be carried out as a one-stage procedure because adhesions developing between the iris and the posterior capsule would otherwise have prevented insertion.[7,11] This made it impossible to insert a lens of suitable power as a secondary procedure. After

Ridley's first report at the Oxford Ophthalmological Congress in 1951, numerous outstanding ophthalmic surgeons followed his example. Among these were Arruga, Barraquer, Binkhorst, Epstein, François, Jonkers, W. Reese, and Weve. Although some achieved initial success, the long-term results were mostly disappointing due to downward decentration, anterior dislocation, and posterior dislocation of the implant. Binkhorst[12] summed it up best by concluding "that this technique is too much of a strain on the surgeon and especially that it is asking too much of the human hand never to fail in completely sparing the delicate suspension system of the zonule and posterior capsule." That some eyes have fared remarkably well is illustrated in Fig. 4-2. The Ridley lens procedure, however, was completely abandoned due to the high incidence of complications resulting from its use. It will be seen later that at least one important aspect of the technique was retained in the most recent methods.

Ridley[13-16] summarized the complications from his original procedure as follows:

1. Some degree of iritis, due mainly to residual material in the eye, and partly to inadequate removal of implant sterilizing solution.
2. Occlusion of the pupil by a dense inflammatory membrane.
3. Late thickening of the posterior capsule in young subjects whose lens cells were still in a state of active growth, necessitating a technically most difficult needling.[17]
4. Loss of the anterior chamber for reasons unknown.
5. Secondary glaucoma due to shallowness of the anterior chamber and a narrow filtration angle.
6. Iris atrophy from pressure by the rim of a badly centered lens was a late complication that might lead to anterior dislocation.
7. Posterior dislocation, occurring in about 6% of cases, was a major catastrophe. Intracapsular extraction and attacks of coughing were especially dangerous in this respect.
8. Extraction of the implant was necessary in 15% of cases.[18]

ANTERIOR CHAMBER LENSES

Anterior chamber lenses with angle fixation

Because of difficulties encountered with secure fixation of the Ridley posterior chamber lens, the next chapter in the modern age of intraocular lenses involved fixation by the chamber angle. Because the appetites of many ophthalmologists for implant surgery had been whetted by Ridley, many anterior chamber lenses and techniques were introduced by numerous surgeons. Baron[19] implanted the first anterior chamber lens on May 13, 1952. He speculated about a lens floating in the anterior chamber ("l'idéal serait d'avoir des lentilles flottantes dans l'humeur aqueuse"), but he, along with others, chose the angle area for support, with rigid or elastic support, with or without transcleral anchoring of the lens. It seems incredible today that so many excellent ophthalmologists were so blinded to the delicacy of the corneal endothelium that they expected these lenses, along with the immediate good results, to last a lifetime. The design of these lenses varied according to whether the supports were rigid or elastic. The most frequently used rigid-supported angle-fixated lens was designed by Strampelli[20,21] (Fig. 4-3). He implanted the first lens of his own design on September 28, 1953. He made the first public report about anterior chamber lenses at the Congress of the Societas Lombardo di Oftalmologica in Pavia on December 8, 1953. Joaquin Barraquer carried out 342 implant operations employing the Strampelli lens, some in phakic eyes suffering from high myopia. Because of the rigid supports, this lens was difficult to center and fixate ideally. Since 1952 Dann-

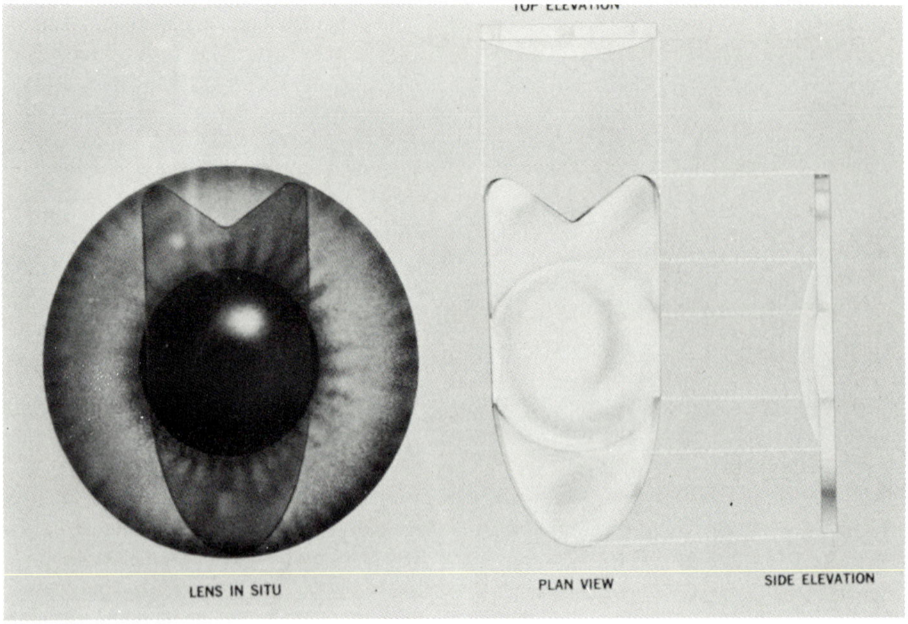

Fig. 4-3. Strampelli nonperforating rigid anterior chamber angle implant. (From Jaffe, N. S.: Cataract surgery and its complications, ed. 2, St. Louis, 1976, The C. V. Mosby Co.)

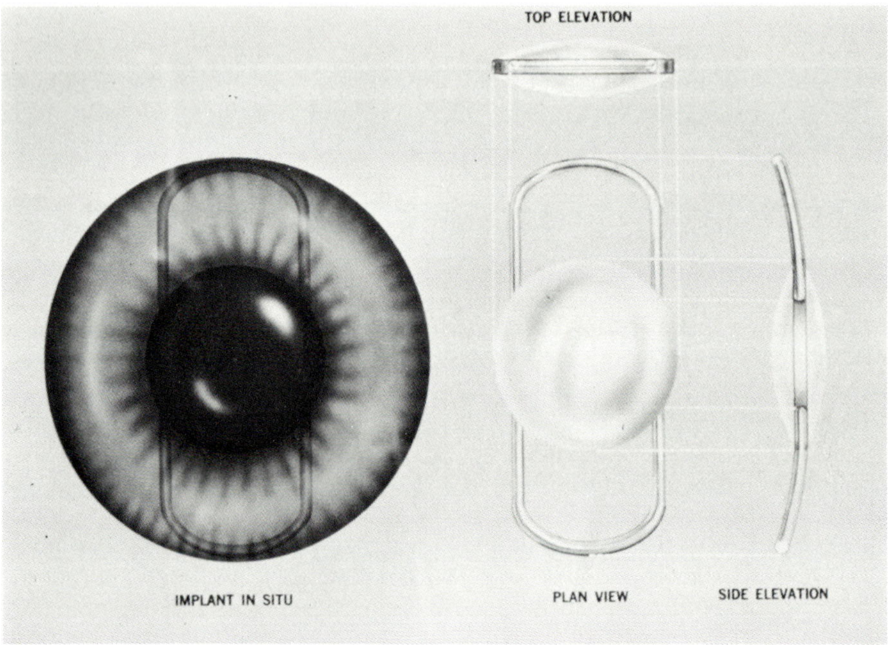

Fig. 4-4. Dannheim nonperforating elastic anterior chamber angle implant. (From Jaffe, N. S.: Cataract surgery and its complications, ed. 2, St. Louis, 1976, The C. V. Mosby Co.)

heim[22] tried to solve the problem of centering the lens in the anterior chamber by means of elastic supporting loops of 0.1 mm Supramid thread (Fig. 4-4). These stabilize the optical portion by means of pressure in the chamber angle.

The first designs of angle-fixated lenses were put into practice by (in alphabetical order) Apollonio, Baron, Barraquer, Bietti, Dannheim, Lieb and Guerry, Ridley, Scharf, Schreck, and Strampelli. Almost universally, the initial results were favorable, but, tragically, disaster lay ahead. Strampelli[23] began to report numerous complications in 1958. However, later that year in Brussels he reported that a new type of late complication had presented itself.[24] After 5 years of quiescence, two-thirds of the eyes operated on in 1953 showed bullous keratopathy. This resulted from late necrosis due to compression of an extreme peripheral part of Descemet's membrane, with imbibition of aqueous into the corneal parenchyma. These lenses lend little margin for error. The length of the implant is vital. A lens that is too large produces deformation of the pupil by pushing the iris up, occasional ocular hypotony due to an inadvertent cyclodialysis, delayed disappearance of loose pigment, and corneal dystrophy.[9,25-27] Too small a lens leads to decentering during eye movements, causing irritation of the ciliary body and the angle structures. This may result in peripheral anterior synechiae, secondary glaucoma, and corneal dystrophy.[9,26-28]

Disturbed by the high incidence of postoperative complications, Strampelli suggested various ways of preventing corneal dystrophy by modifying the haptic portion that appeared to be the source of the trouble. He made the blunted ends come to rest against the sclera by means of a reverse cyclodialysis, thus avoiding any contact with the cornea or trabecular meshwork. He used Dannheim Supramid loops, but observed that they could cause corneal edema if they were not the correct length. Finally he resorted to external fixation by means of Supramid loops

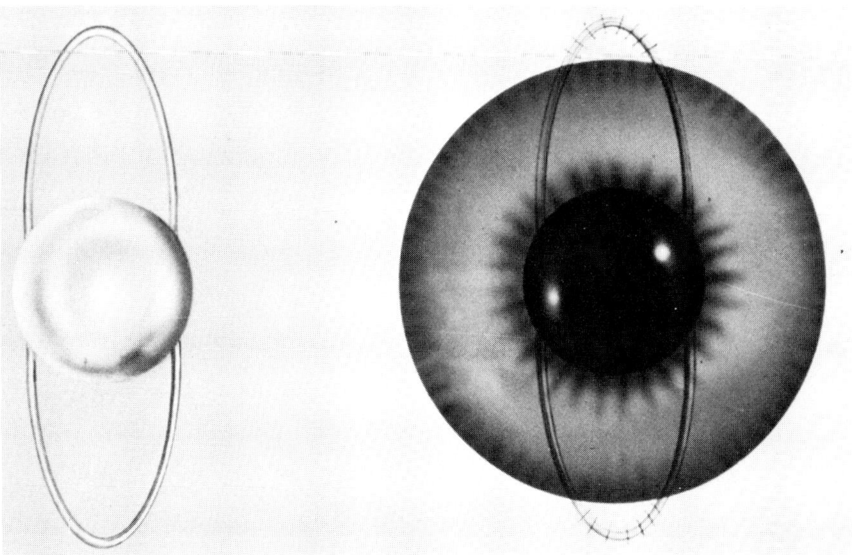

Fig. 4-5. Strampelli perforating external-fixation implant. (From Jaffe, N. S.: Cataract surgery and its complications, ed. 2, St. Louis, 1976, The C. V. Mosby Co.)

perforating the limbus and being sutured to the sclera, but with a conjunctival covering (Fig. 4-5). He first described his external fixation method in 1956.[29-32] The implant had a 5 mm optic portion and was suspended top and bottom by loops 0.12 mm thick. These perforated the sclera at 12 and 6 o'clock and were buried subconjunctivally. The most difficult part of the operation was the determination of the correct amount of tension to be exerted on the loops before suturing.[11] He also employed autoplastic auricular cartilage between the haptic ends and the trabecular meshwork. Fyodorov[33] substituted fibers from the patient's Achilles tendon for the Supramid. Choyce also contributed an external fixation implant (Fig. 4-6).

In spite of numerous modifications, complications did not lessen appreciably. An example of this disastrous episode in implant surgery was the experience of Barraquer, who between 1954 and 1960 implanted 493 lenses. These included 342 Strampelli, 140 Dannheim, 9 Barraquer, and 2 Boberg-Ans lenses implanted after intracapsular or extracapsular extraction or in phakic eyes with high myopia. He eventually found it necessary to remove approximately 250 of the 493 lenses.[34]

Choyce persisted in his use of anterior chamber lenses and now uses a version he refers to as Mark VIII. It is to his credit to have proven that with really sophisticated supports the corneal endothelium could be avoided and that consequently the incidence of endothelial and corneal breakdown could be lowered in a significant way. However, the other anterior chamber lenses have been abandoned. They were complete failures, mainly due to the high percentage of bullous keratopathy. Due to the fact that so many excellent surgeons were involved with these disappointing results, the feeling spread throughout the world that implant surgery was adventuresome and fraught with potential disaster for the eye. It is understandable then that a bias toward later innovations and implant surgeons

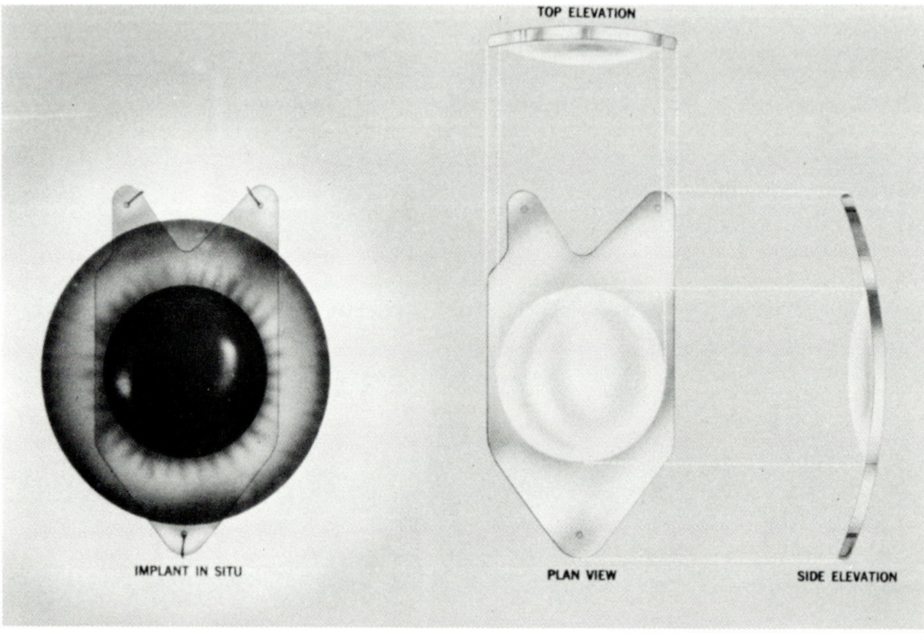

Fig. 4-6. Choyce perforating external-fixation implant. (From Jaffe, N. S.: Cataract surgery and its complications, ed. 2, St. Louis, 1976, The C. V. Mosby Co.)

would occur. To some extent this has persisted.

Anterior chamber lenses with iris fixation or capsular fixation or both

A revival of enthusiasm for lens implant surgery occurred when lenses were designed that depended on the iris for support. The major credit for this renewed interest belongs to Binkhorst, whose experience with Ridley's original posterior chamber lens and the ill-fated anterior chamber angle–supported lenses paralleled those of others.

Epstein and Binkhorst independently directed their efforts to the iris diaphragm as a support for the lens. Schillinger and co-workers[35] performed experimental work in animal eyes. Epstein[36] designed an iris-supported lens shaped like a collar stud and used it in conjunction with an intracapsular extraction in 24 eyes after June 1953. He later abandoned the collar-stud principle and developed his so-called Maltese cross lens, a pupillary plane lens, at first with all solid and later with two solid (placed behind the iris) and two fenestrated (placed anterior to the iris) supports (Fig. 4-7). He inserted 40 of these. An outgrowth of this lens was the Copeland iris-plane lens that has been used extensively in the United States since 1968. This lens is much thinner than the original Epstein Maltese cross lens and has four solid supports. It is shaped like an airplane propeller. Although Epstein first began to use his lens in 1953, he first reported its use in 1959.[36] In the meantime, Binkhorst developed his iris-clip lens in 1957 and used it for the first time on August 11, 1958. He has used it ever since, although variations in the shape, length, and insertions of the loops have occurred. It is a lens with four Supramid loops: the optic portion and the two anterior loops begin on one level, and the two posterior loops at a different level. The entire optic portion rests in a prepupillary position.

The Copeland iris-plane lens is unique among currently used iris-supported lenses. It is the only lens whose optical portion rests exactly in the pupillary plane. This is due to the fact that all four

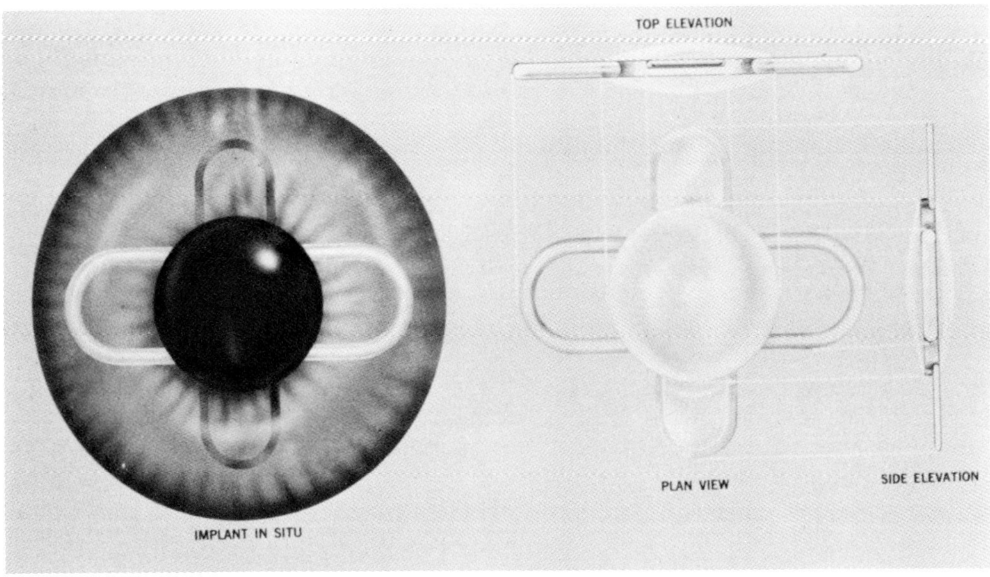

Fig. 4-7. Epstein iris-fixation implant. (From Jaffe, N. S.: Cataract surgery and its complications, ed. 2, St. Louis, 1976, The C. V. Mosby Co.)

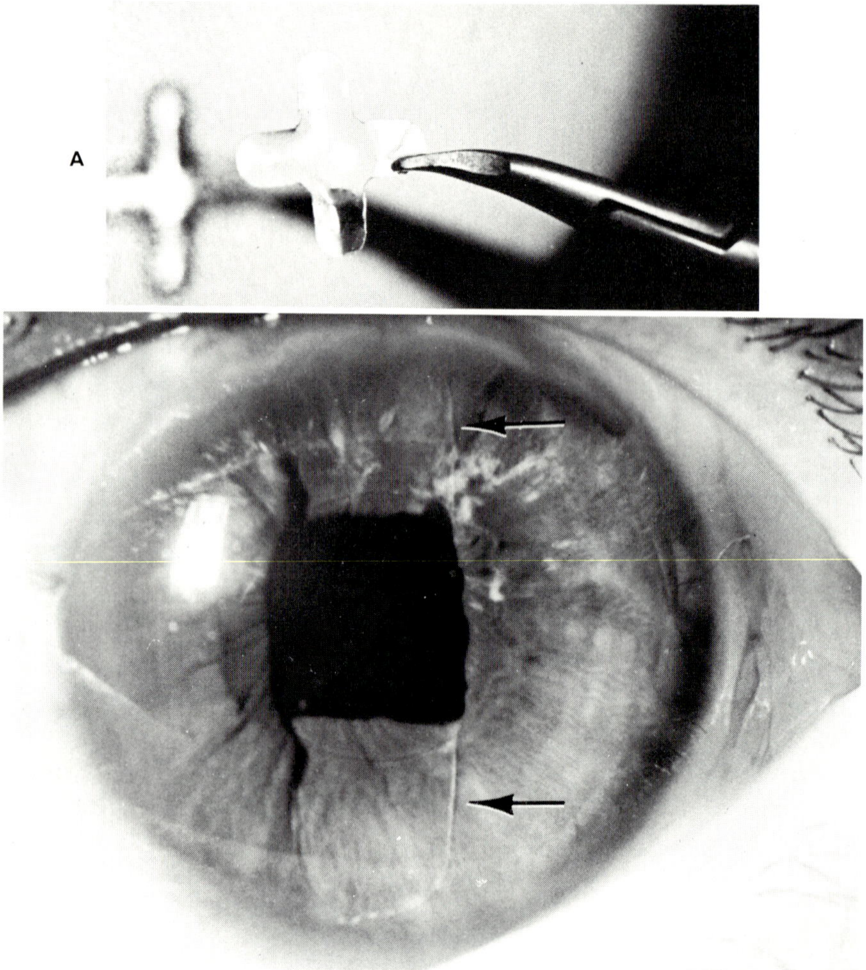

Fig. 4-8. A, Copeland iris-plane lens in needle holder. **B,** Square pupil (4 mm) in aphakic eye with iris-plane lens. Solid haptics *(arrows)* anterior to iris. (From Jaffe, N. S.: Cataract surgery and its complications, ed. 2, St. Louis, 1976, The C. V. Mosby Co.)

supports, which are placed 90° apart, lie in the same plane (Fig. 4-8). It is the only iris-supported lens made entirely of polymethylmethacrylate. The supports of other commonly used lenses are made of other materials such as nylon, polypropylene, platinum, platinum-iridium, and titanium.

The iris-clip lens avoids fixation in the posterior chamber and in the chamber angle. In this way the most important complication arising from positioning the implant behind the iris, namely dislocation, was greatly lessened. In addition, the possibility of corneal damage, the most important complication of anterior chamber angle–supported lenses, was greatly lessened. Fyodorov used the Binkhorst iris-clip lens for the first time in the Soviet Union in 1963, but in 1964 started to use a modification of the iris-clip lens with the anterior and posterior loops at right angles to each other (Fig. 4-9). Since 1968 he has used another modification of the iris-clip lens with three posterior loops and three antennae-like extensions

A

B

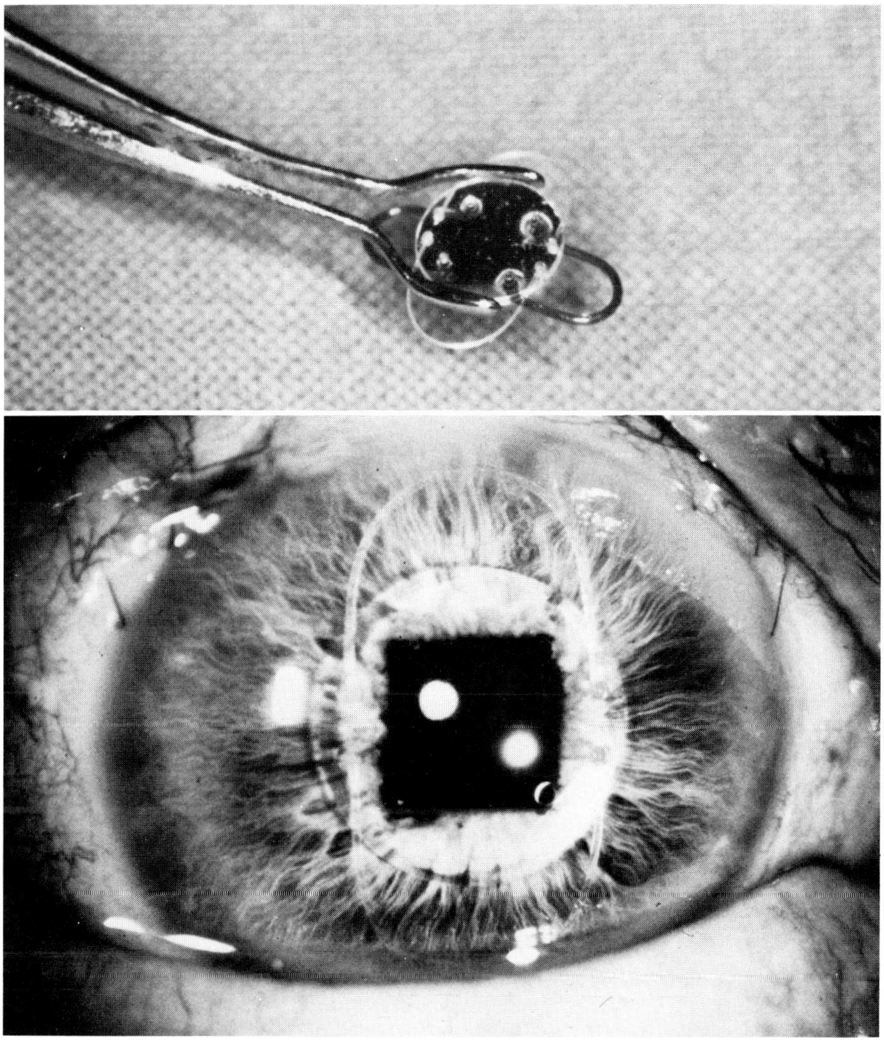

Fig. 4-9. A, Fyodorov-Binkhorst iris-clip implant held in forceps. Posterior haptic supports are dyed a dark color. **B,** Fyodorov-Binkhorst iris-clip implant in situ. (From Jaffe, N. S.: Cataract surgery and its complications, ed. 2, St. Louis, 1976, The C. V. Mosby Co.)

with a small round knob at each end in front of the iris (Fig. 4-10). This has been termed the sputnik lens.

In June 1965 the length of the anterior loops of the iris-clip lens was changed from 7.5 to 8 mm to 9 to 9.5 mm. This was done in order to reduce the number of dislocations (11.5%) that had occurred among the first 208 implants.[37,38] However, this caused an increased incidence of corneal edema. Therefore the original length of 7.5 to 8 mm was restored on January 1, 1970. In November 1971 all loops manufactured were bent backwards at a radius of about 30 mm in order to reduce the risk of corneal touch. For technical reasons the thickness of the anterior loops remained 0.2 mm (Fig. 4-11).

In 1967, at the suggestion of R. D. Binkhorst (brother of C. D. Binkhorst), the optic portion was changed from a biconvex to a simple convexoplano lens because of the following: aqueous flowing through the pupillary aperture would be less easily obstructed, optical computations would be easier and more accurate, and spherical aberration would theoretically be less. Early in 1972 the length of the diagonals of the square formed by the posterior loop attachments was reduced from 4 to 3 mm. This made it possible for the pupil to constrict to a diameter of 3 mm, thus reducing the photophobia that occurred rather often with the earlier 4 mm diameter pupils.

In order to prevent dislocation of the iris-clip lens, miotics were prescribed for every patient. This proved effective, but

A

B

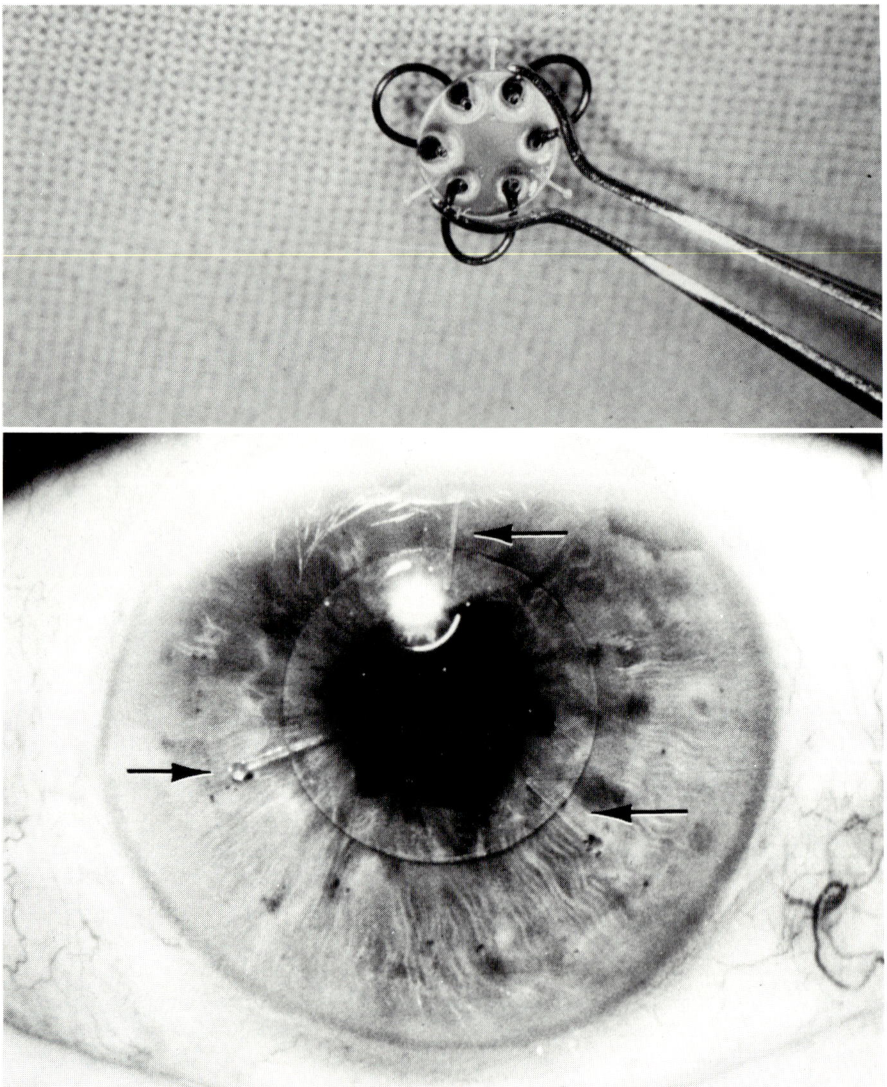

Fig. 4-10. A, Fyodorov sputnik implant held in forceps. Note three posterior loops dyed a dark color and three anterior sticks with rounded knob at end. **B,** Hexagonal pupil (4 mm) in aphakic eye with Fyodorov lens. Three supporting sticks *(arrows)* anterior to iris. (From Jaffe, N. S.: Cataract surgery and its complications, ed. 2, St. Louis, 1976, The C. V. Mosby Co.)

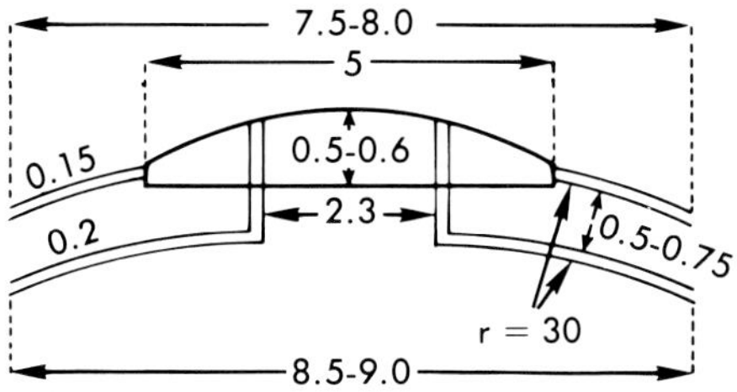

Fig. 4-11. Schema of modern Binkhorst 4-loop iris-clip implant. Note relatively short anterior haptics and posterior curvature of both anterior and posterior nylon haptic supports. (From Jaffe, N. S.: Cataract surgery and its complications, ed. 2, St. Louis, 1976, The C. V. Mosby Co.)

it was not considered the ideal solution, since some patients were not faithfully using the drops. In addition, the pupillary border suffered from indentations and atrophy caused by the posterior loop insertions. Histologic studies showed, among other minor pathologies of the pupillary border, a definite sphincter muscle atrophy in nearly every case. It was clear that a reliable method was needed with which the regular use of miotics could be abandoned and which would permit full pupil dilatation without fear of dislocation. Worst, in February 1969, began to suture the lens on the iris, at first one loop and later the equatorial zone of the lens

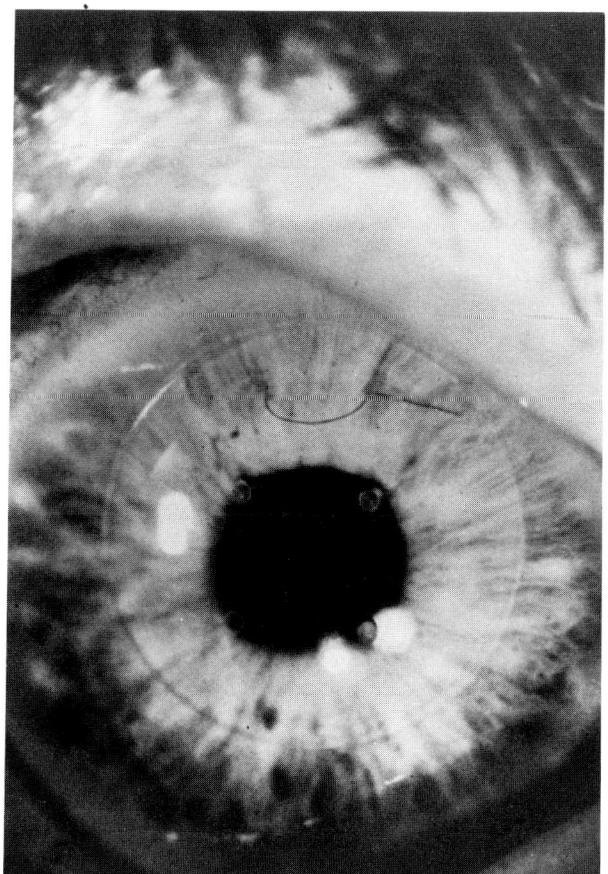

Fig. 4-12. Worst Medallion implant in situ. Note iris suture. (From Jaffe, N. S.: Cataract surgery and its complications, ed. 2, St. Louis, 1976, The C. V. Mosby Co.)

A

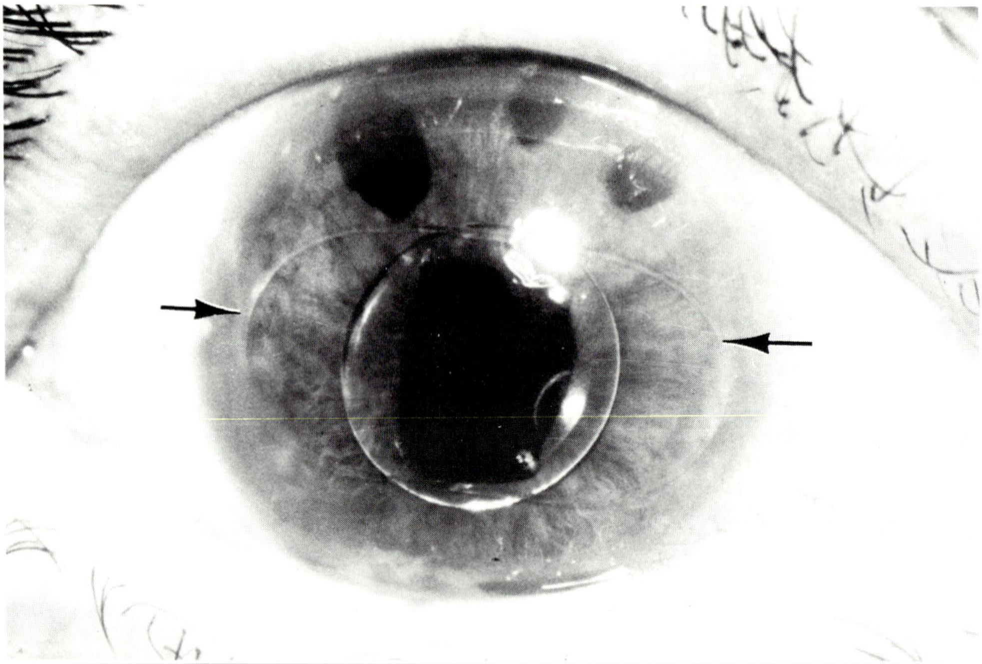

B

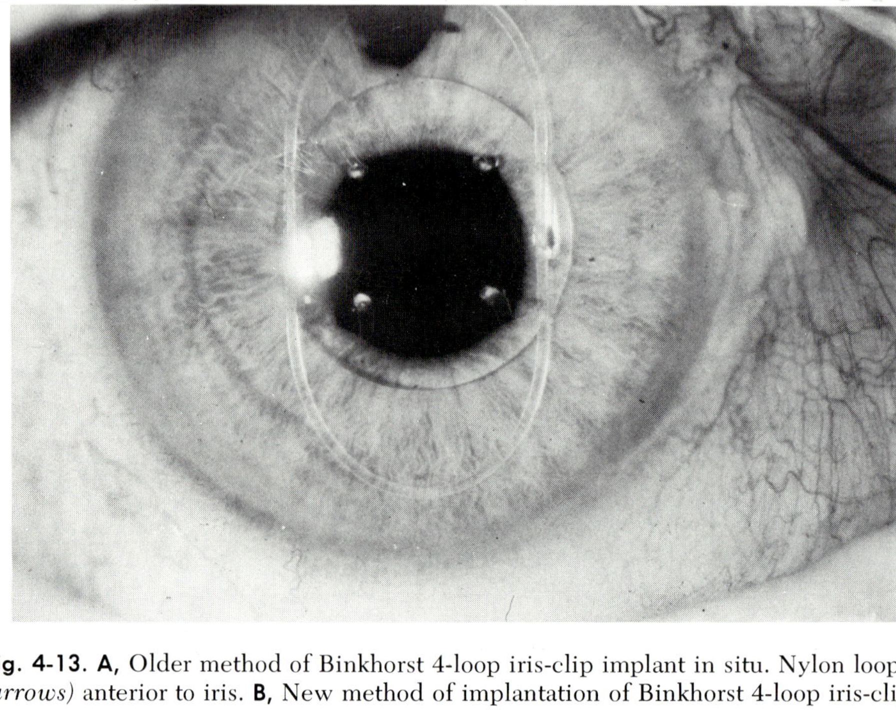

Fig. 4-13. A, Older method of Binkhorst 4-loop iris-clip implant in situ. Nylon loops *(arrows)* anterior to iris. **B,** New method of implantation of Binkhorst 4-loop iris-clip implant. (From Jaffe, N. S.: Cataract surgery and its complications, ed. 2, St. Louis, 1976, The C. V. Mosby Co.)

A

B

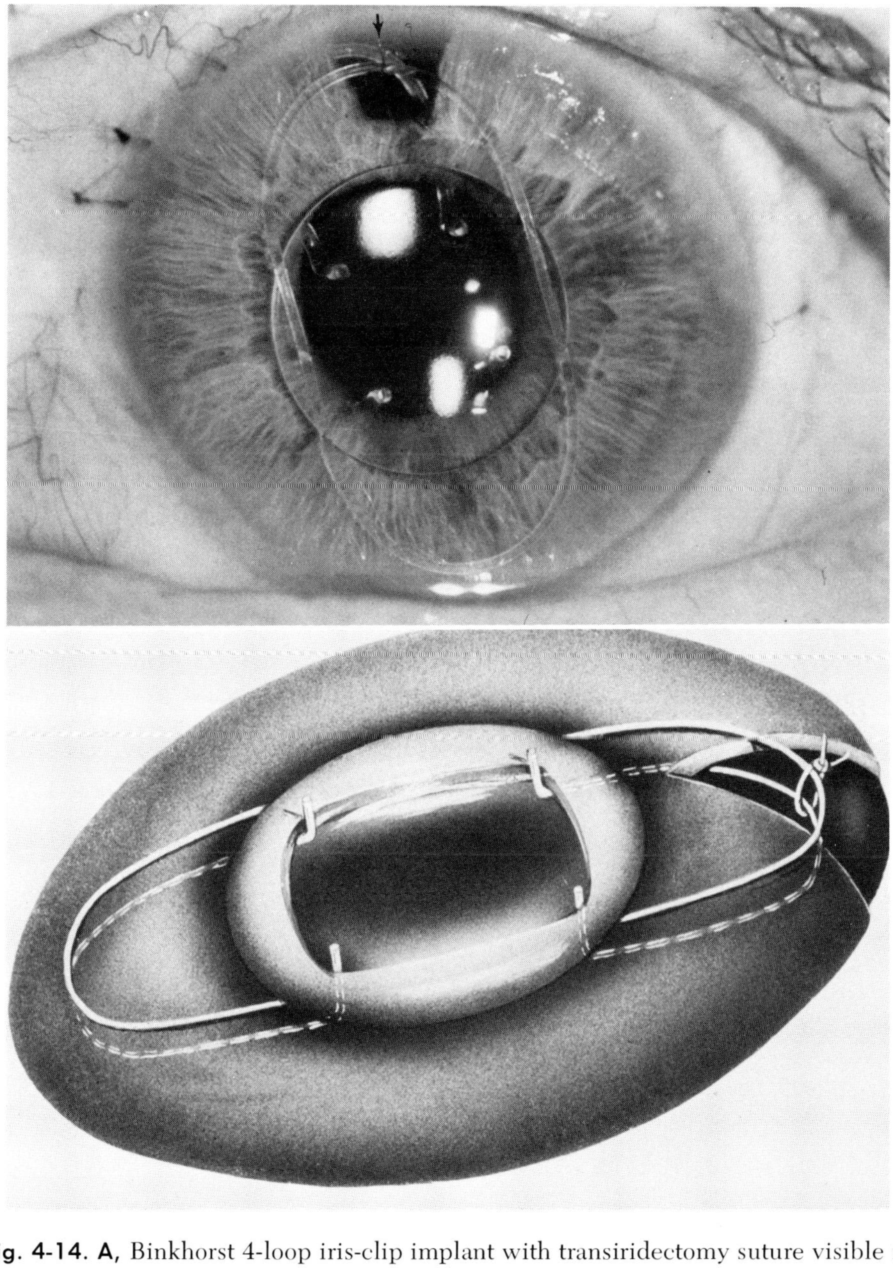

Fig. 4-14. A, Binkhorst 4-loop iris-clip implant with transiridectomy suture visible in peripheral iridectomy *(arrow)*. **B,** Drawing of transiridectomy suture technique. (From Jaffe, N. S.: Cataract surgery and its complications, ed. 2, St. Louis, 1976, The C. V. Mosby Co.)

body. This led him to the development of an enlarged lens body with two holes in the upper segment to pass a monofilament Perlon suture (Fig. 4-12). His lens therefore contained no anterior loops. This became known as the Medallion lens, which was inserted for the first time on December 18, 1970. Subsequently Binkhorst changed his surgical technique so that the iris-clip lens was placed in the vertical, rather than the horizontal, position (Fig. 4-13). This made it possible to connect both upper loops in a peripheral iris coloboma (transiridectomy fixation) with a monofilament nylon suture (Fig. 4-14). This permits the lens to remain centric during pupillary dilatation, whereas lenses with an iris suture ride high during dilatation. Binkhorst commenced this technique in March 1970. Another advantage of the vertical position of the iris-clip lens is the lessened possibility of corneal contact during ocular movements. Horizontal movements of the eye are definitely more frequent than vertical movements. Horizontal movements of the eye cause a horizontally placed lens to swing, thus increasing the possibility of periodic corneal touch.

In December 1973 Worst announced that he had partially abandoned the iris stitch technique because of unreliability of the nylon. He developed a transiridectomy hooking technique with a fingerlike extension mounted at the edge of the lens body (safety pin principle). Worst's Medallion lens can be used with both an intracapsular and extracapsular cataract extraction.

The possibility of capsular support, as

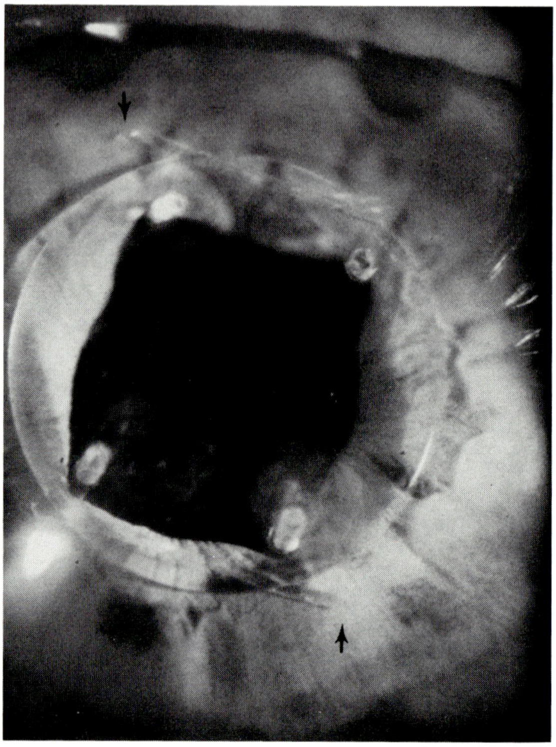

Fig. 4-15. Binkhorst 2-loop iridocapsular implant made from 4-loop implant by cutting off anterior loops *(arrows)*. (From Jaffe, N. S.: Cataract surgery and its complications, ed. 2, St. Louis, 1976, The C. V. Mosby Co.)

originally used by Ridley, had been abandoned until in December 1963 Binkhorst inserted an iris-clip lens after an extracapsular extraction of a traumatic cataract. This was followed by other such procedures. The posterior loops got embedded in adhesions between iris and posterior capsule. Lenses thus supported could not move around inside the eye. The anterior loops lost their function under these circumstances (Fig. 4-15). Thus a 2-loop iridocapsular lens (containing only posterior loops) was designed and used for the first time on September 16, 1965. The first iridocapsular lens proper, having only two platinum-iridium loops, was inserted on October 27, 1965. It was inserted into a traumatic aphakic eye with a capsular membrane. The 2-loop iridocapsular lens was designed especially for children.[39] At present it is used for patients of any age, after extracapsular cataract surgery in one stage, as well as in two-stage procedures[40] (Figs. 4-16 and 4-17). Since the fixation is predominantly capsular, the term iridocapsular is actually a misnomer. Whereas the central area of the membrane, consisting only of the posterior lens capsule, should be as clear as possible, it is advisable to leave a few cortical remnants of the lens at the periphery behind the iris. This promotes the development of iridocapsular adhesions embedding parts of

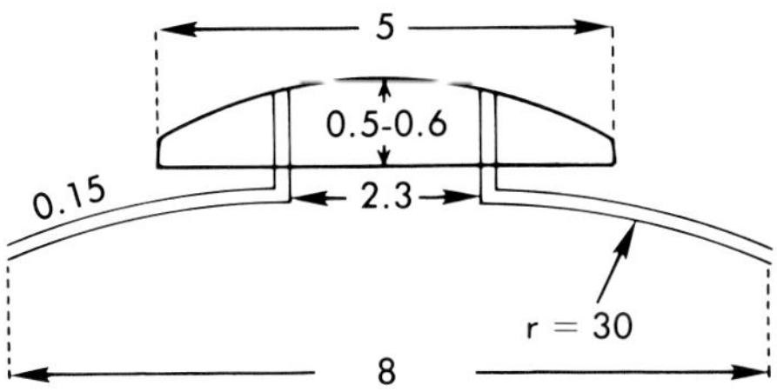

Fig. 4-16. Schema of modern Binkhorst 2-loop iridocapsular implant. Supporting loops are made of platinum-iridium. (From Jaffe, N. S.: Cataract surgery and its complications, ed. 2, St. Louis, 1976, The C. V. Mosby Co.)

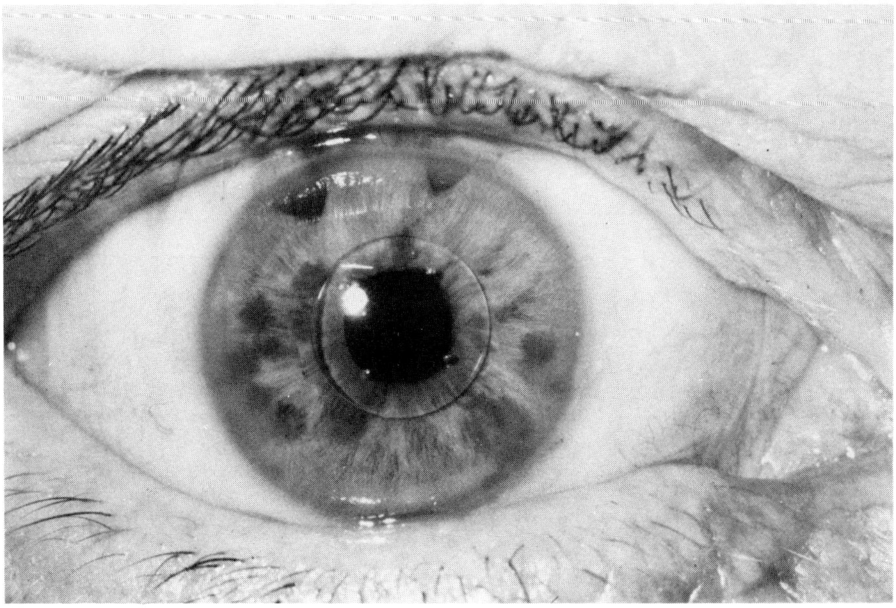

Fig. 4-17. Binkhorst 2-loop iridocapsular implant in situ. (From Jaffe, N. S.: Cataract surgery and its complications, ed. 2, St. Louis, 1976, The C. V. Mosby Co.)

the wire loops and giving extra stability to the implant as well as preventing undesirable mydriasis. Binkhorst currently favors the iridocapsular lens for routine use, reserving the iris-clip lens for special occasions: (1) dislocation of the crystalline lens; (2) fixation in the iridocapsular cleft cannot be expected to take place, for example, in cases of milky cataract, aphakia after intracapsular lens extraction, or secondary implantation without synechiae; and (3) the patient prefers intracapsular extraction because restoration of visual acuity is usually more rapid.

Binkhorst's change in preference for the iridocapsular over the iris-clip lens was favored by the establishment of absolute security for the corneal endothelium by combining the advantages of the iridocapsular lens with those of extracapsular extraction.[40,41] According to Binkhorst, the advantages include a smaller incision, safer surgery due to less bulging of the vitreous, and fewer cases of maculopathy. A definite disadvantage of extracapsular cataract extraction was found to be the occurrence of secondary cataract. The frequency of needling may, however, decrease considerably with increasing experience, especially in elderly patients.[41,42]

SUMMARY

The history of intraocular lenses is replete with innovations, some successful and some unsuccessful. It would be foolhardy to ignore the early disasters and dismiss them as expected occurrences in the development of a new modality. These sequential events should remind us to accept changes with caution. For, after all, the implant is intended to remain safely in situ for the remainder of the patient's life.

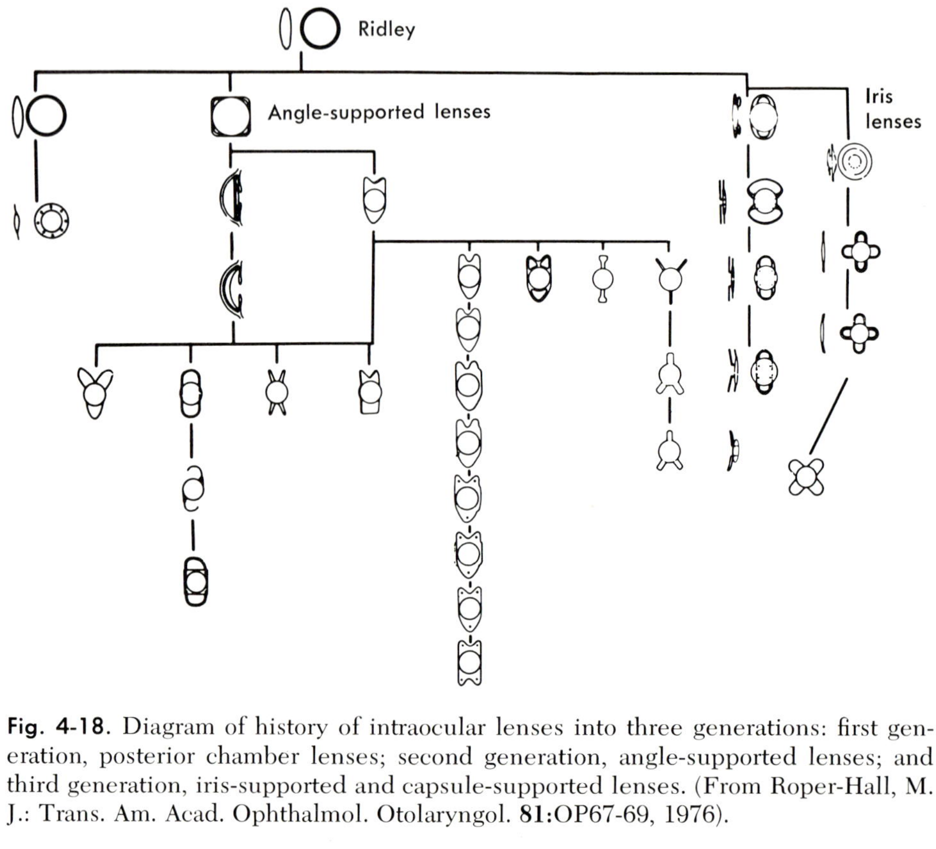

Fig. 4-18. Diagram of history of intraocular lenses into three generations: first generation, posterior chamber lenses; second generation, angle-supported lenses; and third generation, iris-supported and capsule-supported lenses. (From Roper-Hall, M. J.: Trans. Am. Acad. Ophthalmol. Otolaryngol. **81**:OP67-69, 1976).

One cannot leave this subject without noting that there is a trend to return to capsular fixation, which was Ridley's original concept. One can only marvel at the difference in sophistication between Ridley's original posterior chamber lens and a modern iridocapsular lens as to implant design and technique of implantation. There is also a tendency to divide the history of intraocular lenses into three eras, usually referred to as generations. The first generation was limited to the Ridley posterior chamber lens, the second generation to the anterior chamber angle–fixated lenses, and the third generation to iris-supported and iridocapsular lenses (Fig. 4-18). One thing is certain. This is not the last generation.

REFERENCES

1. Taieb, A.: Des mémoires de Casanova à l'opération de Ridley, Arch. Ophtalmol. **15:**501-503, 1955.
2. Münchow, W.: Zur Geschichte der intraokularen Korrektur der Aphakie, Klin. Monatsbl. Augenheilkd. **145:**771-777, 1964.
3. Ascher, K. W.: Prosthetophakia two hundred years ago, Am. J. Ophthalmol. **59:**445-446, 1965.
4. Marchi, W., cited by Strampelli, B.: L'evolution des lentilles plastiques de chambre antérieure. Dernières acquisitions techniques, An. Inst. Barraquer **3**(4):519-530, 1962.
5. Ridley, H.: Intra-ocular acrylic lenses, Trans. Ophthalmol. Soc. U.K. **71:**617-621, 1951.
6. Ridley, H.: Further observations on intraocular acrylic lenses in cataract surgery, J. Int. Coll. Surg. **18:**825-833, 1952.
7. Ridley, H.: Intra-ocular acrylic lenses after cataract extraction, Lancet **1:**118-121, 1952.
8. Ridley, H.: Intra-ocular acrylic lenses. A recent development in the surgery of cataract, Br. J. Ophthalmol. **36:**113-122, 1952.
9. Schreck, E.: Erfahrungen mit über 150 Vorderkammerlinsen eines eigenen Modells, Acta Conc. Ophthalmol. Belgica **2:**1699-1705, 1958.
10. Binkhorst, C. D.: Some thoughts on the fixation of intraocular lenses. First International Symposium on Artificial Lens Implantation, Utrecht, April 1974. Edited by A. T. M. van Balen, The Netherlands, 1975, Dr. W. Junk N. V., Publishers, pp. 99-128.
11. Choyce, D. P.: Intra-ocular lenses and implants (adapted from a thesis), London, 1964, H. K. Lewis.
12. Binkhorst, C. D.: De implantatie van kunststoflenzen in het oog. Een nieuwe fixatiemethode: de pupillens of iris-cliplens, Ned. Tijdschr. Geneeskd. **103:**1289-1294, 1959.
13. Ridley, H.: Further observations on intraocular acrylic lenses in cataract surgery, Trans. Am. Acad. Ophthalmol. Otolaryngol. **57:**98-106, 1953.
14. Ridley, H.: Further experiences of intra-ocular acrylic lens surgery, Br. J. Ophthalmol. **38:** 156-162, 1954.
15. Ridley, H.: Cataract surgery with particular reference to intraocular lenticular implants of various types, Trans. Ophthalmol. Soc. U.K. **78:**585-592, 1958.
16. Ridley, H.: Intra-ocular acrylic lenses: 10 years' development, Br. J. Ophthalmol. **44:**705-712, 1960.
17. Guerry, D.: Present status of the anterior chamber lens, Am. J. Ophthalmol. **50:**250-258, 1960.
18. Ridley, H.: Personal communication to J. G. F. Worst, 1970.
19. Baron, A.: Tolerance de l'oeil a la matiere plastique. Protheses optiques cristalliniennes, Bull. Soc. Ophtalmol. Fr. **9:**982-988, 1953.
20. Strampelli, B.: Sopportabilità di lenti acriliche in camera anteriore nella afachia e nei vizi di refrazione, Ann. Ottal. **80:**75-82, 1954.
21. Strampelli, B.: Due anni di esperienza con le lenti camerulari, Atti Soc. Oftal. Ital. **15:**427-433, 1955.
22. Dannheim, H.: Vorderkammerlinse mit elastischen Halteschlingen, Ges. Heidelberg **60:** 267-268, 1956.
23. Strampelli, B.: Complications de l'opération de Strampelli, L'Année Ther. Clin. Ophtalmol. **9:**349-370, 1958.
24. Strampelli, B.: Les lentilles camérulaires après six années d'experience, Acta Conc. Ophthalmol. Belgica **2:**1692-1698, 1958.
25. Barraquer, J.: Lentilles plastiques dans la chambre antérieure: indications, technique, expérience personnelle sur cent cas, Bull. Soc. Belge Ophtalmol. **114:**503-516, 1956.
26. Barraquer, J.: Complicaciones de la inclusion segun los diversos tipos de lentes, An. Inst. Barraquer **3**(4):588-592, 1962.
27. Schreck, E.: Linsenimplantation nach Staroperation. In Rohrschneider, W., editor: Augenheilkunde in Klinik und Praxis, Stuttgart, Germany, 1958, Ferdinand Enke Verlag, pp. 151-163.
28. Choyce, D. P.: Correction of uni-ocular aphakia by means of anterior chamber acrylic implants, Acta Conc. Ophthalmol. Belgica **2:**1705-1708, 1958.
29. Strampelli, B.: Fissazione di lenti camerulari mediante filo di supramis, Atti Soc. Oftalmol. Ital. **17:**669-682, 1957.
30. Strampelli, B.: Anterior chamber lenses, Arch. Ophthalmol. **66:**12-17, 1961.
31. Strampelli, B.: Anterior chamber lenses. In

Fasanella, R. M., editor: Modern advances in cataract surgery, Philadelphia, 1963, J. B. Lippincott Co.

32. Strampelli, B., Marchi, W., and Valvo, A.: Lentine in camera anteriore con fissazione esterna (10 anni di esperienza clinica), Ann. Ottal. **94**:9-42, 1968.
33. Fyodorov, S. N.: Scientific research in behalf of the medical practice (interview, translation), Nauka i zjiznj (Science and Life) **8**:93-95, 1972.
34. Nordlohne, M. E.: The intraocular implant lens: development and results with special reference to the Binkhorst lens, The Hague, 1975, Dr. W. Junk N. V., Publishers, p. 23.
35. Schillinger, R. J., Shearer, R. V., and Levy, O. R.: Animal experiments with a new type of intraocular acrylic lens, Arch. Ophthalmol. **59**: 423-434, 1958.
36. Epstein, E.: Modified Ridley lenses, Br. J. Ophthalmol. **43**:29-33, 1959.
37. Binkhorst, C. D., and Léonard, P. A. M.: Results in 208 iris-clip pseudophakos implantations, Am. J. Ophthalmol. **64**:947-956, 1967.
38. Binkhorst, C. D., and Léonard, P. A. M.: Implantation of the iris-clip pseudophakos: results in the first 208 cases, Perspect. Ophthalmol. **1**:195-214, 1968.
39. Binkhorst, C. D., and Gobin, M. H. M. A.: Pseudophakia after lens injury in children, Ophthalmologica **154**:81-87, 1967.
40. Binkhorst, C. D., Kats, A., and Léonard, P. A. M.: Extracapsular pseudophakia: results in 100 two-loop iridocapsular lens implantations, Am. J. Ophthalmol. **73**:625-636, 1972.
41. Binkhorst, C. D.: The iridocapsular (two-loop) lens and the iris clip (four-loop) lens in pseudophakia, Trans. Am. Acad. Ophthalmol. Otolaryngol. **77**:589-617, 1973.
42. Binkhorst, C. D.: Praxis und theorie der "Iris Klipp Linse" und der "Irido-Kapsular Linse." Sitzungsber. 125. Vers. Ver. Rhein.-Westfäl. Augenärzte Bonn. Grafischer Betr. Gebr. Zimmermann, Balve/Sauerland, 1972.

CHAPTER 5

Guidelines for intraocular lens implantation

Although it is a fact that well over 100,000 pseudophakoi have been implanted to date in the United States by more than 1000 implant surgeons, there still exists controversy over the safety of the procedure as regards both the lens and the surgery. In general the results have been spectacular, but there have also been disasters. Some of the problems are due less to the intraocular lens implant itself than to poor selection of patients and to inadequately trained surgeons. Therefore it would appear reasonable to establish a suggested set of guidelines for intraocular lens implant surgery, particularly for the neophyte. As skill and experience progress, these guidelines can and should be altered. These guidelines should be oriented not toward the outstanding technical surgeon but rather to the mainstream of ophthalmic surgeons. The indications and contraindications for implant surgery discussed here are not intended to reflect unfavorably on those used by other surgeons. Pending long-term clinical experience, the approach is designed to emphasize caution.

INDICATIONS

Indications may be classified into three categories: general, special, and specific.

General indications

1. Intraocular lens implants are most easily inserted and are most successful in older patients and initially should be restricted to the elderly.
2. Intraocular lenses are implanted only in eyes of younger patients who are not likely to succeed with a contact lens.
3. Intraocular implants should initially be restricted to one eye, unless the needs of the patient dictate otherwise.

The reasons for restricting implants to the elderly should be apparent. Older people adapt poorly to spectacles for aphakia and to contact lenses. In addition, more hard data need to be obtained about the long-term safety of polymethylmethacrylate, polyamide, polypropylene, platinum-iridium alloy, titanium, and the additives that comprise an implant within the eye. If a young patient can be reasonably expected to manage the wearing of a contact lens, an implant is generally not performed by many. The surgery for routine cataract surgery without an implant is far less burdensome, and certain postoperative complications such as dislocation of the implant or an intraocular lens membrane are not encountered.

Why is surgery on one eye often sufficient? Many patients who achieve good vision with a pseudophakos can manage well with one eye even if the opposite eye is nearly blind. They do not have to cope with the problems of spatial disorientation, pincushion distortion, and the ring scotoma inherent in cataract spectacle lenses, and they do not require the dexterity and central vision necessary to manage contact lens wear. It should be obvious that these statements do not apply to all patients. Any ophthalmologist knows patients who manage extremely well after routine cataract surgery in only one eye where a contact lens is used in spite of poor vision in the second eye. He also is aware of many patients who complain bitterly about the loss of binocularity. The same applies to the use of an implant in one eye. Some patients find unilateral surgery adequate for their needs, others do not.

Special indications

1. There are certain occupational drawbacks to contact lens wear, for example, in ranchers, miners, and divers. In addition, contact lenses may disqualify some people for certain occupations (for example, pilots). Ophthalmologists who treat such patients are familiar with the difficulties of contact wear. Ophthalmologists who do not treat persons in these categories may not be overly sympathetic to the occupational handicaps of a contact lens.

2. It is well known that we usually have been unsuccessful in the prevention of amblyopia in children ages 3 to 8 years who sustain a traumatic cataract. In spite of successful cataract removal and diligent contact lens wear, these eyes usually become amblyopic. The use of an intraocular lens in this situation has been studied widely in the Netherlands. American ophthalmologists have only limited experience in this situation. This subject is discussed more fully in Chapter 11.

Specific indications

1. An elderly patient who has an advanced cataract in one eye and visual acuity of 20/40 to 20/60 in the other eye basically has a unilateral cataract. The patient may perform poorly in bright sunlight and may have lost his license to drive an automobile. The same indication might also include those patients who have even better vision than this in the better eye but who have an advanced cataract that interferes with their activities.

2. The same indication exists in slightly younger people with infirmities such as rheumatoid arthritis, parkinsonism, hemiplegia, or mental retardation. These patients are poor candidates for contact lenses, although there may be a poor but partially satisfactory solution in bilateral cataract surgery corrected with spectacles.

3. An elderly patient who has disabling cataracts in both eyes, with a visual acuity of, for example, 20/100 in each eye, appears to manage satisfactorily if implant surgery is performed in one eye. From what has been discussed above, they manage well because they are not confronted with the obstacles of the spectacle correction of aphakia. There is some controversy in this indication. Some ophthalmologists prefer to do surgery in both eyes while others favor surgery in one eye only. If surgery is undertaken in both eyes, it would appear prudent to leave a reasonable period of time between the two operations. Certainly one should be more conservative in this regard than for the management of bilateral cataracts where routine cataract surgery is performed. The trend in the United States in the latter situation appears to be toward cataract surgery within a brief period of time (for example, 1 week). There are still enough uncertainties in implant surgery that a longer interval of time between operations would be in the best interest of the patient. This interval should be longer for patients who are younger. In patients over 80 years of age the interval can be shortened. However, in patients of this age range it is questionable whether bilateral surgery is indicated in all cases. Again, this is a judgment decision.

4. It is well known that patients having extensive bilateral macular degeneration and later developing advanced cataracts in both eyes perform poorly after cataract extraction where spectacles are used. The loss of peripheral field represents a severe obstacle to these patients, since this is the only field of vision they possess. In addition, they have insufficient central vision to manage a contact lens. When

such patients undergo lens implant surgery successfully, they represent some of the happiest patients one might encounter. In spite of the absence of a central visual field, they are delighted by the improvement of vision after implant surgery.

5. An elderly patient has worn a contact lens for unilateral aphakia for many years but is faced with a nearly mature cataract in the second eye. This prevents him from managing the contact lens in the first eye. Most patients who wear a contact lens successfully after a cataract extraction in one eye do just about as well as a patient who has a successful lens implantation in one eye. However, the management of the contact lens requires a certain amount of vision in the opposite eye. If the cataract in the opposite eye advances sufficiently, the patient may have some difficulty with the contact lens in the aphakic eye. Therefore a lens implant in the second eye is usually a very satisfactory solution for this problem.

It is repeated that these indications cannot be imposed on all surgeons. In the end the surgeon is expected to exercise his own judgment in the best interest of his patient. There is a marked difference in the surgical abilities of different surgeons and a marked difference in their basic attitude toward indications and contraindications. Therefore what has been stated above can only be called a set of guidelines and not a strict list of indications.

To illustrate some of these indications, consider the following actual situations.

SITUATION: An elderly patient has aphakia in the first eye and wears a contact lens.

TREATMENT: An implant may be used in the second eye if the cataract in the second eye interferes with the patient's ability to manage the contact lens in the first eye. If the patient is doing well with the contact lens, no surgery need be done in the second eye no matter what the status of the cataract.

SITUATION: A patient has aphakia in the first eye, has adapted well to spectacles, and likes them.

TREATMENT: Routine intracapsular cataract extraction is indicated in the second eye; spectacles are prescribed for both eyes.

SITUATION: A successful implant has been performed in the first eye of a patient under 70 years of age.

TREATMENT: No implant is indicated for the second eye unless the cataract disturbs the patient. The surgeon may then choose between an implant in the second eye or a routine cataract extraction with contact lens correction.

SITUATION: A successful implant has been performed in the first eye of a patient over 70 years of age.

TREATMENT: No implant is indicated for the second eye in many cases. Alternate choices could be an implant for the second eye in a patient over 70 years of age with a reasonable follow-up period in the first eye or a shorter postoperative period if the patient is over 80 years of age.

SITUATION: The patient has aphakia in the first eye and has not successfully adapted to spectacles or to a contact lens.

TREATMENT: Routine cataract extraction is preferred for the second eye with spectacles prescribed for both eyes. At this time a secondary implant in the first eye is still considered risky because the risks are greater than with primary implantation. This problem really gets to the heart of the problem of secondary implantation (Chapter 10). Since so many patients who wear a spectacle in the first eye after cataract extraction are unhappy with this method of optical correction of aphakia, there is a great danger of an epidemic of secondary implantations. It has been demonstrated that there is a significant risk of complications in secondarily implanted iris-supported pseudophakoi. The most reasonable solution might be the use of a Choyce Mark VIII implant. However, the surgeon must weigh the possibility that even though the patient cannot tolerate the method of optical correction of aphakia in the first eye, there is danger of reducing the vision in this eye by secondary implantation. Again, this is a judgment decision to be made by the surgeon. Some patients appear to benefit when the cataract is removed from the second eye, and the patient is given spectacles for both eyes. However, this is not a satisfactory solution for all patients. If secondary implantation is performed in the first eye, the patient must be fully informed as to the risk of reducing the functional status of that eye in spite of the fact that he has not been able to use the first eye with either a spectacle or a contact lens. If the patient if fully informed and is really intolerant of the spectacle or contact lens, a secondary implantation may prove to be the procedure of choice. However, this situation has not been followed for any long period of time in the United States. Therefore the procedure is still in a period of clinical evaluation.

Another important judgment decision is whether an extracapsular cataract extraction lowers the incidence of cystoid macular edema and retinal detachment seen after a routine intracapsular cataract extraction. To date, there are no extensive age-matched series that support this view. Proponents of planned extracapsular extraction, whether by phacoemulsification or by the conventional method, usually reserve this technique for younger cataract patients. However, according to the criteria used by most implant surgeons, these patients would not qualify for an implant, since they could reasonably be expected to manage contact lens wear.

CONTRAINDICATIONS

Indications for pseudophakos implantation having been enumerated, contraindications may now be considered. In a controversial area such as lens implant surgery, it is not surprising that there would be more contraindications than indications. Some of these contraindications appear to be well defined. Others are questionable at this time.

1. The patient does not want an implant or expresses anxiety over the procedure. Anything less than a perfect result in such a patient is an invitation to a medicolegal adventure.
2. Axial myopia greater than 7 D. The advantages of an implant are minimal in this situation since the residual refractive error is small.
3. A poor result was obtained with an implant in the first eye.
4. The patient has only one eye with potentially good vision. It is hoped that contraindications 3 and 4 would be universally accepted by implant surgeons.
5. The patient is young. The definition of young is a judgment decision to be made by the surgeon. Most significant is the surgeon's impression as to whether the patient could be reasonably expected to manage a contact lens.
6. Postoperative follow-up is impossible. The patient who lives far from the nearest implant surgeon may receive inadequate management of late complications from ophthalmologists inexperienced in implant surgery.
7. Severe senile macular choroidal degeneration is present without a nearly mature cataract in both eyes. Such a patient will derive little benefit from implant surgery.
8. Endothelial corneal dystrophy is present. Implant surgery requires greater intraocular manipulation than a routine cataract extraction. Therefore there is a much greater likelihood of postoperative corneal edema.
9. Proliferative diabetic retinopathy is present. Cystoid macular edema and other postoperative complications are more likely in these eyes.
10. Uncontrolled glaucoma is present (Chapter 10). Postoperative inflammation with its effects on the anterior chamber angles may be disastrous for such eyes.
11. There has been previous retinal detachment. Since vitreous problems are

more likely in implant surgery than in routine cataract surgery, there is a greater risk of redetachment. In addition, if extensive synechiae of the iris to a pseudophakos occur or if a membrane develops over the surface of the implant, visualization of small breaks in the retinal periphery is more difficult.

12. Congenital cataracts, especially of the rubelliform type, are present. With the exception of postnatal zonular cataracts, many of these eyes could not be expected to tolerate or benefit from an intraocular lens implant.

13. Cataract is associated with other abnormalities such as recurrent iritis, essential iris atrophy, or atopic dermatitis.

Although it is conceded that the technical abilities of some intraocular implant surgeons may make some of these contraindications appear unusually conservative, the human eye should not be an arena for surgical heroics. Since it is likely that more surgeons will engage in intraocular implant surgery, and therefore more eyes will be subjected to the procedure, the conservative approach to indications and contraindications should reasonably be expected to be in the best interests of our patients.

In these days of increasing peer review, it is becoming mandatory to formulate a reasonable set of guidelines that would be universally accepted. Greater permissiveness in selection of patients should be guided only by additional favorable experience. It should be apparent that a less conservative approach to lens implant surgery should only be undertaken after surgical education and patient experience has significantly increased.

CHAPTER 6

Preoperative estimation of intraocular implant lens power

In the early days of intraocular lens surgery the lens was implanted secondarily, that is, some time after the cataract extraction. This enabled the surgeon to determine first the aphakic refraction and then select a suitable power intraocular lens. This was the principal justification for a second surgical procedure. One would expect that this would offer a highly accurate method of refractive correction. This proved not to be the case, since it was reported[1,2] that residual anisometropia and aniseikonia occurred to a significant degree in a group of patients thus corrected. These errors were attributed to the fact that neither the refracting power of the cornea nor the anterior chamber depth were included in the calculations.

When the transition from angle-supported lenses to iris-supported lenses occurred, primary implantation became the method of choice. The Choyce Mark VIII angle-supported lens is currently also implanted in a one-stage operation. This places a greater burden on the surgeon to predict a suitable power pseudophakos. He has two methods available to him:

1. Estimations based on the basic refraction of the eye, that is, the refraction prior to the development of cataract

2. Estimations based on sophisticated measurements: axial length of the globe, the refractive power or radius of curvature of the cornea, and anterior chamber depth

ESTIMATIONS OF INTRAOCULAR LENS POWER BASED ON THE BASIC REFRACTION OF THE EYE

The majority of patients who undergo lens implant surgery in the United States receive implants whose power is estimated from the basic refraction of the eye (spherical equivalent). Experience has shown that when the basic refraction is accurate, a reasonable prediction of implant power is possible. However, there are many pitfalls in estimating the basic refraction. A reliable history of the refractive status before the onset of cataract is not always available. If lenticular myopia occurs, this is irrelevant to the basic refraction. If a reliable history is not available, it is impossible to assess the degree of myopia attributable to the crystalline lens. An old pair of spectacles may yield misleading information. The patient may have a high degree of unilateral myopia that is not reflected in his spectacle lenses. Conversely, there may be a high degree of unilateral hypermetropia or astigmatism not corrected because of the high degree of anisometropia or because of amblyopia. Therefore additional history is required. An inquiry should be made as to the patient's vision in youth. Were glasses required for distance vision? Were reading glasses required during the usual presbyopic years? It would be useful to know that the patient did not require glasses to see the blackboard during his school years or to drive an automobile, or that his first pair of glasses were for close vision at the age of 45 years and later in life he needed glasses for distance but not for reading. This is typical of emmetropia, which gives way to lenticular myopia in later life.

There are other sources of possible error. The power of the crystalline lens is unrelated to the refraction. The normal range of powers of the crystalline lens have been established, and the absence of correlation between the power of the crystalline lens and the refraction has been emphasized.[3,4] The main components of the refraction of the eye—power of the cornea, depth of the anterior chamber, power of the lens, and axial length of the eye—show relatively little correlation in emmetropia as well as ametropia. Sorsby[4] has reported the following values for these major components in 107 emmetropic eyes:

	Corneal power (D)	Lens power (D)	Anterior chamber depth (mm)	Axial length (mm)
Range	39.0-47.6	15.5-23.9	2.5-4.2	22.3-26.0
Mean	43.1	19.7	3.5	24.2
Standard deviation	1.62	1.62	0.34	0.85

It is clearly evident then that the emmetropic eye is a finely correlated functional apparatus built of widely varying components. Therefore the removal from the eye of a crystalline lens whose power is at either extreme of the range (15.5 to 23.9 D) may alter the refraction by significantly different amounts. Thus an error is possible if it is assumed that a standard power pseudophakos exists that will retain emmetropia in an emmetropic eye after lens implantation. Mean values for corneal power, lens power, and anterior chamber depth may be found in extreme refractive errors. Thus corneal power may be 43.1 D in an eye with +10 D hypermetropia or −10 D myopia. One or more of the other components of the refraction must vary from their mean values to create these extreme refractive errors. The only exception is that the mean value for axial length is rarely seen in extreme refractive errors.

To achieve emmetropia or the same preoperative basic refractive error, the power of the pseudophakos should be less than that of the crystalline lens, since the pseudophakos is in a more forward position than the crystalline lens. This means that the equivalent planes of the pseudophakic eye are further forward than those of the phakic eye.

An 18 D intraocular lens tends to restore the basic refraction, that is, the refraction prior to the development of cataract. It then becomes necessary to estimate the lens power required to achieve a desired postoperative refractive error. It is incorrect to assume a 1:1 relationship; that is, a +19 D pseudophakos placed in an emmetropic eye does not result in 1 D of residual spectacle myopia. Since the residual refractive error is corrected by a spectacle lens worn at a vertex distance of about 12 mm, a change in lens power within the eye has a slightly different effectivity.

A satisfactory rule is to add 1.25 D to 18 D for each diopter of hypermetropia to be corrected and to subtract 1.25 D from 18 D for each diopter of myopia to be corrected. Stated in another way, given the basic refraction, we add to or subtract from 18 the number of diopters of hypermetropia or myopia to be corrected times 1.25. This also tells us that for each diopter of intraocular lens power change there results only 0.8 D change in the basic refraction (see table on p. 60).

This method is not foolproof even if the basic refraction is accurately known (no small task in itself). Recall that Sorsby's survey of emmetropic eyes revealed a mean crystalline lens power of 19.7 D with a standard deviation of 1.62. Thus an error of some magnitude could result from assuming a lens of average power. A thorough analysis of biometric data reveals that for each diopter of basic refrac-

Basic refraction (D)	Emmetropizing pseudophakos power (D)
+5.00	24.25
+4.00	23.00
+3.00	21.75
+2.00	20.50
+1.00	19.25
0.00	18.00
−1.00	16.75
−2.00	15.50
−3.00	14.25
−4.00	13.00
−5.00	11.75

tion to be changed, 1.1 to 1.4 D must be added to or subtracted from 18 D. Therefore using the 1.25 rule may lead to additional error. It is also possible that further sophistication in biometric technology will prove the 18 D value for achieving the basic refraction to be erroneous. However, at our current state of knowledge, if the basic refraction is known with a reasonable degree of accuracy, a target error of greater than 2 D will rarely occur.

ESTIMATIONS OF INTRAOCULAR LENS POWER BASED ON SOPHISTICATED MEASUREMENTS

It is theoretically possible to reach a highly accurate estimate of intraocular lens power by making sophisticated measurements of the various components of the basic refraction and incorporating this data into one of several formulas. The degree of accuracy of this method is still unsettled. There are no large documented series published that support, on a clinical level, the dependability of this approach. There are inherent errors in the precision of the testing equipment and some unavoidable changes in this data postoperatively. This will be discussed below. In spite of these drawbacks, this method has great merit. It is impossible for a highly myopic eye (axial myopia) to escape detection. In addition, further application of this technique will lead to greater accuracy.

The feasibility of adapting the power of the intraocular lens to each individual depends on three measurements: (1) refracting power of the cornea, (2) depth of the anterior chamber or, more accurately, the distance between the anterior surface of the cornea and the anterior surface of the pseudophakos at the optical axis, and (3) axial length of the eye or the distance from the anterior surface of the cornea to the fovea.

Refracting power of the cornea

The refracting power of the cornea is measured with the keratometer or ophthalmometer. In order to obtain a spherical equivalent, the two principal meridians are averaged. One popular formula utilizes the dioptric power, while another uses the radius of curvature of the anterior corneal surface. It should be recalled that, in contradistinction to the ophthalmoscope and the retinoscope, the keratometer measures the radius of curvature of a reflecting surface rather than the dioptric power of a refracting surface. If the dioptric power appears on the dial of a particular keratometer, it is only because an arbitrary overall index of refraction of the interface has been adopted. There are some sources of error that can be minimized. The average of at least three readings in each principal meridian is recorded. Some keratometers have a fixation light that can be seen by a patient with a nearly mature cataract. With some it is necessary to improvise to obtain central fixation. Another possible source of error is a postoperative change in corneal curvature. Although the surgically induced astigmatism can be considerable on occasion, there is usually little change in average corneal curvature using modern techniques of wound incision and closure. One suggested formula[5] allows for a slight postoperative flattening of the cornea by using a refractive index of 4/3 for the cornea. This compensates for a postoperative increase in the radius of corneal curvature of about 0.08 mm. Keratometric measurement errors are rarely of high magnitude. An error of 0.1 mm in radius curvature results in a refractive error of approximately 0.5 D.

Anterior chamber depth

Estimation of anterior chamber depth is subject to more variability than the other measurements. It has been consistently reported that there is a constant decrease in anterior chamber depth with age. This has been attributed to increasing lens thickness. This is of lessened importance in the aphakic state where anterior chamber depth averages about 4 mm. However, this measures the distance between the anterior corneal surface and the anterior iris surface at the pupillary border. The formulas for intraocular lens power utilize the corneal vertex distance of the pseudophakos, which is about 0.5 mm less. Therefore many currently used methods employ an empiric value of 3.5 mm for anterior chamber depth. An accurate measure of axial anterior chamber depth can be made preoperatively with the Jaeger method, using an attachment to the Haag-Streit or the Zeiss slit lamp. Anterior chamber depth may also be estimated by assuming it to be the height of a spherical segment, the radius of which is equal to the radius of curvature of the cornea, and the internal diameter of which is 1 mm longer than that of the visible external diameter of the cornea. These values are then substituted into the following formula:

$$K = r - \sqrt{r^2 - \frac{d^2}{4}}$$

K = Anterior chamber depth
r = Radius of curvature of cornea
d = Diameter of visible external part of cornea + 1 mm

An error of 0.1 mm in estimating the pseudophakic anterior chamber depth would result in a refractive error of about 0.1 D.

Axial length

Axial length measurements currently employ ultrasonography. The equipment

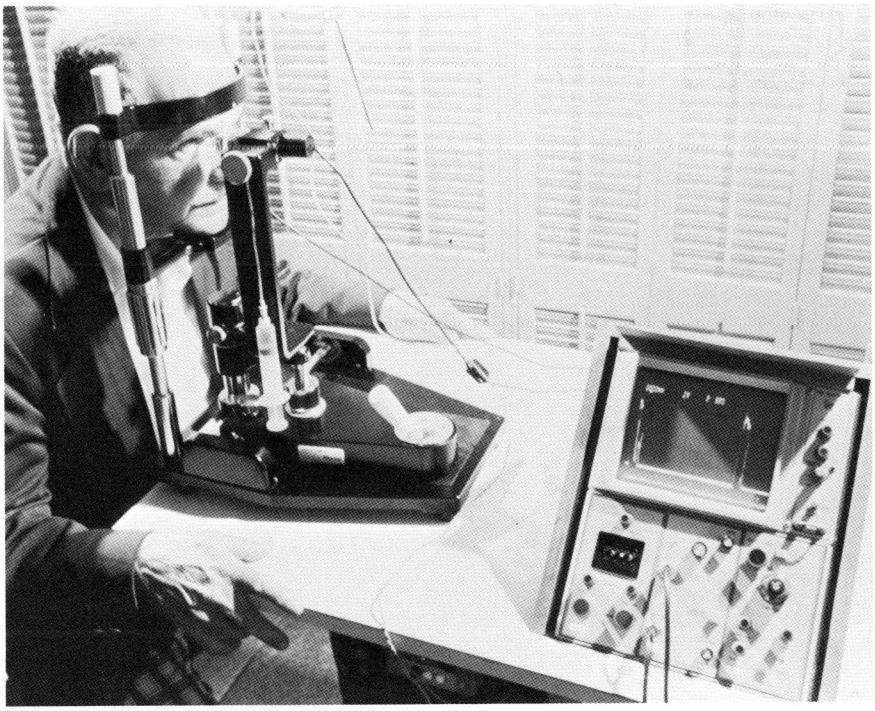

Fig. 6-1. Determination of axial length by A-scan ultrasonography using Digital Biometric Ruler. (Sonometrics Systems, Inc., 2067 Broadway, New York, N.Y. 10023.)

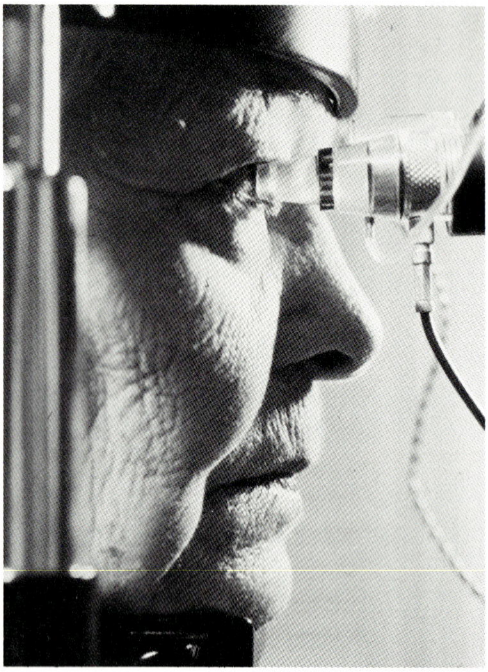

Fig. 6-2. Coupling device (filled with fluid) makes contact with cornea in much the same manner as an applanation tonometer. (Sonometrics Systems, Inc., 2067 Broadway, New York, N.Y. 10023.)

is expensive. Biometric techniques employ A-scan ultrasonography. Various methods of providing the sound coupling path between the transducer and the eye are available according to the equipment used. This may be a Steri-Drape water bath, a contact lens, or a crystal transducer that resembles the prism of an applanation tonometer (Figs. 6-1 and 6-2). A high degree of accuracy in estimating axial length is mandatory if this is used in calculating intraocular lens power. An error of 1 mm in measurement leads to a miscalculation of 2.5 to 3.5 D, which is considerable. If an ultrasound frequency of 20 MHz or more is used, it may be possible to achieve an accuracy of about 0.1 mm. Aside from instrument error, another possible source of error is a change in axial length postoperatively. This is probably not highly significant, but it has not yet been investigated fully.

Formulas for calculating intraocular lens power

There are several formulas available for the purpose of calculating the power of the intraocular lens. Their differences are based on a few minor variables resulting from voids in our complete understanding of the optical system of an eye containing an intraocular lens.

Colenbrander[6] has studied such a system and has offered a formula for arriving at the power of an iris-clip lens, giving a sharp image on the retina without the use of spectacles, that is, the power of the iris-clip lens required to produce emmetropia. The formulas to be presented use similar symbols to designate the various components of such an optical system. The Colenbrander formula is

$$D = \frac{n}{a - d - 0.00005} - \frac{n}{\frac{n}{Dc} - d - 0.00005}$$

D = Refracting power of the iris-clip lens in diopters
n = Refractive index of aqueous and vitreous (1.336)
d = Distance from the anterior surface of the cornea to the anterior surface of the iris-clip lens at the optical axis
a = Axial length of the eye
Dc = Refracting power of the cornea in diopters

The reader is referred to Colenbrander's article for the derivation of his formula.

Fyodorov and co-workers[7] have offered the following formula:

$$D = \frac{n - a\,Dc}{(a - d)\left(1 - \frac{d\,Dc}{n}\right)}$$

Richard Binkhorst[5] has suggested the following formula:

$$D = \frac{1336\,(4r - a)}{(a - d)\,(4r - d)}$$

r = Radius of curvature of the anterior surface of the cornea in millimeters

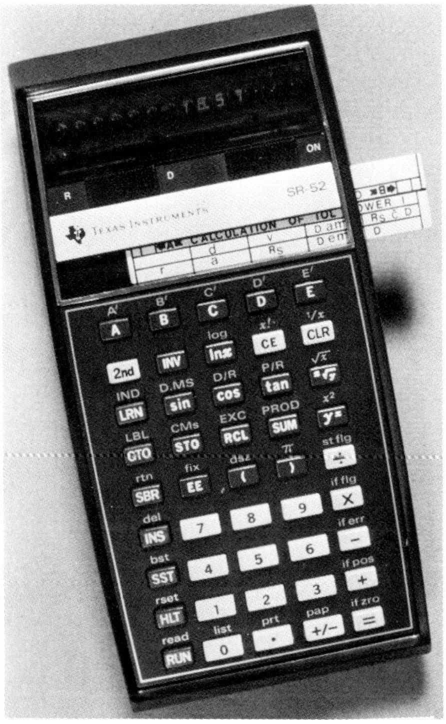

Fig. 6-3. Texas Instruments SR-52 programmable calculator used for preoperative determination of pseudophakos power.

Binkhorst has made available an Intraocular Lens Power Calculation Kit that describes a variety of calculations that can be made on a relatively inexpensive programmable calculator (for example, Texas Instruments SR-52 [Fig. 6-3] and Hewlett-Packard HP-65). Once the basic measurements of corneal curvature, axial length, and anterior chamber depth have been made, several complex calculations can be performed in a matter of seconds.

The following four calculations may be made by inserting the programmed strip of tape into the calculator.

1. Intraocular lens power required to create emmetropia
2. Intraocular lens power required to create any refractive error at any vertex distance
3. The refractive error, at any vertex distance, to be expected with an intraocular lens of known power
4. The aphakic refraction, at any vertex distance, for an eye without an intraocular lens

The formula to create emmetropia has been described above. To compute the intraocular lens power required to create any refractive error, at any vertex distance, the following formula is used:

$$D = \frac{1336\,\{4r - a - [v\,(4r - a) + 0.003\,a\,r]\,Rs\}}{a - d\,\{4r - d - [v\,(4r - d) + 0.003\,d\,r]\,Rs\}}$$

Rs = Spectacle refraction in diopters
v = Vertex distance in millimeters

The formula to compute the refractive error, at any vertex distance, to be expected with an intraocular lens of known power is shown below.

This formula also makes it possible to calculate the aphakic refraction, at any vertex distance, to be expected without an intraocular lens.

Since the average of the keratometer readings is used, any intraocular lens power is calculated to produce a spherical equivalent refraction, be this emmetropia or a refractive error. Likewise, any calculated refraction is a spherical equivalent.

To illustrate the simplicity of making these complex calculations on a Texas Instruments SR-52 calculator, the following sample problems are given.

PROBLEM □ Find the intraocular lens power required to make an eye with the following data emmetropic: (1) average of keratometer readings = 7.81 mm; (2) axial length = 23.87 mm; (3) postoperative anterior chamber depth = 3.5 mm.

$$Rs = \frac{1336\,(4r - a) - D\,(a - d)\,(4r - d)}{1336\,[v\,(4r - a) + 0.003\,a\,r] - D\,(a - d)\,[v\,(4r - d) + 0.003\,d\,r]}$$

D = Dioptric power in aqueous of the intraocular lens

SOLUTION
7.81 A* 23.87 B 3.5 B¹
D = 17.43

PROBLEM □ Find the intraocular lens power required to make the same eye 2.25 D myopic at a vertex of 12 mm.

SOLUTION
7.81 A 23.87 B 3.5 B¹ −2.25 C 12 C¹
D¹ = 20.19

PROBLEM □ Find the refractive error, at a vertex distance of 12 mm, which a 20.5 D intraocular lens would produce in the same eye.

SOLUTION
7-81 A 23-87 B 3.5 B¹ 12 C¹ 20.5 E
E¹ = −2.51

PROBLEM □ Find the aphakic refraction, at a vertex distance of 12 mm, for the same eye without an intraocular lens.

SOLUTION
7.81 A 23.87 B 12 C¹ O E
E¹ = 11.38

GOALS OF PREOPERATIVE ESTIMATION OF LENS POWER

While it is often desirable, emmetropia may not be the ideal postoperative refraction in all patients who undergo intraocular lens implant surgery. To appreciate this the implant surgeon should have a basic understanding of the altered optics in an eye with an intraocular lens. This involves the principles of telescopic magnification. The intraocular implant lens occupies a more anterior position than the crystalline lens. Thus if the intraocular lens does not have enough refracting power to restore emmetropia, there will be a resulting hypermetropic pseudophakic refraction. This deficit in refracting power of the intraocular lens plus the required hypermetropic spectacle correction form a Galilean telescope. Each diopter of spectacle correction represents an image size magnification of 2%. Conversely, if the intraocular lens has an excess of refracting power and thus renders a previously emmetropic eye myopic, an inverted Galilean telescope is introduced. Each diopter of myopia required causes an image size minification of 2%. Another factor must be considered. The iris-clip and Medallion lenses cause an image size magnification of 3.25%, the iridocapsular lens slightly less, and the iris-plane lens possibly the least. Thus it can be easily seen that if residual hypermetropia is significant, the image size can exceed that caused by contact lens correction of aphakia.

It has been stated[5] that when a 0.5 mm thick convexoplano lens, its anterior vertex 3.5 mm from the anterior vertex of the cornea, is substituted for the lens of the schematic eye, the magnification of the retinal image would be 3.25%, if the eye is made emmetropic. To restore the original image size the eye would have to be made 1.7 D myopic with the correction placed at the anterior focus. Similarly the axially ametropic schematic eye would have to be made 1.7 D more myopic or less hypermetropic to restore the original image size, again with the spectacle corrections at the anterior focal points.

C. D. Binkhorst[8] has described a method for determining the iseikonic pseudophakos for the schematic eye. Iseikonia between the schematic pseudophakic eye and the schematic phakic eye exists when the focal lengths of both eyes are identical. The following relationship is used for the focal length.

$$f_E = \frac{fc\, f_L}{f_L + fc^1 - d}$$

f_E = Anterior focal length of complete eye (−17.055 mm)
fc = Anterior focal length of cornea (−23.227 mm)
fc^1 = Posterior focal length of cornea (31.031 mm)
d = Distance of first equivalent plane of pseudophakos from second equivalent plane of cornea (3.5506 mm)
f_L = Focal length of pseudophakos

The value for d is calculated by assuming a corneal vertex distance (v) of 3.5 mm. The second equivalent plane of the cornea equals −0.0506 mm. Therefore the distance (d) of the first equivalent plane of the pseudophakos from the sec-

*The letters following the numbers (A, B, B¹, and so on) in this and the following sample problems indicate keys on the calculator to be pressed.

ond equivalent plane of the cornea equals 3.5506 mm.

The focal length of the schematic iseikonic pseudophakos (f_L) turns out to be 75.921 mm, which gives a radius of the anterior surface (r_1) of 8.751 mm and an equivalent power of the pseudophakos (F_L) of 17.6 D. In arriving at these figures, note that

$$r_1 = \left(\frac{1.49 - 1.336}{1.336}\right)$$

and

$$F_L = \left(\frac{1.449 - 1.336}{r_1}\right)$$

Therefore a pseudophakos with power of 17.6 D at a corneal vertex distance of 3.5 mm is iseikonic with Gullstrand's schematic crystalline lens of 19.11 D.[9]

Since the pseudophakos is in a more forward position than the crystalline lens, the equivalent planes of the pseudophakic eye are further forward than those of the phakic eye. If the focal lengths are the same, this results in a more forward position of the posterior focal point and plus ametropia.

For the schematic pseudophakic eye one can calculate the anterior displacement of the second equivalent plane and the correlated myopia as follows: the distance of the second equivalent plane of the pseudophakos from its posterior surface is

$$(-n_1)\left(\frac{t}{n_2}\right)\left(\frac{F_L^1}{F_L}\right) = 0.448 \text{ mm}$$

in which t is the center thickness of the pseudophakos (0.5 mm), n_1 is the refractive index of the aqueous (1.336), n_2 is the refractive index of the pseudophakos (1.490), and F_L^1 equals F_L. The corneal vertex distance of the second equivalent plane of the pseudophakic eye is therefore 3.552 − 2.607 = 0.945 mm.

Compared with the corneal vertex distance of the second equivalent plane in Gullstrand's schematic phakic eye of 1.602 mm, the second equivalent plane of the schematic iseikonic eye is in a 0.657 mm more forward position. Calculation with Newton's object image relation $(x \times x^1 = f \times f^1)$ shows that this corresponds with a 1.69 D myopia at the anterior focal point.

These estimations are for the schematic eye that represents the mean values of the components of refraction. However, as discussed previously, the components of the refracting system of the eye have been shown to have a normal distribution with considerable variation. For example, one eye may be emmetropic with a relatively long axial length but a flatter than average cornea. Another may have a shorter than average axial length, an average corneal curvature, but a crystalline lens of high refracting power. The possibilities are considerable in emmetropia as well as ametropia. It should then be apparent that the 3.25% magnification of the retinal image is an average figure for the emmetropic eye. Taking the total variation of the components of emmetropic eyes into account, this range would be from 2.6% to 3.9%. Likewise there would be a range of myopia, from 1.15 to 2.35 D, with the correction at the anterior focus, required to restore the original image size in previously emmetropic eyes.[5] The same range of magnification would apply for ametropia if the intraocular lens were meant to restore the original ametropia, and the range within which these eyes would have to be made more myopic or less hypermetropic would be the same. These figures must be varied slightly according to whether an iris-clip, iridocapsular, or iris-plane lens is used.

Ideally there should be neither anisometropia nor aniseikonia. However, from the above discussion it is apparent that, with currently used intraocular lenses, *there can be no isometropia without aniseikonia and no iseikonia without anisometropia.*

The method just described to achieve iseikonia by changing the refraction of the pseudophakic eye a certain amount to the myopic side is subject to some errors, since it does not take into account the variation of the components of the refracting system of the eye. C. D. Binkhorst[8] has shown that his method of using a standard 19.5 D pseudophakos is subject to these errors and has suggested a method of producing iseikonia based on data obtained from both eyes. This will especially be more accurate in cases of anisometropia, whether absolute or relative. Absolute anisometropia, which refers to unequal refraction of the two eyes, is particularly common in the higher degrees of refractive errors. Relative anisometropia, which refers to equal refraction of the two eyes, but with differences in their components, would remain unrecognized unless the components of both eyes are determined.

R. D. Binkhorst[5] has described a method that takes the variation of the components of the two eyes into account in the calculation of the intraocular lens power required to produce iseikonia in unilateral pseudophakia. As stated earlier by C. D. Binkhorst,[8] the aim is to equalize the focal lengths of the two eyes. The calculation is carried out in three steps:

1. In the first step the focal length of the crystalline lens in the fellow eye is determined with the following formula:

$$F = \frac{(a - ACD - 2.21)\left(\dfrac{1336}{Dc + Rc} - ACD - 2.08\right)}{\dfrac{1336}{Dc + Rc} - a + 2.21 - 2.08}$$

F = Focal length of the crystalline lens in millimeters
a = Axial length in millimeters
ACD = Anterior chamber depth in millimeters
Dc = Dioptric power of the cornea
Rc = Refraction at the cornea in diopters
2.08 and 2.21 = Respective schematic values for the distances of the anterior and posterior principal planes for the crystalline lens from its anterior vertex in millimeters

Given the thickness and the refractive indexes of a lens and the surrounding medium, the location of the principal planes depends almost entirely on the ratio of the radii of curvature. The power of the lens has a negligible influence. The value for *Rc*, the refraction at the cornea, can be found in a table of contact lens powers corresponding to the spectacle refraction at various vertex distances, or it can be calculated as follows:

$$Rc = \frac{Rs}{1 - vRs}$$

Rs = Spectacle refraction in diopters
v = Vertex distance in meters

2. With the value for the focal length of the crystalline lens (*F*), the anterior focal length of the fellow eye can now be calculated:

$$F_1 = \frac{1000\,F}{Dc\,[F - (ACD + 2.08)] + 1336}$$

F_1 = Anterior focal length of fellow eye in millimeters

3. The pseudophakic eye must be given the same focal length. This is accomplished by calculating the intraocular lens power as follows:

$$D = \frac{1336\left(\dfrac{3r}{F_1} - 1\right)}{4r - d}$$

D = Dioptric power in aqueous of the intraocular lens
F_1 = Anterior focal length in millimeters
r = Radius of curvature of the anterior surface of the cornea in millimeters
d = Distance between the anterior vertex of the cornea and the intraocular lens in millimeters

The refractive index used for the cornea is 1.3375 for the fellow eye and 4/3 for the eye to be made pseudophakic.

In this calculation the axial length of the eye to be made pseudophakic is not taken into account. The two eyes having the same focal length would have the same image size if the corrections were placed at their respective anterior focal points. Since usually the spectacle correction is closer to the eye than the anterior focus and since usually the refraction of the pseudophakic eye will be less hypermetropic or more myopic than the fellow eye, there is still a problem with the image size. The image will usually be slightly larger in the pseudophakic eye than in the fellow eye. To calculate the intraocular lens power, which would compensate for these factors in a given situation, is a very complicated procedure. In general the intraocular lens would have to be 0.25 to 0.5 D stronger. This correction can be added to the calculated intraocular lens power; for intraocular lens implants available in 0.5 D steps, the next step up should be used.

As with the calculations described on p. 62, R. D. Binkhorst has programmed these calculations for the Texas Instruments SR-52 and Hewlett-Packard HP-65 calculators.

PROBLEM □ Find the intraocular lens power required to produce iseikonia using the following data (with the Texas Instruments SR-52 calculator).

Fellow eye
Average of keratometer readings = 7.85 mm
Axial length = 23.28 mm
Anterior chamber depth = 3.65 mm
Thickness of crystalline lens = 3.82 mm
Spherical equivalent refraction = +1 D
Vertex distance = 13 mm

Eye to be made pseudophakic
Average of keratometer readings = 7.87 mm
Postoperative anterior chamber depth = 3.5 mm

SOLUTION
7.85 A* 23.28 A¹ 3.65 B 3.82 B¹ +1 C
13 C¹ 7.87 D 3.5 D¹
E = 21.25 D

Comprehension of the above formulas and their derivation may not appeal to most ophthalmologists. Most intraocular lens implant surgeons still use standard power lenses, some select lens powers based on the basic refraction, and only a minority resort to sophisticated measurements and utilize the formulas discussed above. With increasing accuracy and simplicity of A-scan ultrasound equipment and with the availability of relatively inexpensive calculators, it is likely that this trend will change.

The implant surgeon must decide when to make a pseudophakic eye emmetropic and when to make it ametropic. It is difficult to set rigid rules for this decision, since implant surgeons use varying guidelines for indications and contraindications for implant surgery.

When should emmetropia be the goal?

1. When bilateral pseudophakia is planned. There is no useful purpose in aiming for myopia if the opposite eye has a visually disturbing cataract. The surgeon may elect to implant a lens in the second eye at a later date. Therefore emmetropia in both eyes would be a more satisfactory goal. If the first eye is made myopic, the second eye should be made the same so as to avoid aniseikonia. Frequently the cataract in the second eye is sufficiently advanced so that binocular vision is so rudimentary that the goal of iseikonia is unrealistic. Another factor to be considered is the possibility of increasing lenticular myopia in the second eye. It is probably wise not to correct this changing refractive error.

2. Hypermetropia of 1.5 to 2.5 D in a useful fellow eye. This is a frequent situation, since a small to moderate degree of hypermetropia is near the peak of the population curve of refractive errors. It is possible that the fellow eye may not have a cataract, or if it does, it may not change for many years.

3. Known or suspected absence of binocular vision. The indication for emmetropia is particularly valid in high ametropia.

4. When surgery on one eye is planned. Many elderly patients who have undergone a successful lens implantation find that this is entirely adequate for their needs. Since they have none of the visual handicaps of unilateral aphakia, surgery on the second eye is often unnecessary.

5. When senile macular choroidal degeneration is present in both eyes. There

---

*The letters following the numbers (A, A¹, B, and so on) in this sample problem indicate keys on the calculator to be pressed.

is a lessened demand for iseikonia in these patients.

6. When a contact lens is used in the fellow eye in patients with higher amounts of hypermetropia or myopia. However, it may be argued that if a patient can successfully manage a contact lens in a phakic eye, why bother with an implant in the cataractous eye? A routine cataract extraction with contact lens correction is probably a better choice.

7. When a contact lens is used in an aphakic fellow eye. To achieve iseikonia with an implant in the second eye would necessitate making the pseudophakic eye several diopters hyperopic, a high price to pay. Bilateral contact lens correction would of course achieve iseikonia. If, however, an implant is preferred and that eye is made emmetropic, the aniseikonia is less than in unilateral aphakia corrected with a contact lens and a normal fellow eye. The implant provides some magnification and lessens some of the image size disparity between the two eyes.

When should ametropia be the goal?

The only indication to make the pseudophakic eye ametropic exists in unilateral pseudophakia. The rationale for this is the avoidance of aniseikonia, which has been discussed earlier. The only important exceptions are hypermetropia of 1.5 to 2.5 D in the fellow eye and where surgery on only one eye is planned in patients with bilateral cataracts or absence of binocular vision.

It was stated on p. 64 that the schematic eye requires 1.7 D myopia to restore the original image size if the spectacle correction is worn at the anterior focal point (about 17 mm). Thus an acceptable method would be to change the refraction of the pseudophakic eye 2.25 D for the iris-clip lens, 2.1 D for the iridocapsular lens, and 2 D for the iris-plane (Copeland) lens. The discrepancy is because of the vertex distance of the spectacle correction (about 12 mm), which is always within the anterior focal point.

SUMMARY

The true potential of intraocular implant lenses can only be realized if the implant surgeon understands the principles outlined in this chapter and makes an appropriate selection of the power of the implant in each situation. Increasing sophistication in the techniques of measuring the various components of the refraction is also necessary to achieve this potential.

REFERENCES

1. Troutman, R. C.: Artiphakia and aniseikonia, Trans. Am. Ophthalmol. Soc. **60**:590-658, 1962.
2. Troutman, R. C.: Artiphakia and aniseikonia, Am. J. Ophthalmol. **56**:602-639, Oct. 1963.
3. Stenström, S.: Untersuchungen über die Variation und Kovariation der optischen Elemente des menschlichen Auges, Acta Ophthalmol. [Suppl.] (Kbh) vol. 26, 1946.
4. Sorsby, A.: Epidemiology of refraction, Int. Ophthalmol. Clin. **11**:1-18, 1971.
5. Binkhorst, R. D.: The optical design of intraocular lens implants, Ophthalmic Surg. **6**:17-31, 1975.
6. Colenbrander, M. C.: Calculation of the power of an iris clip lens for distance vision, Br. J. Ophthalmol. **57**:735-740, 1973.
7. Fyodorov, S. N., Galin, M. A., and Linksz, A.: Calculation of the optical power of intraocular lenses, Invest. Ophthalmol. **14**:625-628, Aug. 1975.
8. Binkhorst, C. D.: Power of the prepupillary pseudophakos, Br. J. Ophthalmol. **56**:332-337, 1972.
9. Duke-Elder, S.: System of ophthalmology, vol. 5, St. Louis, 1970, The C. V. Mosby Co., p. 119.

CHAPTER 7

Sterilization of lens implants

A variety of terms has been applied to the attempt to reduce or prevent microbiologic contamination of medical products or devices. These terms, which include antisepsis, disinfection, and sterilization, to mention but a few, have a long and noble history but are no longer useful expressions for the physician implanting intraocular lenses. The physician needs to know whether the lens is free of organisms but must also know if the sterilizing system alters the lens, whether long-term degradation products result, and whether the process of sterilization creates a noninert material.

Gaseous and liquid chemical systems currently are used to sterilize intraocular lenses. Sodium hydroxide and ethylene oxide respectively appear to satisfy the necessary criteria for efficacy and safety as outlined above. This chapter will review why these agents are in use, the evidence for their efficacy and safety, and consider some of the shortcomings of other forms of sterilization.

The term sterilization means that all forms of microbial life are destroyed.[1] This must include bacterial spores that are resistive to many forms of sterilization even though the parent vegetative bacteria remain quite sensitive to the same system. For example, tetanus spores are resistive to many commonly used agents, while the bacillus itself is killed by low concentrations of virtually every disinfectant. Spores have been cultured from detergents used in operating rooms, while the vegetative forms have been easily killed by the same material. Consequently, assessment of the effectiveness of sterilization takes into account the ability to eliminate all forms of a given organism, the ease with which this occurs, and the probability that sterilization has been effected.

One method of expressing the effectiveness of sterilization is the use of the term "inactivation factor." If, for example, an article contained 10^3 organisms prior to sterilization and 10^{10} articles need to be examined after sterilization to find one organism, the inactivation factor for the sterilization process would be 10^{13}. This is a quantitative method to express sterilization efficiency for a given process versus a given organism. Another method for such expression, which takes into account the probability of effecting sterilization (after all, sterilization is a probability function) as determined from growth and death curves of organisms, is the decimal reduction time or D number, an approach that traces its origin to the food industry.[2] An understanding of the D number is essential to present-day concepts of sterilization.

Microbial cells have rapid growth rates, and this rate may be expressed in terms of the number of generations (a generation is the doubling of the cell number) created per hour. Simple organisms (unicellular) multiply by geometric progression, and plotting such exponential growth on a semilogarithmic scale against time for short periods results in a straight line, the slope of which reflects the growth rate of the population of organisms. However, the growth curve of organisms after long periods in culture indicates that full replicative potential is not exhibited due to depletion of nutriment, death of organisms, changes in pH and so on. The various components of the growth and death cycles of bacterial cultures are of importance for a variety of reasons, not the least of which is the fact that positive cultures are more difficult to obtain in certain phases of the growth curve though the organism is still living. Microbial death is difficult to ascertain if it is defined as an irreversible state in which the processes necessary for growth and replication are not operant. It is more correctly represented by a probability function; that is, a sterilization process is a probability function quantitated by the number of surviving organisms. One method of expressing this function is the term value (from decimal reduction time), which is the time required to destroy 90% of the organisms by a given method of sterilization. With respect to the organism, it is convenient to express the resistance of an organism in terms of its D_{10} value, which means the time necessary to reduce a given population of organisms to 10% of its original number (destruction or inactivation of 90% of the original population). Conversely, since growth of organisms is essentially exponential, the D value also represents the time necessary for the survivor curve to traverse one log cycle.

The U. S. Food and Drug Administration in its published guidelines for intraocular lenses uses D values because this approach permits the theoretical calculation of a single surviving organism from a terminal sterilization process. This agency believes that, by at least two suggested testing criteria, methods of sterilizing intraocular lenses should have a probability that 10^6 lenses would be gone through before a single viable organism would be found.

THERMAL STERILIZATION

Proteins and nucleic acids are rapidly denatured between 50° and 90° C. This means that the fine colloidal protein state is coagulated, making the constituent materials nonfunctional. The degree of denaturation is a function of accessibility to the heat source. Barriers to heat conductivity and a host of other factors mandate higher temperatures than those sufficient for microbial cultures. Dry heat sterilization (160° C for 1 hour or 190° C for 1½ minutes) causes physical alteration in polymethylmethacrylate, which depolymerizes at such temperatures and alters its physical form. Consequently, this approach has never been used commercially. Moist heat, well known in hospitals as saturated steam under pressure, is the most common and most dependable means of destroying all forms of microbial life. It is the moist heat, not the pressure, that is the sterilizing medium for this process. Although a prevacuum improves efficiency by cutting down sterilizing time, the steam temperature of at least 135° C exceeds the softening point of acrylics, making this method inadequate for intraocular lenses.

IRRADIATION

Both high (gamma and electron) and low (ultraviolet) energy radiation have been employed for sterilizing acrylics, though a dearth of basic microbiologic studies with intraocular lenses and these forms of sterilization is available.[3] Ultraviolet (250 nm) possesses sufficient energy to sterilize certain smooth surfaces but would not appear to be adequate for the convoluted and tunneled bases of certain intraocular lenses. Further, this particular wavelength is absorbed by polymethylmethacrylate and theoretically has a degrading influence on the plastic.

Gamma irradiation usually employs cobalt 60 or occasionally cesium 137. Gamma rays have enormous penetration and are most suitable for large and dense products. High-energy electrons emitted by a cathode ray gun have low penetration and very rapid sterilizing ability. However, these forms of sterilization alter the bonding and polymer structure of polymethylmethacrylate, which tends to yellow with low doses and becomes progressively brittle. Further, the chemical reactions that may be caused with oversterilization (greater than 2.5 Mrads) lead to free radical formation and highly active breakdown products of polymethylmethacrylate, which may induce serious inflammatory sequelae. One lot of cobalt 60–sterilized lenses from Europe had to be withdrawn in the United States due to these circumstances.

CHEMICAL DISINFECTION

Liquid germicides have enormous application for reducing organism counts on surfaces in and about surgical areas, but have had progressively less application in the sterilizing of materials, devices, and instruments involved in ocular surgery. Besides the problem of efficacy for certain members of this group, the potential for tissue toxicity has severely restricted the use of liquid germicides potentially available for intraocular application.

Quaternary ammonium compounds, often used in the past because of their blandness, have little use in sterilizing intraocular lenses. Cationic agents conceivably can be absorbed to the acid surface of acrylic, since in theory a certain degree of surface hydrolysis must occur while intraocular lenses are in solution. Perhaps this explains why lenses originally sterilized with tetradecyltrimethyl ammonium bromide were highly irritating in the anterior chamber. Anionic detergents, which would have no potential for absorption on the surface of acrylic, appear to be inert and have been used as the initial cleaning material for the Ridley method of sterilization, but have not been used as sterilizing agents. Nonionic detergents of this group of compounds will penetrate into the plastic and provide the problem of uncontrolled elution, making this group potentially dangerous as well as ineffective. For the same reason, high concentrations of acid such as HCl, which would contain significant unionized fractions, would penetrate the lens surface readily and mandate a knowledge of complete elution times before such lenses could be used intraocularly.[4]

The Frederick Ridley method for chemically sterilizing intraocular lenses, introduced in 1957, has stood the test of time and with only slight variation fulfills the criteria for a safe and effective method of sterilization.[5-7]

Based on previous work by Hobbs and Wilson and Tilley that 10% NaOH had a sterilizing effect even on the spores of *Bacillus subtilis* at 30° C in 30 minutes, Ridley reasoned that the smooth surfaces of those lenses available in 1957 would similarly be sterilized.[8] Since 10% caustic soda is intensely anionic, its diffusion into acrylic is negligible. It does not harm the plastic and is easily removed from the surface by washing. Ridley recommended that after 1 hour in 10% NaOH the lenses be stored in 0.1% NaOH. He concluded that this concentration of NaOH is a "safe storage medium for several months at room temperatures."[5]

Prior to use in the operating room, lenses stored in 0.1% NaOH are washed copiously with a large volume of 0.5% $NaHCO_3$. The action of bicarbonate is to form an inert bicarbonate-carbonate buffer, ridding the lens of any residual NaOH.

Ridley noted that the concentration of 0.1% NaOH slowly decreased with time at room temperature and very rapidly at 40° C. He postulated that perhaps dilute caustic soda slowly liberated copolymerized methacrylic acid, which "used up" available alkali. For this reason he recommended that lenses stored in 0.1% NaOH for 3 months be resterilized and reissued for use.

We have attempted to analyze the steps of the Ridley method on high levels of contamination using lenses with loop supports that less readily permit access of NaOH to the convoluted interiors of drilled holes. Using 10^6 organisms of a variety including *B subtilis*, it was found that sterilization was not achieved unless lenses were stored in 10% NaOH for at least 3 hours. Further, for a similar inoculum, lenses were not sterilized in 0.1% even after 3 months. For much smaller inocula, the Ridley system is effective. It would appear, then, that simple 10% NaOH meets FDA requirements, eliminates the potential for contamination by handling, and is indeed a terminal sterilization system. Adequate rinsing would appear necessary for loop-supported lenses and is easily achieved during the interval of commencing a case and inserting a lens.

GAS STERILIZATION

A variety of gaseous agents have been used for sterilizing purposes since ancient times. Burning of oils and sulfur and the use of formaldehyde all have in common gaseous sterilization. In recent years propylene oxide, betapropiolactone, and particularly ethylene oxide have come into widespread use, particularly for the sterilization of plastic materials.[9] Ethylene oxide

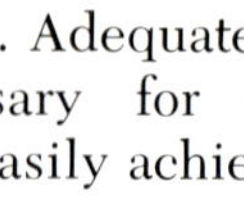

is the simplest of the cyclic ethers and has been in use for many years as a disinfectant but only in recent years as a gaseous sterilizing agent. Its primary action is one of alkylation or esterification of acids, and ether or thioether formation with proteins. Thus, one form of the bactericidal effect of ethylene oxide on a sulfhydryl-containing protein necessary for bacterial function would be

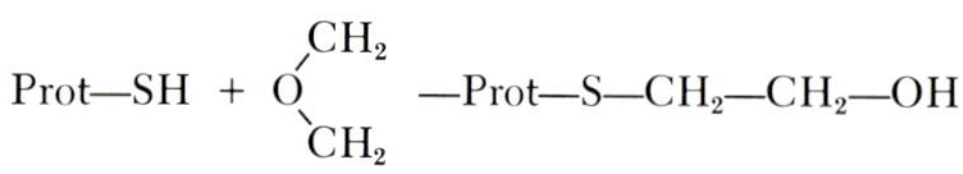

alkylating the protein SH grouping and rendering it inactive.

Ethylene oxide boils at 11° C, is a gas at normal temperatures, and is violently explosive in all mixtures with air from 3% to 80%. For this reason it has been used mixed with carbon dioxide, nitrogen, freon, or other inert gases. After its use it is rendered harmless by passing it through a gas absorber. For safety, pure gas sterilization is run at subatmospheric pressures, but the mixtures, which are explosion proof, can be run above atmospheric pressure.

Ethylene oxide does not react with plastics and does not affect their physical or chemical properties. However, certain plastics will retain ethylene oxide or one or more of its reactive products and must therefore be purged of these materials. Ethylene glycol will be formed by ethylene oxide and water and ethylene chlorhydrin with ethylene oxide and chloride ion. These two agents, and particularly the latter, are highly tissue toxic and must be eliminated during the purge period. Twenty-five parts per million of the trio of these constituents are considered within appropriate safety limits.

The great advantage of ethylene oxide is the ability to sterilize plastic products that would be altered by the more available and familiar steam sterilization process or that require the inconvenient multifaceted steps of the original Ridley NaOH sterilization. Consequently many optical products, endoscopes in particular, are sterilized by this route. Further, since the penetrance of the gas is excellent for nonpolar barriers such as polymethylmethacrylate, and residual materials are easily ascertained by gas chromatography, it is an ideal agent for intraocular lenses.

REFERENCES

1. Stuart, L. S.: Introduction to antimicrobial testing methods. In Lawrence, C. L., and Block, S. S., editors: Disinfection, sterilization, and preservation, Philadelphia, 1968, Lea & Febiger, p. 110.
2. Katzin, L. I., Sandholzer, L. A., and Strong, M. E.: Application of the decimal reduction time principle to a study of the resistance of coliform bacteria to pasteurization, J. Bacteriol. **45**:265-272, 1943.
3. Binkhorst, C. D., and Flu, F. P.: Sterilization of

intraocular acrylic lens prosthesis with ultraviolet rays, Br. J. Ophthalmol. **40**:665, 1956.
4. Ridley, F.: Intraocular acrylic implants. A recent development in the surgery of cataracts, Br. J. Ophthalmol. **36**:113, 1952.
5. Ridley, F.: Safety requirements for acrylic implants, Br. J. Ophthalmol. **41**:359, 1957.
6. Reddish, G. F.: Antiseptics, disinfectants, fungicides and sterilization, Philadelphia, 1954, Lea & Febiger, p. 25.
7. Galin, M. A., and Turkish, L.: Sodium hydroxide sterilization of acrylic intraocular lenses, Am. J. Ophthalmol. In press.
8. Hobbs, B. C., and Wilson, G. S.: The disinfectant activity of caustic soda, J. Hyg. (Camb.) **42**:436, 1942.
9. Lebovits, A.: Permeability of polymers to gases, vapors and liquids, Mod. Plastics **43**:139-146, 1966.

CHAPTER 8

Surgical techniques

When a surgeon begins lens implant surgery, he should not make too many changes initially in his standard technique. Experience will lead him to decide if a fornix-based or limbus-based flap is more desirable. The merits of absorbable and nonabsorbable sutures may have to be considered. Some surgeons find preplaced sutures in lens implant surgery a nuisance; others believe they are a necessity. Beyond debate is the advantage of a concave anterior hyaloid face following intracapsular cataract extractions. It is possible to achieve this in a high percentage of cases by applying digital pressure for a longer period than is customary for an intracapsular cataract extraction without lens implantation. Most surgeons have little experience with 7 to 10 minutes of digital pressure. The globe appears well sunken into the orbit, the cornea feels soft to palpation, and the Schiøtz tonometric reading is between 15 scale units and off the scale with a 5.5 g weight. It is easier to achieve profound hypotony in elderly patients in whom vitreous degeneration is common and in whom scleral rigidity permits the vitreous to fall back after lens extraction. In recent years there has been a tendency to rely more on digital pressure than on hyperosmotic agents. The latter must be used with caution because of their cardiovascular side effects in elderly patients. The rapidity of the fall in intraocular pressure with digital pressure is a fairly reliable indicator of vitreous and orbital decompression.

In both intracapsular and extracapsular lens implant surgery a viable iris is essential. The iris must dilate sufficiently for cataract extraction and yet constrict promptly to center and secure the implant. Iris sphincter damage is unimportant in routine cataract surgery, but in implant surgery it should be avoided. The anterior chamber should be kept clear of blood. Blood on the iris inhibits pupillary constriction and may obstruct the view as the implant is inserted. An excessively concave iris diaphragm is advantageous inasmuch as it accompanies a concave hyaloid face, but the iris should be floated forward with balanced saline solution before the implant is inserted.

The surgeon should reconsider his routine postoperative orders. If it is the custom to maximally dilate the pupil after cataract extraction, then the orders should be revised. Maximum pupillary dilatation in the immediate postoperative period can lead to lens implant dislocation. Lastly, and of great importance, the surgeon should be sure of the quality and sterility of the implant being used.

BINKHORST IRIS-CLIP (4-LOOP) IMPLANT

Description

The design of this implant varies slightly from one manufacturer to another, especially as to the materials used in the loops (haptics). Common to all is a pair of anterior and posterior loops that are nearly but not quite parallel to each other. The most frequently used 4-loop implant, as manufactured by Morcher (Stuttgart, W. Germany), has anterior and posterior loops made of the same material, Supramid (nylon 6). The loops are

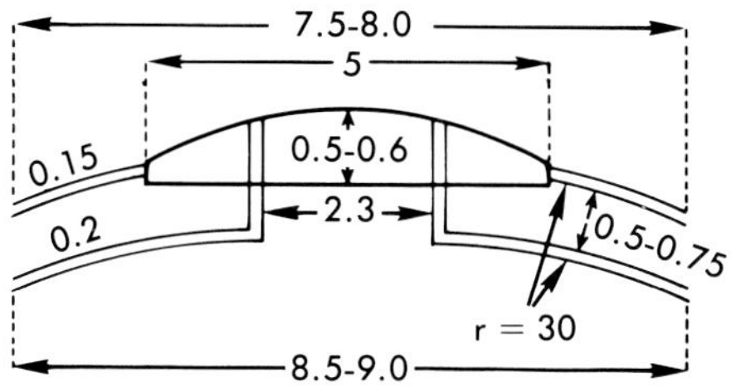

Fig. 8-1. Schema of current Binkhorst 4-loop iris-clip implant, as manufactured by Morcher, W. Germany. (From Jaffe, N. S.: Cataract surgery and its complications, ed. 2, St. Louis, 1976, The C. V. Mosby Co.)

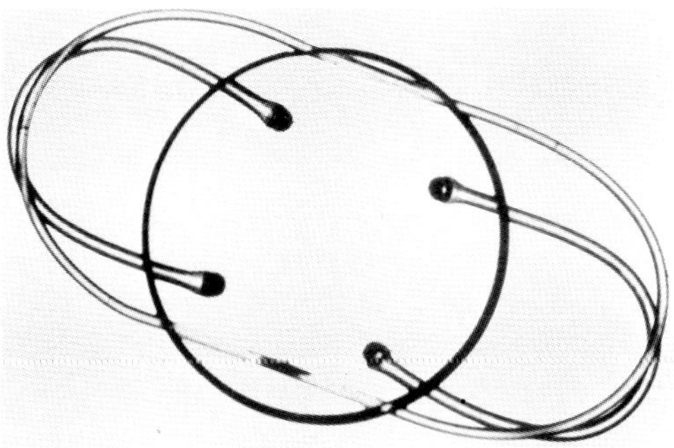

Fig. 8-2. Binkhorst 4-loop iris-clip implant (Morcher) slightly rotated. Note that anterior loops are fused together within implant.

all angled backward (posteriorly) at an angle of 10° to 15° (Fig. 8-1). This is done to conform to the anterior surface of the iris diaphragm and to lessen the possibility of contact with the cornea. The anterior loops are situated in the plane of the optical portion of the implant. They pass completely through the outer edge of the optical portion and join at one point within it (Fig. 8-2). Other manufacturers have the anterior loops attach in four places to the optical portion by passing a short distance into the optic. The anterior loops are 7.5 to 8.0 mm from end to end. This is shorter than the posterior loops, which are 8.5 to 9.0 mm long. The anterior loops are wider than the posterior loops by a small amount. The separation between the anterior and posterior loops is 0.5 to 0.75 mm in order to permit easy passage of the iris between the pairs of loops (Fig. 8-3). All four ends of the posterior loops project from the posterior surface of the optical portion for a short distance perpendicular to the plane of the optical portion and then bend either superiorly or inferiorly at an angle of about 90°. The thickness of the anterior loops is 0.1 mm and the posterior loops 0.2 mm with the Morcher implant.

Other manufacturers use different materials for one or both pairs of loops. One manufacturer uses platinum-iridium wire for both anterior and posterior loops. The anterior loops are cosmetically undesirable, and metal loops add to the weight of the implant. Other manufacturers use nylon anterior loops and metal posterior loops. There is a trend toward substituting titanium for platinum-iridium. Titanium is lighter and more resistant to corrosion, although corrosion has not yet been recognized with intraocular lenses. Though the weight of titanium in air is approximately equivalent to Supramid, it is four times heavier in aqueous. The weight of this implant is important because it is supported entirely by the iris. The weight of most 4-loop implants ranges from 12 to 15 mg in air. One manufacturer's model decreased from 24 to 13 mg when titanium was substituted for platinum-iridium.

Another manufacturer has made an implant with loops entirely of polymethylmethacrylate so that only one material is used. There is no documented long-term experience with this model. Polypropylene loops are now being used. This has the advantage of durability and lightness, the implant weighing 9 mg in air.

The optical portion of all implants consists entirely of polymethylmethacrylate because of its optical properties, as discussed in Chapter 2. Its diameter is 5 mm and its center thickness is about 0.5 mm (slightly greater with some manufacturers). The position of the posterior loop attachments determines the diameter of

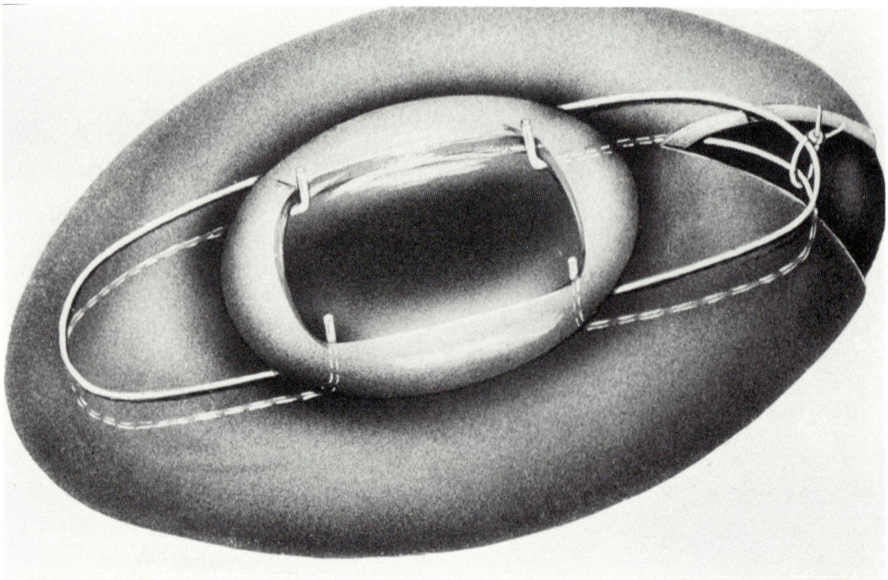

Fig. 8-3. Schema showing relationship of iris to Binkhorst 4-loop iris-clip implant. (From Jaffe, N. S.: Cataract surgery and its complications, ed. 2, St. Louis, 1976, The C. V. Mosby Co.)

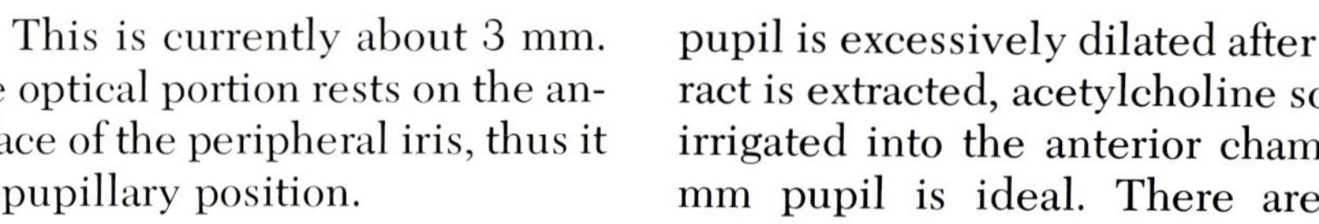

Fig. 8-4. Binkhorst-Jaffe cross-action implantation forceps.

the pupil. This is currently about 3 mm. The entire optical portion rests on the anterior surface of the peripheral iris, thus it is in a prepupillary position.

Surgical technique

The preparation of the implant in the operating room before insertion into the eye differs according to the method of sterilization and packaging used by each manufacturer.

The usual technique of intracapsular cataract extraction is performed with special attention being directed to vitreous and orbital decompression as well as to hemostasis (wet-field coagulator). If the pupil is excessively dilated after the cataract is extracted, acetylcholine solution is irrigated into the anterior chamber. A 4 mm pupil is ideal. There are several satisfactory forceps for holding the 4-loop implant. The most commonly used is that designed by C. D. Binkhorst (Fig. 8-4). It is a cross-action forceps with jaws designed to grasp the optical portion of the implant. It is supplied with a cannula so that the anterior chamber may be irrigated as the implant enters the anterior chamber. This protects against contact with the corneal endothelium and lessens the risk of rupture of the anterior hyaloid membrane. The implant may also be

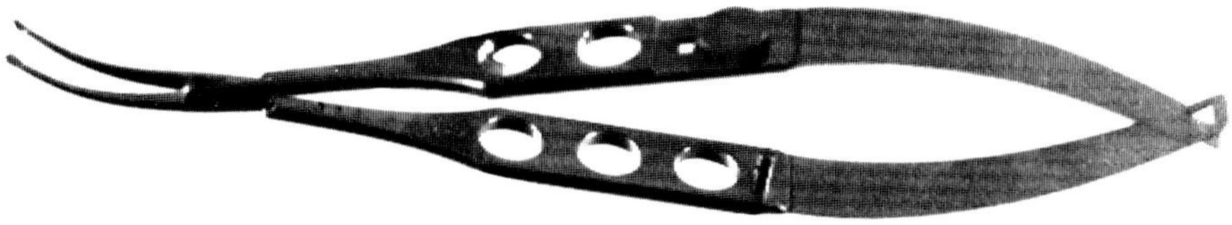

Fig. 8-5. Shepard lens implantation forceps.

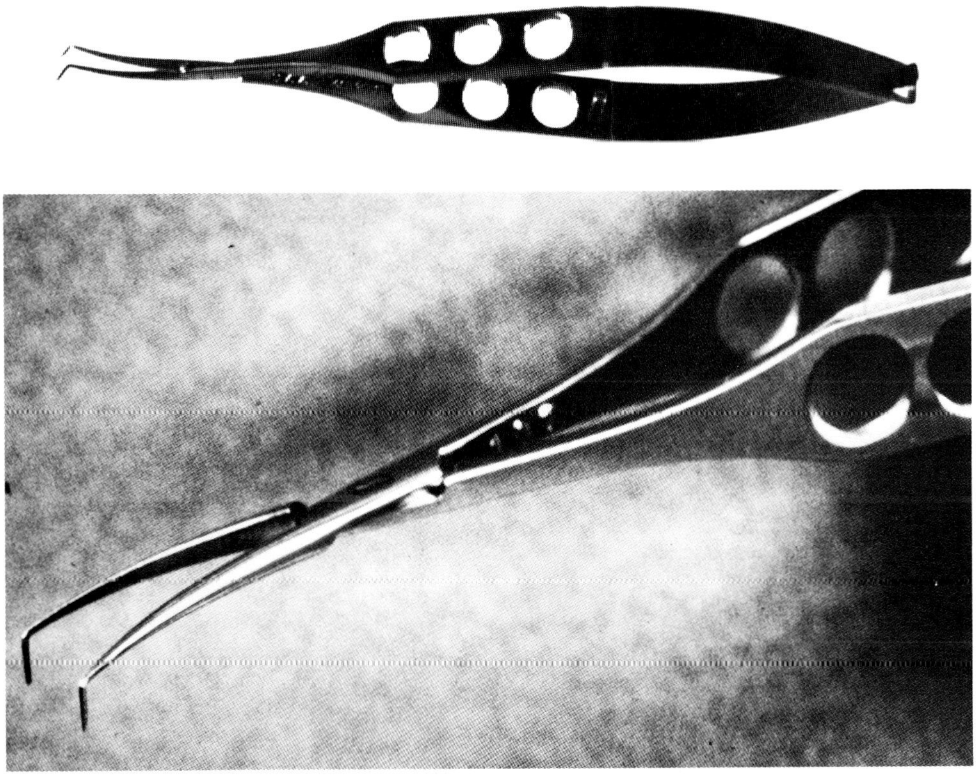

Fig. 8-6. Clayman lens implantation forceps.

grasped by a Shepard forceps (Fig. 8-5), which also may be supplied with a cannula and a lock as well. This forceps grasps the edge of the optical portion of the implant at the 12 o'clock position. A Clayman forceps (Fig. 8-6) grasps the optical portion at the insertion of the right, superior, anterior loop and is useful for one of the techniques described below.

In the classical Binkhorst technique the implant enters the anterior chamber as the cornea is gently lifted. The assistant irrigates balanced salt solution through the cannula portion of the forceps as the cornea resumes its natural position. The pair of inferior loops is threaded onto the iris at 6 o'clock. This is the origin of the name "iris clip" for the 4-loop implant. "Clip" is probably not a good term, but it is understood that the iris fits between the anterior and posterior loops. The implant is released by the cross-action Binkhorst forceps. The forceps are removed from the anterior chamber, leav-

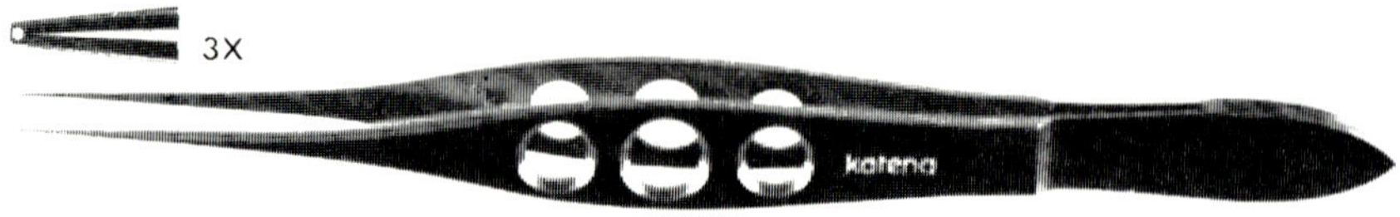

Fig. 8-7. Pierse forceps.

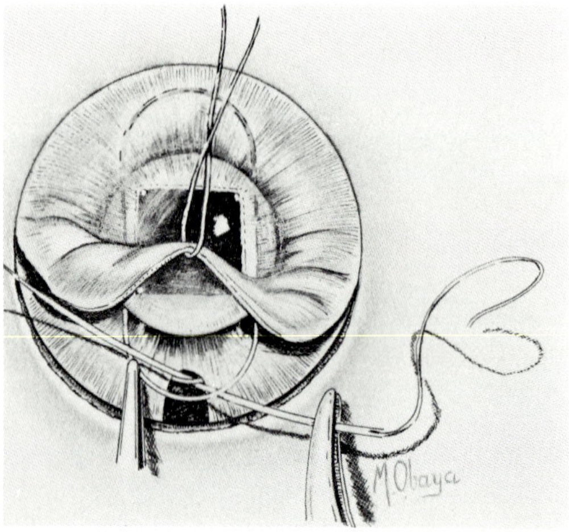

Fig. 8-8. Technique of passing transiridectomy suture. Illustrated is a special order long needle. (Courtesy Ethicon, Inc.)

ing both superior loops anterior to the iris. A dull-tipped iris hook is used to retract the iris sphincter at 12 o'clock and thread it between the superior loops, while the implant is held back with an iris repositor that has been passed between the superior loops. Binkhorst recommends performing the peripheral iridectomy at this point. The iridectomy should extend from the midstromal area to the iris base. It is placed at 12 o'clock so that the posterior loop is visible through the coloboma. It is a matter of choice whether the peripheral iridectomy is performed before the lens extraction or after the implant is in position. With the implant in position, the transiridectomy suture is placed. The anterior loop is lifted slightly with a pair of fine forceps (for example, Hoskins No. 19 or Pierse forceps [Fig. 8-7]) so that the posterior loop is clearly visible in the iris coloboma. A monofilament nylon or polypropylene suture (9-0 or 10-0) swaged on to a special long, blunt, tapered needle (Ethicon, Inc., Somerville, N.J.) is passed through the loops from bottom up (Fig. 8-8). The long length of the needle enables the surgeon to drop it outside the eye on the left side (if the surgeon is right handed). The suture is tied around the two superior loops at 12 o'clock in a manner so as to leave a space between the ends of the superior loops. This permits dilation of the pupil without the implant being updrawn to 12 o'clock. The suture engages no portion of the iris, hence it is called a transiridectomy suture. The wound is then closed in the usual manner.

The following two variations of this technique have been useful and may appeal to some implant surgeons.

Jaffe modification. The Jaffe modification of the Binkhorst technique differs from what has been described above in three important respects. The peripheral iridectomy is performed before the lens extraction. After the lens is clipped onto the iris at 6 o'clock and the implant forceps removed from the eye, a very fine Jaffe spatula (Fig. 8-9) is placed between the two superior loops. The optical part of the implant is displaced toward 6 o'clock. This displacement is often sufficient to have both superior loops pass beyond the iris sphincter at 12 o'clock. By depressing the posterior loop and discontinuing the inferior displacement of the implant, the iris will spontaneously pass between the two superior loops. If the loops cannot be made to clear the iris at 12 o'clock, the iris is gently grasped with Pierse forceps held

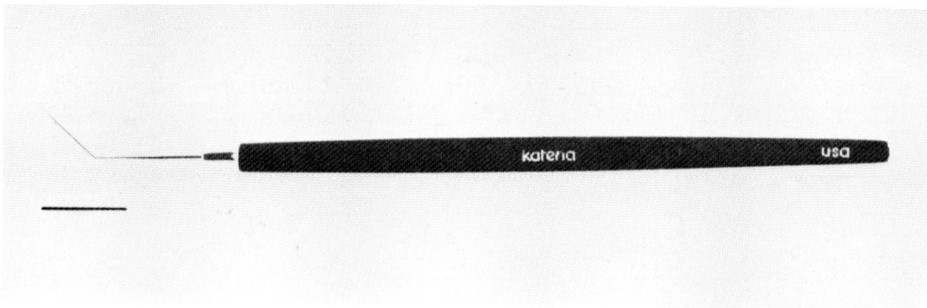

Fig. 8-9. Jaffe lens spatula.

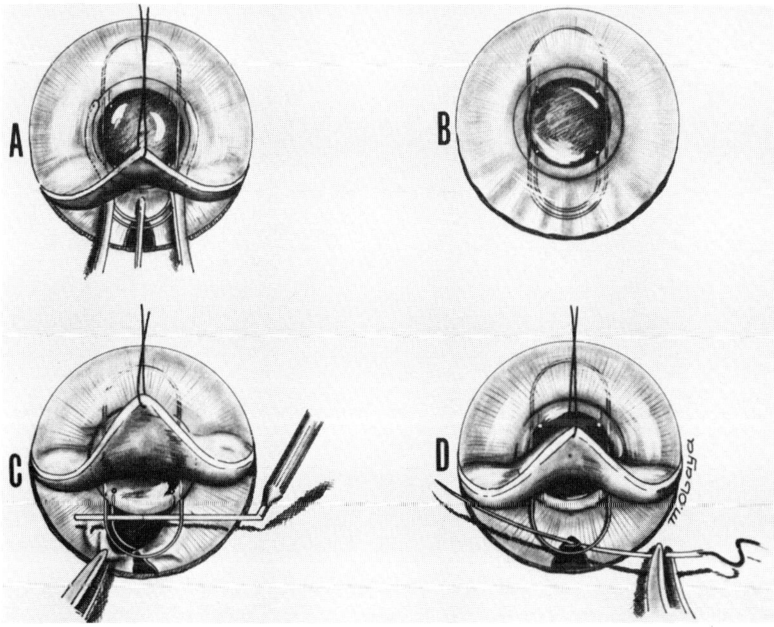

Fig. 8-10. A to **D,** Jaffe technique of Binkhorst 4-loop iris-clip implant insertion. (From Jaffe, N. S.: Cataract surgery and its complications, ed. 2, St. Louis, 1976, The C. V. Mosby Co.)

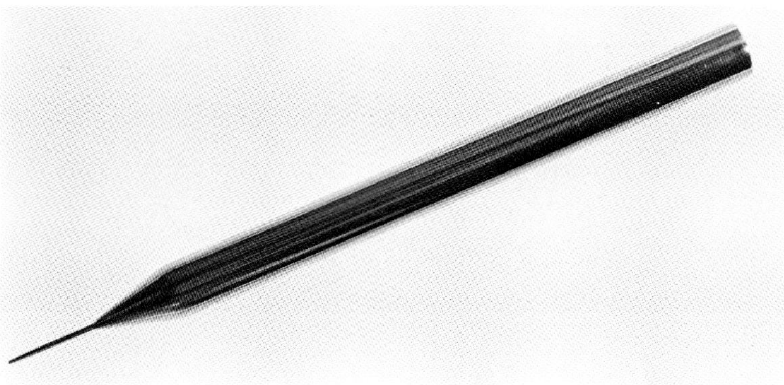

Fig. 8-11. Beauchamp Magnesure.

in the surgeon's other hand and passed between the two loops. An iris hook is not used (Fig. 8-10). The third modification is the placement of the transiridectomy suture. This is performed with the use of the Beauchamp Magnesure (Clinitex, Danvers, Mass.). This is a simple magnet about the size of a ball-point pen. It has a fine, rounded tip (Fig. 8-11). The suture material favored is 10-0 polypropylene (Prolene, Ethicon, Inc., Somerville, N.J.), which, unlike nylon, is a true nonabsorbable material. The needle of the suture is cut, leaving a 2 mm portion attached to the suture. This remaining portion of the needle is held by the assistant with fine

A

B

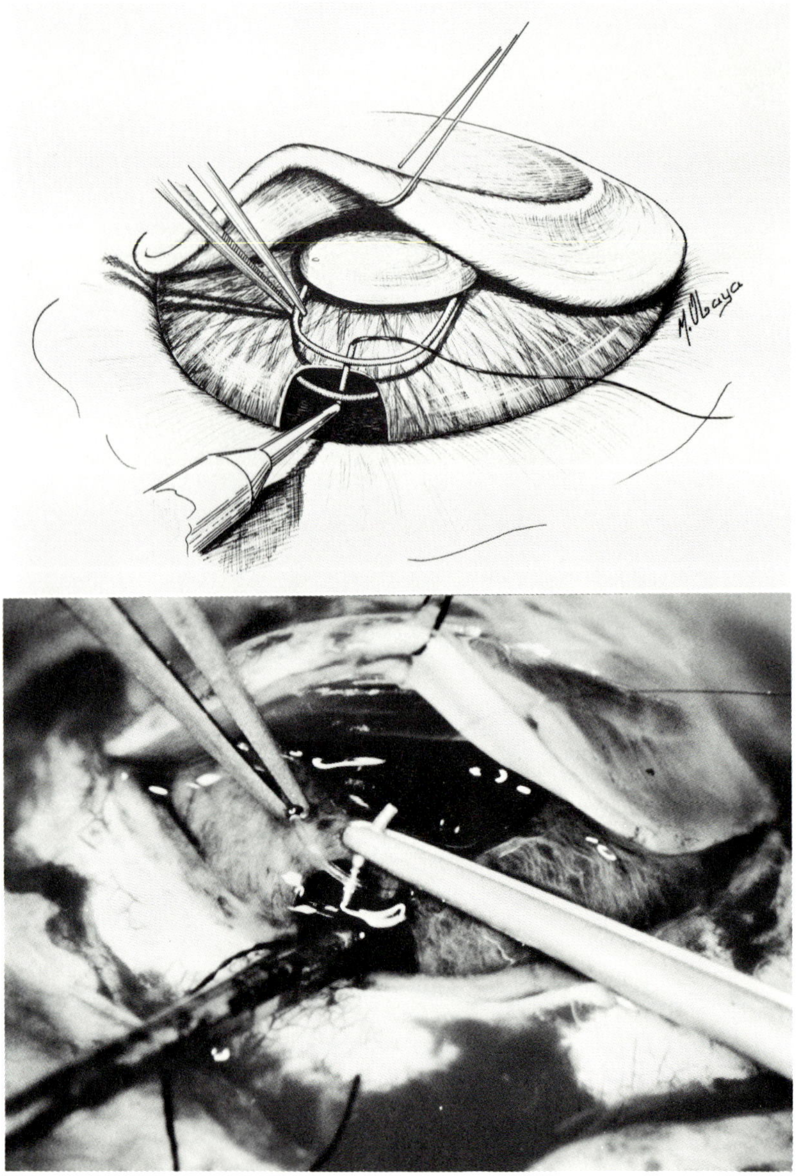

Fig. 8-12. Transiridectomy technique using Beauchamp Magnesure. (**A** from Beauchamp, J. O., Clayman, H. M., and Jaffe, N. S.: Am. J. Ophthalmol. **82**:795, 1976.)

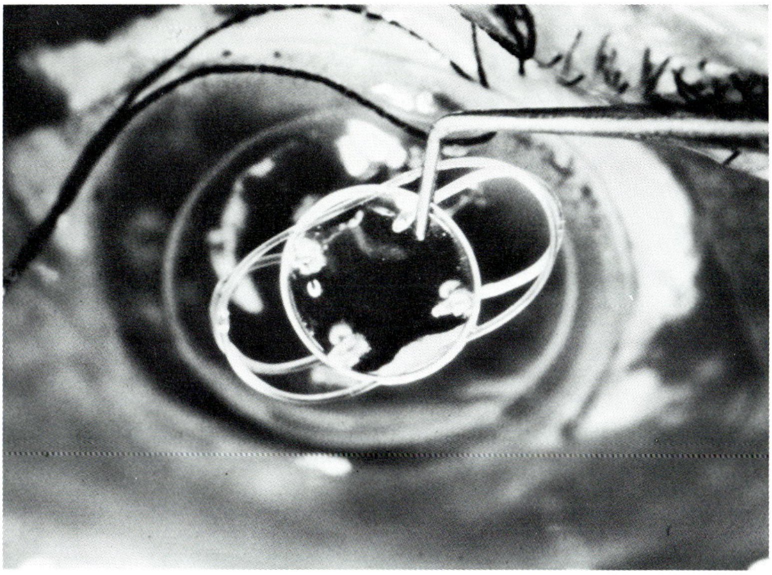

Fig. 8-13. Method of holding implant with Clayman forceps. (From Clayman, H. M.: Trans. Am. Acad. Ophthalmol. Otolaryngol. 83:147-148, 1977.)

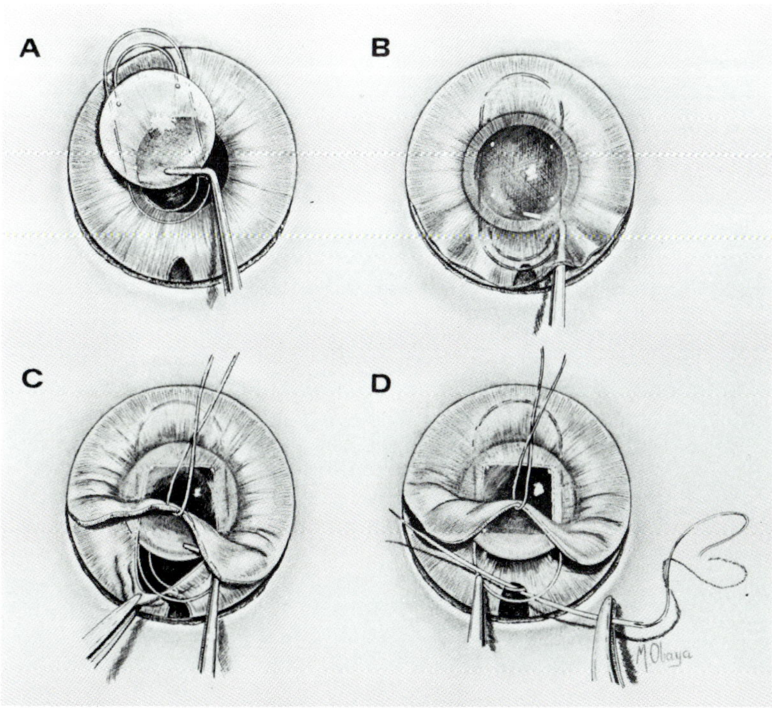

Fig. 8-14. Clayman technique of Binkhorst 4-loop iris-clip implant insertion. **A,** Implant grasped at optic where right arm of superior loop originates. **B,** Implant inserted into anterior chamber with inferior loops straddling iris. **C,** *Still* holding implant, iris is placed between superior loops with forceps. **D,** Transiridectomy suture is passed.

nonmagnetic tissue forceps (Storz, St. Louis, Mo.). The surgeon elevates the superior anterior loop, which makes the posterior loop present through the iridectomy. With the opposite hand he passes the tip of the magnet just behind the posterior loop. The assistant makes contact between the tip of the magnet and the shortened piece of the suture needle through the openings in the loops (Fig. 8-12). When contact is made with the magnet, the assistant releases the shortened needle and the surgeon pulls the suture to one side out of the eye. It is important to pull to one side and not toward 12 o'clock so as to avoid pulling the loops off the iris at 6 o'clock. The suture is tied around the loops in the usual manner and cut at the knot. In this method the suture is passed through the loops from top to bottom, while in the Binkhorst method it is passed from bottom up. This technique has been used successfully in several hundred cases. The main drawback is that the magnet may magnetize instruments in its vicinity. This is easily corrected with an instrument demagnetizer.

Clayman modification. The Clayman modification of the Binkhorst technique is a one-step implantation technique. The implant is grasped by the optic at the insertion of the right, anterior, superior loop using Clayman forceps (Katena Products, Inc., E. Hanover, N.J. [Fig. 8-13]). The lens is inserted into the anterior chamber and clipped onto the inferior iris. While the implant is still being held, the iris is grasped at 1 o'clock with Pierse forceps and placed between the superior haptics (Fig. 8-14). Clayman prefers performing the peripheral iridectomy before the lens extraction. The trans-iridectomy suture is placed with the Beauchamp Magnesure or with a long taper needle (see Fig. 8-8), using 10-0 polypropylene suture material.

When working with the microscope,

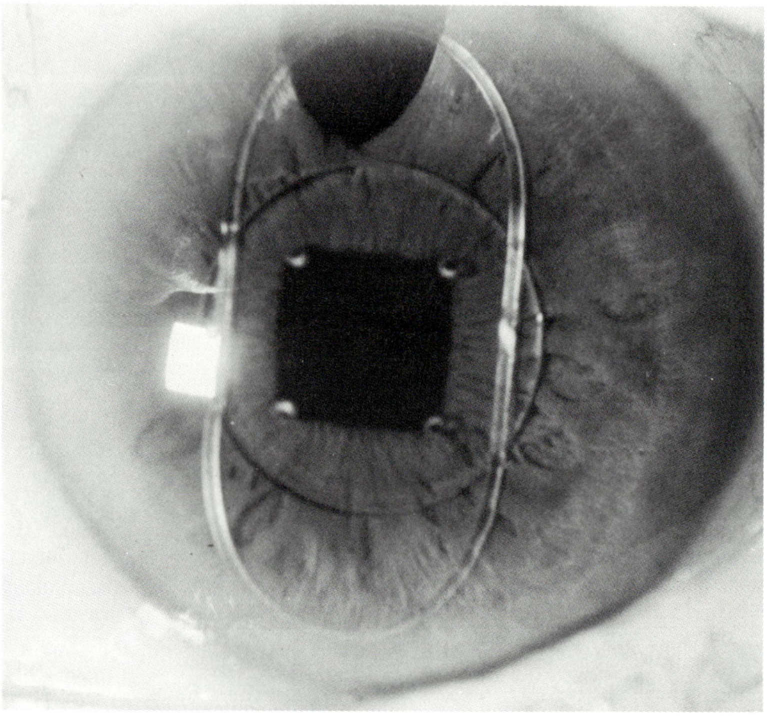

Fig 8-15. Binkhorst 4-loop iris-clip lens implant in situ.

the surgeon may find it more convenient to orient the loops in the 1 to 7 axis, rather than 6 to 12. In this case the peripheral iridectomy is placed at 1 o'clock. The Clayman modification is simple but is more difficult than the Binkhorst and Jaffe methods when there is any vitreous bulge.

Thus the 4-loop Binkhorst implant is oriented in the vertical position, which lessens the possibility of loop contact with the cornea during horizontal ocular movements (Fig. 8-15). The loops are shorter than an earlier model, and a transiridectomy suture is used to lessen the possibility of dislocation. This implant may also be used in conjunction with an extracapsular cataract extraction, since there is less likelihood of dislocation than with the iridocapsular implant.

If the transiridectomy suture is omitted, the only change in the above routine is the placement of the iridectomy openings. Two small peripheral iridectomies or iridotomies are made at 10 and 2 o'clock instead of a large iridectomy at 12 o'clock.

BINKHORST IRIDOCAPSULAR (2-LOOP) LENS IMPLANT

Description

Figure 8-16 is a schema of the Binkhorst iridocapsular lens implant as manufactured by Morcher (p. 74). The implant consists of an optic 5 mm in diameter and 0.5 to 0.6 mm thick. Two loops originate

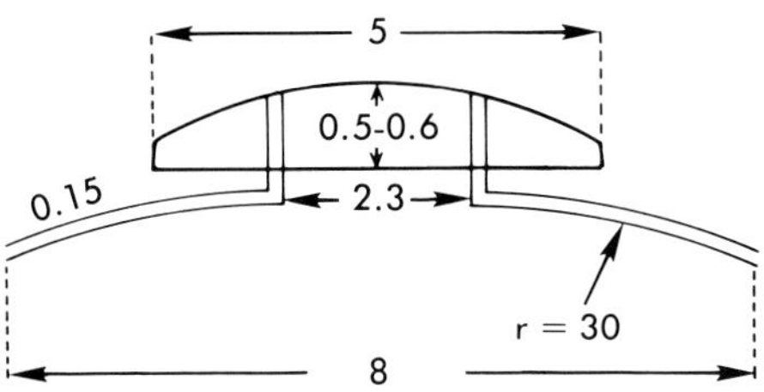

Fig. 8-16. Schema of Binkhorst iridocapsular implant. (From Jaffe, N. S.: Cataract surgery and its complications, ed. 2, St. Louis, 1976, The C. V. Mosby Co.)

from the posterior surface of the implant and are angled posteriorly at about 10° to 15°. The loops are 0.15 mm thick, and their total diameter is 8 mm from tip to tip.

The optic is manufactured of polymethylmethacrylate, and the loops pass vertically into four drill holes in its back surface. As with the Binkhorst iris-clip model, the loop material varies between manufacturers. The lens is available with Supramid (nylon 6), platinum-iridium, titanium, polymethylmethacrylate, and polypropylene loops. The weight varies with the materials used, and assuming equivalent quality, the lighter the implant, the better. The angulation of the loops posteriorly approximates the configuration of the iris contour. The loops are designed to rest posteriorly on the posterior capsule, while the optic is prepupillary. In the model made by Morcher the optic is convexoplano. This may vary with manufacturer; Rayner of England, for example, produces a biconvex lens.

If one considers this implant inserted in an eye in the 6 to 12 o'clock axis (Fig. 8-17), then the horizontal diameter of the implant is that of the optic, namely, 5 mm. The point is that this implant has the potential of being inserted through a small incision of about 6 to 7 mm, an advantage particularly relevant to the automated techniques of extracapsular surgery. The implant should never be inserted after an intracapsular cataract extraction, as the lack of posterior capsule and anterior loops would make the implant especially vulnerable to posterior dislocation.

Surgical technique

The packaging of the lens depends on the manufacturer's sterilizing technique. The implant should be removed from its container, inspected, and washed with balanced saline. The instruments required depend on which technique of extracapsular cataract surgery is used.

In the standard extracapsular cataract extraction technique the anterior capsu-

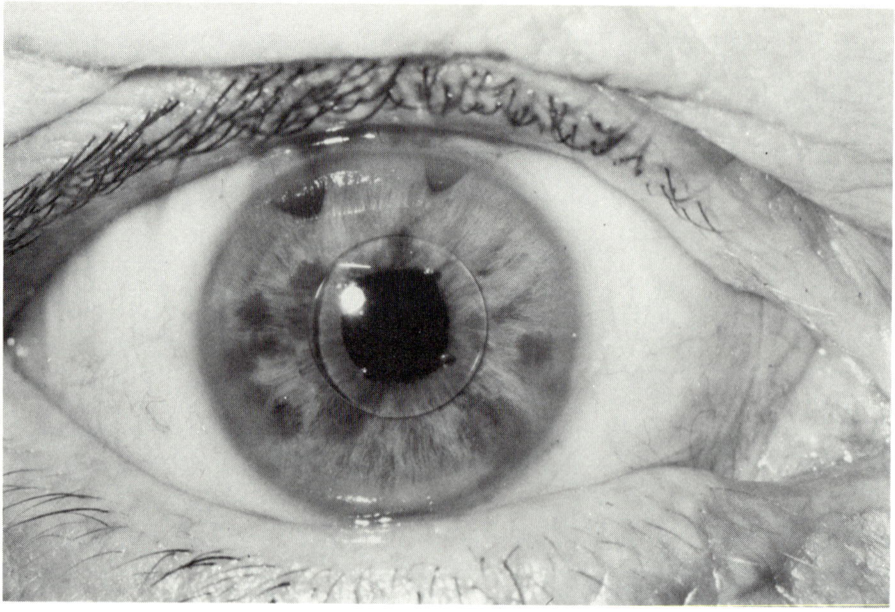

Fig. 8-17. Binkhorst iridocapsular lens implant in situ with posterior loops in vertical position. (From Jaffe, N. S.: Cataract surgery and its complications, ed. 2, St. Louis, 1976, The C. V. Mosby Co.)

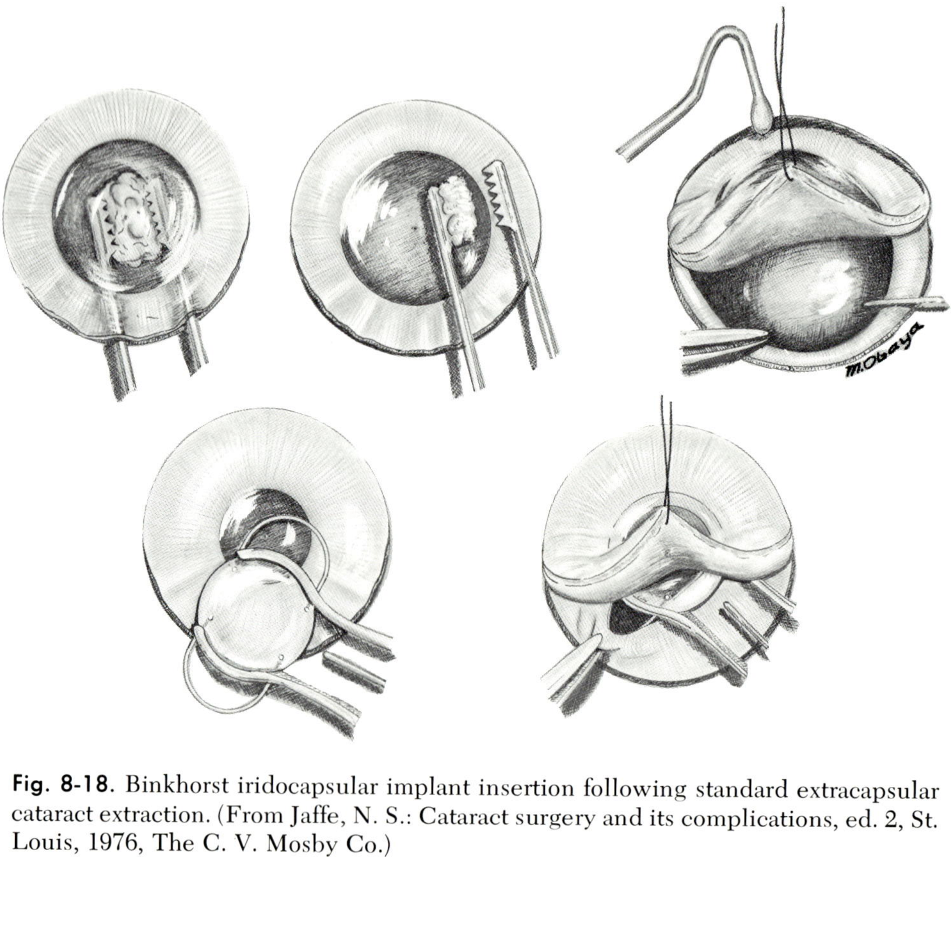

Fig. 8-18. Binkhorst iridocapsular implant insertion following standard extracapsular cataract extraction. (From Jaffe, N. S.: Cataract surgery and its complications, ed. 2, St. Louis, 1976, The C. V. Mosby Co.)

lotomy is performed with toothed capsular forceps such as the Schweiger forceps. The jaws of the forceps should be spread no greater than 6 mm in order to avoid too large a capsulectomy, which might tear the posterior capsule. The nucleus is then expressed and the cortical remnants are irrigated and aspirated. A special curved irrigating cannula can be used for the cortical remnants in the superior cul-de-sac. Usually the pupil will constrict spontaneously after repeated irrigation and aspiration. The implant is then grasped with the cross-action Binkhorst irrigating lens implant forceps and inserted in the vertical or oblique axis with the inferior loop under the lower iris. The implant is released from the forceps, which are then removed from the anterior chamber. A fine spatula is used to steady the implant, and the superior iris is lifted with a fine, dull-tipped hook over the superior loop. Alternately, still holding the implant in the cross-action forceps, the iris is grasped and lifted over the superior loop. The cross-action forceps are then released (Fig. 8-18), and iridectomies are then performed. Topical miotic eyedrops are used for the first 72 hours to center and im-

A

B

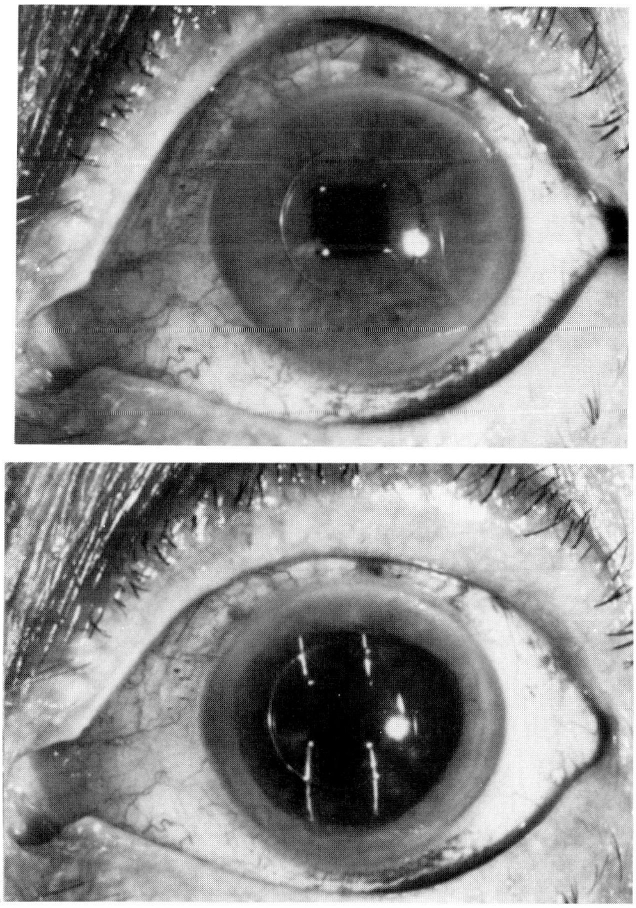

Fig 8-19. Patient 4 days postoperatively. **A,** Undilated pupil. **B,** Same eye dilated, note capsular fixation. (From Jaffe, N. S.: Cataract surgery and its complications, ed. 2, St. Louis, 1976, The C. V. Mosby Co.)

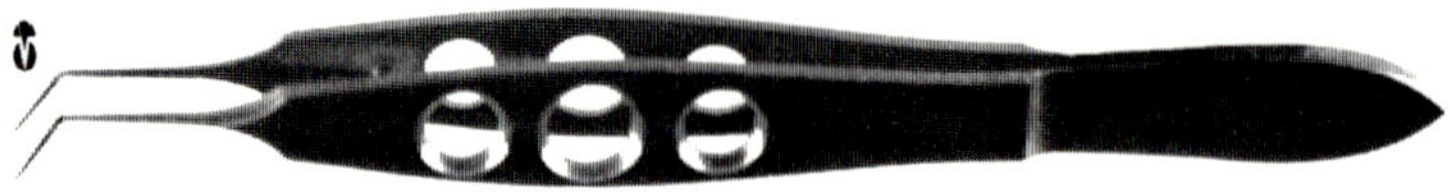

Fig. 8-20. McPherson forceps.

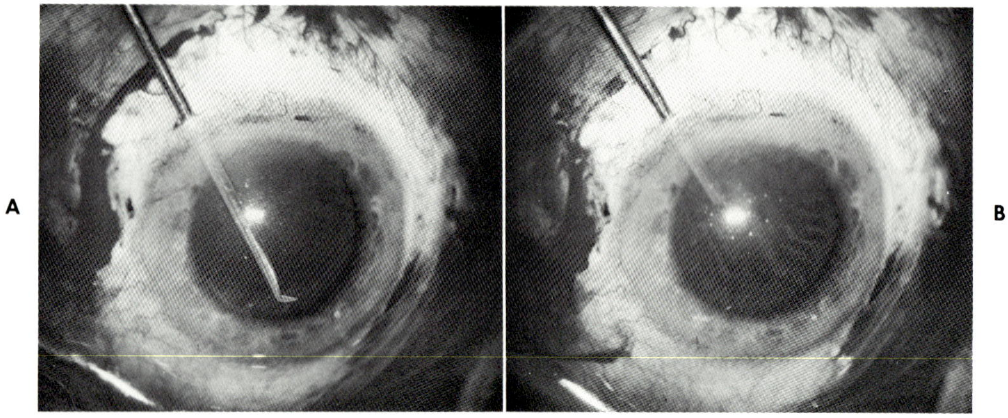

Fig. 8-21. A, Twenty-two-gauge needle with tip bent to form cystotome. **B,** Circular anterior capsulectomy in "can-opener"pattern.

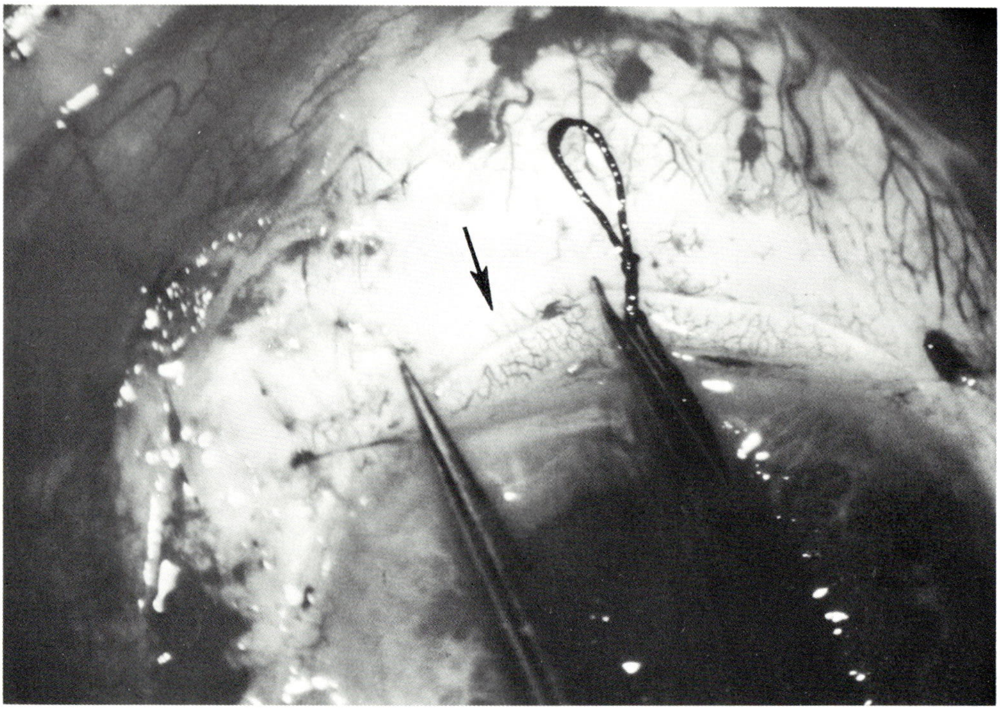

Fig. 8-22. Incision temporarily closed, leaving 3mm opening *(arrow)* for irrigation-aspiration tip.

mobilize the lens, after which mydriatics are used to break iris adhesions. Alternate miosis and mydriasis is continued in the early postoperative period until capsular fixation without iris adhesion is obtained. If capsular fixation has not yet been achieved, the implant will decenter inferiorly with pupillary dilation. Miotic therapy should be continued for several more days before redilating the pupil.

In the classic technique the incision should be large enough to permit expression of the nucleus. The Binkhorst cross-action forceps are difficult to maneuver through a small incision. Accordingly, a 150° (15 to 16 mm) corneal scleral section is advised.

Fig. 8-19 shows a patient 4 days postoperatively undilated and dilated. Note that the pupil dilates widely and symmetrically, revealing a lens implant adherent to the posterior capsule. The central posterior capsule is clear, but cortical remnants are visible in the periphery. We believe capsular fixation to be a function of the capsule rather than a function of the loop material.

Phacoemulsification is described elsewhere (p. 135) but presents a paradox inasmuch as the nucleus is irrigated and aspirated through a 3 mm incision following ultrasonic emulsification, the incision then being enlarged to 6 to 7 mm to permit insertion of the Binkhorst iridocapsular lens implant. Small incision insertion requires special instrumentation such as the McPherson forceps (Fig. 8-20), a fine iris hook, and a lens glide (p. 168).

A transitional technique between the

A

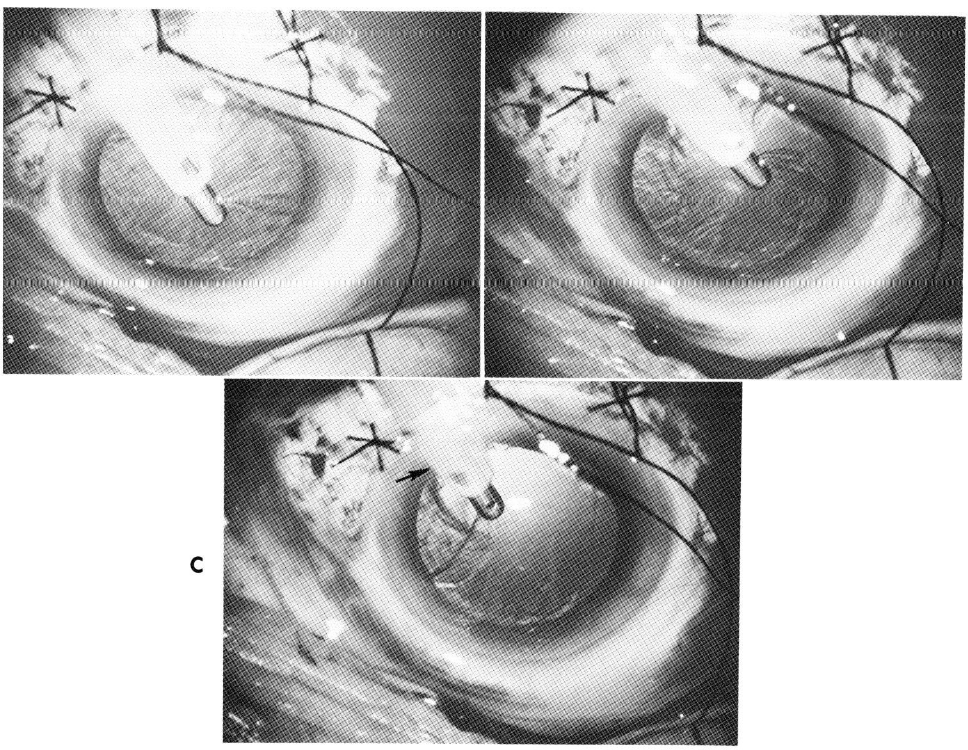

B

C

Fig. 8-23. Irrigation-aspiration of cortical remnants. **A,** Cortex drawn into aspirating device. **B,** Clear posterior capsule visible as cortex aspirated. **C,** Note cortex being drawn into aspirating aperture. Anterior chamber is kept formed by irrigation through plastic sleeve on tip *(arrow)*.

classic extracapsular extraction and phacoemulsification is possible with a number of currently available irrigation and aspiration devices. The Cavitron 800 is an example. This machine has gravity irrigation and aspiration from a positive flow pump. A Kelman cystotome or a 22-gauge needle with a bent tip is connected to the irrigation line. A 3 mm incision is made in the surgical limbus at the 11 o'clock position, and the cystotome is introduced through the opening (Fig. 8-21). An anterior capsulotomy is performed. The incision is opened to 150°, and the nucleus is expressed. The wound is now temporarily closed, leaving a 3 mm opening through which the irrigation-aspiration tip is introduced (Fig. 8-22). Cortical remnants are now aspirated with concomitant irrigation keeping the anterior chamber formed (Fig. 8-23). The irrigation line also fits onto an instrument for cleaning the posterior capsule (for example, Kratz scratcher [Fig. 8-24]). The wound is then opened wide enough to permit the insertion of the lens implant in either the classical or small incision techniques.

There is no unanimity on the management of the posterior capsule. Some surgeons believe that a capsulotomy should not be performed as part of the primary procedure. They feel that the opening in the posterior capsule is unpredictable and are unwilling to accept the anterior hyaloid as support for a lens without anterior loops to prevent posterior dislocation. Other surgeons point to the high incidence of secondary membranes following extracapsular surgery and routinely do a posterior capsulotomy in the belief that they are obviating a later subsequent procedure.

There are cases of failure of capsular fixation and also rupture of the capsule with subsequent dislocation of the lens. Posterior dislocation into the vitreous cavity is a serious complication. Some

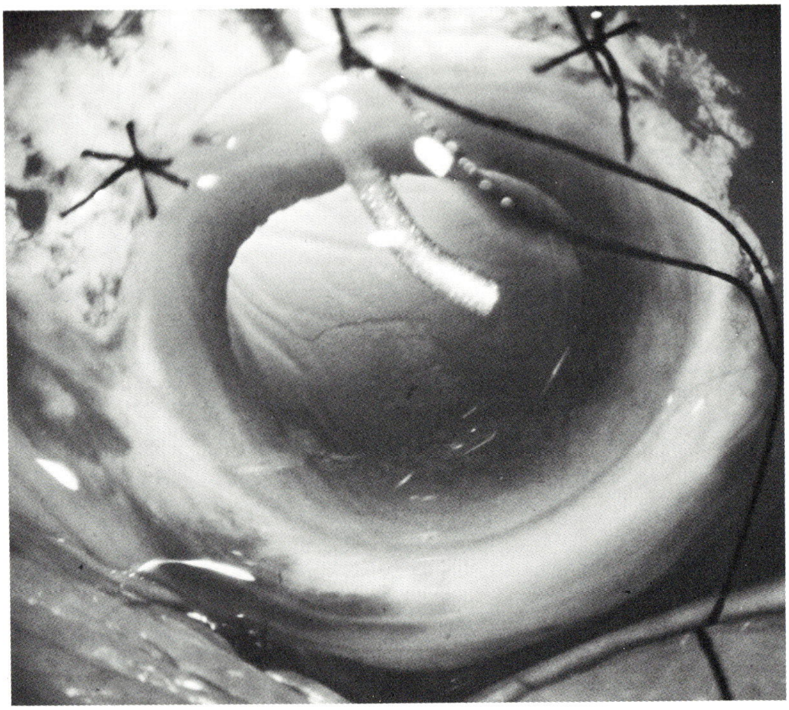

Fig. 8-24. Kratz scratcher used to clean posterior capsule.

surgeons minimize the incidence of dislocation by placing a suture through the iris stroma or iridectomy, then through the superior loop of the implant and out through the adjacent iris stroma, where the suture is tied and trimmed. The net effect is to suspend the superior haptic from the back surface of the iris in the event of inadequate fixation. This probably is a prudent maneuver, which is technically feasible even through small incisions. An alternative method is the use of a 4-loop Binkhorst (iris-clip) implant with an extracapsular extraction without a fixation suture.

FYODOROV SPUTNIK LENS IMPLANT

Description

The current Fyodorov sputnik lens implant evolved from a 4-loop model (p. 42) through a transitional 2-loop 3-strut design to the current lens (Fig. 8-25). This

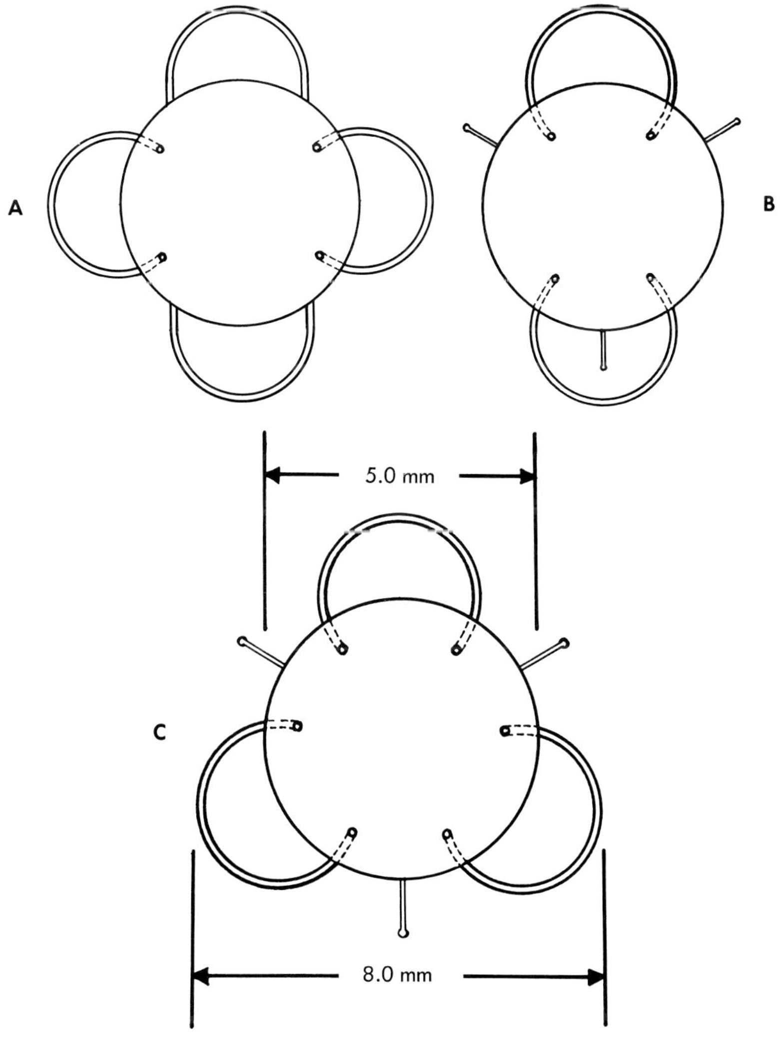

Fig. 8-25. Schemas showing transition from Fyodorov-Binkhorst 4-loop lens to Fyodorov sputnik, 3-strut, 3-loop lens. **A,** Fyodorov-Binkhorst lens. **B,** Transitional Fyodorov 3-strut, 2-loop sputnik lens. **C,** Current Fyodorov 3-strut, 3-loop sputnik lens.

lens has three posterior loops and three anterior struts. The total loop diameter is 8 mm. Its polymethylmethacrylate optical section is 5 mm in diameter with a center thickness of 0.32 mm and edge thickness of 0.15 mm. The nylon loops are 0.12 mm in diameter, and the implant weighs 7.5 mg in air and 0.6 mg in aqueous. As of this writing the Fyodorov sputnik lens of Russian manufacture is unique in having its power in aqueous engraved on its surface by hand prior to sterilization. The Russian lenses are sterilized by the Frederick Ridley caustic soda method (p. 71); the lenses are also manufactured elsewhere, and sterilization techniques vary.

Surgical technique

It is possible, particularly in elderly patients with a concave iris diaphragm, after intracapsular cataract extraction to implant this lens by an open-sky method. These maneuvers are possible as well after an extracapsular extraction but are more difficult if the object of the maneuver is to place the lens in the capsular bag (Fig. 8-26). The lens, however, is used for both types of cataract extraction.

For the open-sky method the lens is best held with an edge holder (Fig. 8-27) between two struts. One loop, usually the inferior one, is inserted beneath the iris and the lens moved horizontally medially and laterally until the remaining two loops pop into place. This type of maneuver requires at least a 6 mm pupil and is more readily performed with an even more dilated pupil. The open-sky method may be carried out using a forceps that grasps the optical portion of the lens as well, but the subsequent maneuvers are slightly more difficult to perform than with an edge holder. If a non-edge holder is employed, it should not be at right angles to the lens, as the surgeon will block his own microscope view with his hand.

In a flat to mildly convex iris diaphragm or in extracapsular extractions it is wisest to position the lens in its final appropriate iris relationships using closed eye maneuvers. The lens is held either centrally or at its edge, and the inferior loop is positioned behind the iris. All preplaced sutures are drawn tight, and the wound is made watertight with additional sutures if necessary. It is essential to avoid lens

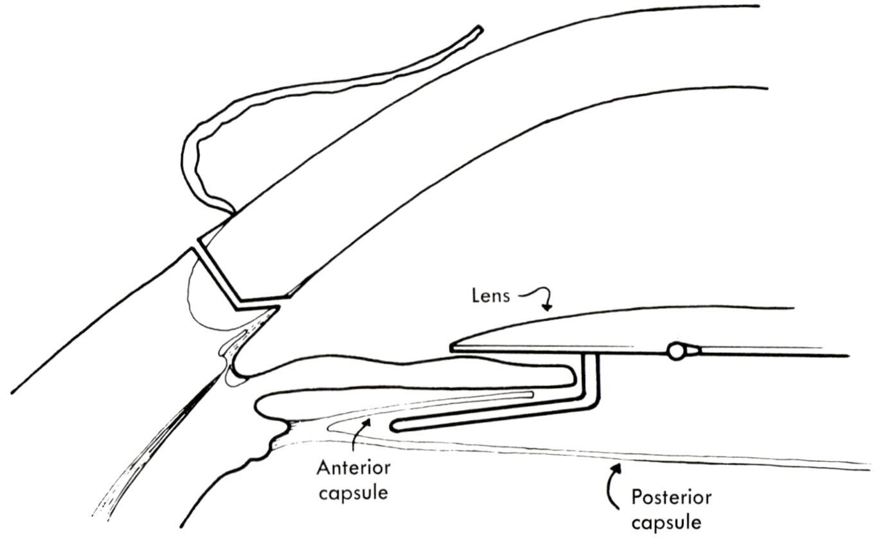

Fig. 8-26. Schema of posterior loop of Fyodorov sputnik lens in capsular bag after extracapsular extraction.

endothelial touch during insertion or subsequent maneuvers. The former may strip Descemet's membrane, and both may reduce the endothelial population to critical survival population densities. The use of preplaced sutures helps reduce this potential by eliminating corneal manipulation once the cataract is out and the implant in. The increased annoyance of suture loops potentially being caught on the implant while it is being inserted or on instruments is easily preventable and will more than justify the time necessary to convert to preplaced sutures for those physicians unfamiliar with them.

The watertight chamber should be deepened with fluid or air; fluid more readily leaks out, but air more readily obscures the surgeon's view. The lens, which is far from the cornea, is now slid into position in a variety of ways, all depending on pupillary size. A widely dilated pupil should always be avoided and never pharmacologically created. A 5 to 6 mm pupil is ideal. A thin spatula is particularly suitable for these maneuvers. This instrument, 0.5 mm in diameter, is introduced into the closed chamber and slid anterior to one malpositioned loop until it abuts on the vertical component of the posterior loop. The lens is then slid away from the pupil until the iris just covers the loop, and the lens literally

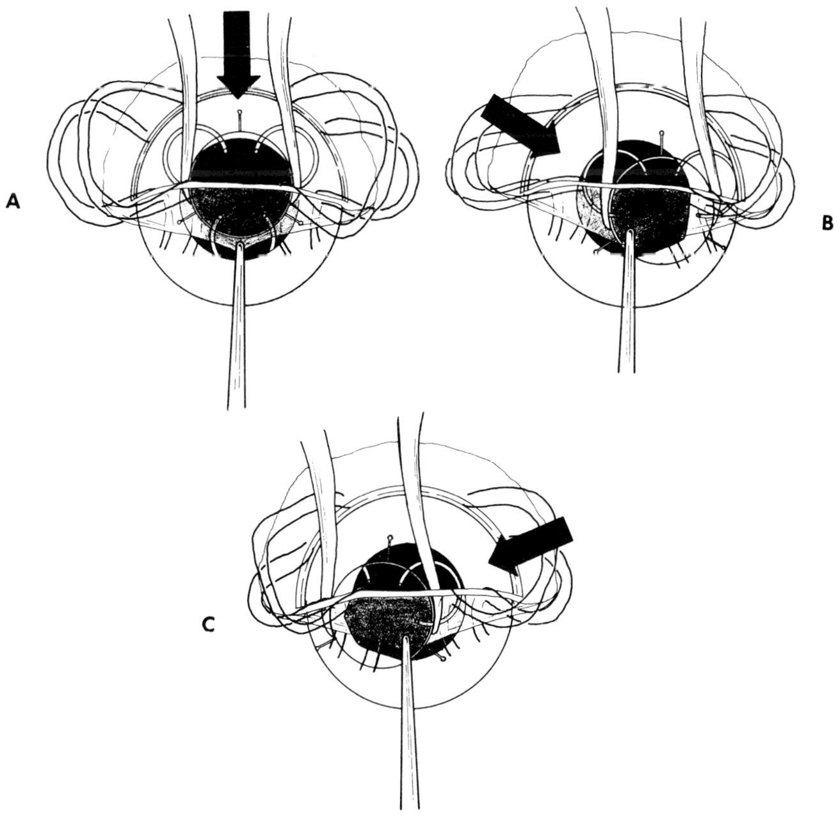

Fig. 8-27. Technique of Fyodorov sputnik lens insertion using open-sky method. **A,** Implant is held with special forceps. Straight forceps below retracts cornea. Inferior loop is inserted under iris. **B,** Right loop is passed under iris. **C,** Left loop is passed under iris.

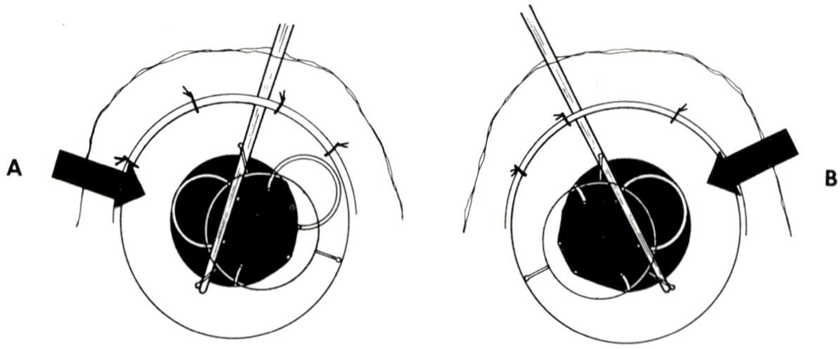

Fig. 8-28. Closed-eye technique of Fyodorov sputnik lens insertion. Fine spatula is inserted through incision to position horizontal loops behind iris.

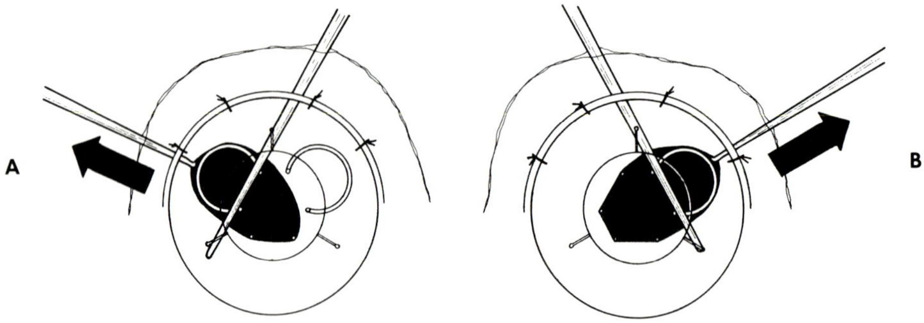

Fig. 8-29. Closed-eye technique of Fyodorov sputnik lens insertion with small pupil. Fine hook is used in conjunction with spatula.

pops into position. As the lens moves from side to side against the pupil, a chord of sphincter is formed (Fig. 8-28). This is always a pleasant sight and acknowledges that the loops are being positioned appropriately. Once the third loop is correctly positioned, the pupil will assume a hexagonal shape.

For pupils approximately 4 mm in size it is often necessary to employ a small, blunt hook like a shepherd's crook as well as the spatula (Fig. 8-29). The hook should first be tried in the iris stroma to attempt to pull the iris to one side as the lens is slid toward the other side with the spatula. This will usually create an oblique pupillary opening sufficient to permit the loop to pop into position. If the pupil is quite small, it is necessary to grasp the iris sphincter with the crook of the hook and lift the iris over the pos-

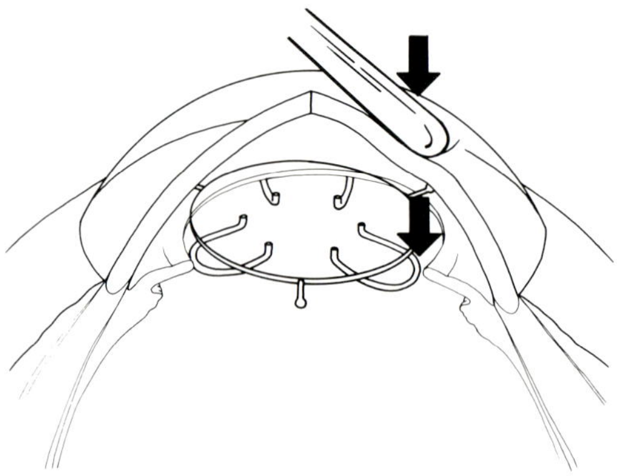

Fig. 8-30. Insertion of Fyodorov sputnik lens implant under air bubble, using closed-eye technique with convex hyaloid face.

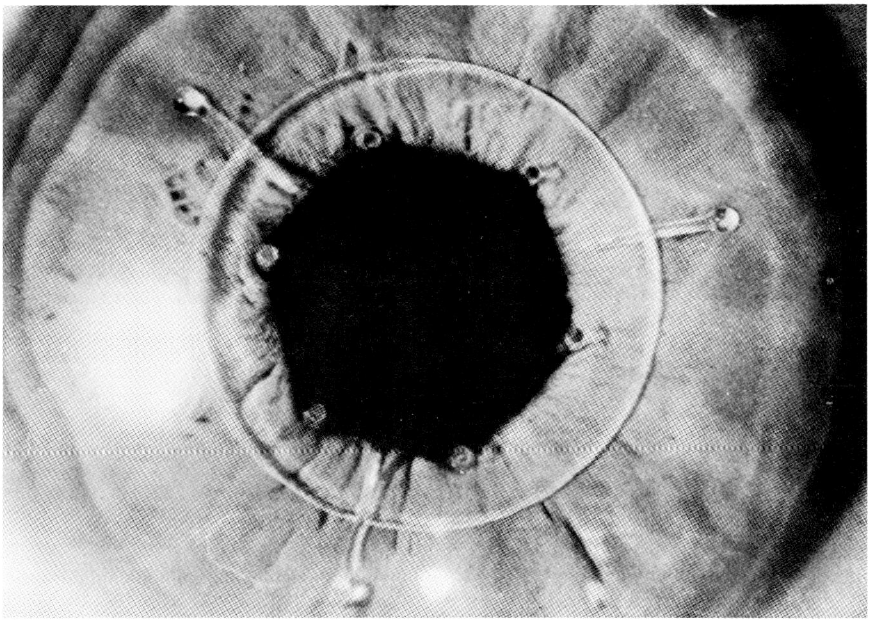

Fig. 8-31. Fyodorov sputnik lens in situ.

terior loop as the lens is again moved away from the direction of the hook with a spatula. Such hooking maneuvers are difficult and may catch the vitreous face, as may any movement of the lens loops unless the loops are floated into position in the closed eye with slow, deliberate, gentle movements.

If the iris diaphragm is moderately to severely convex after the cataract has been extracted, one must consider the wisdom of lens insertion if steps cannot be taken to overcome the virtual assurance of vitreous face rupture during lens placement and manipulation. If it is possible to place the lens into the anterior chamber and the pupil is 6 to 7 mm in size, one may minimize the potential for vitreous extrusion in such circumstances by not placing any loops behind the iris at the time of lens placement. The wound should be sealed and the chamber formed. Fig. 8-30 demonstrates the maneuvers that now permit lens loop placement without entering the eye. Pressing on the corneal surface of a watertight chamber, particularly if a large air bubble is present, will compress the chamber content and push the lens posteriorly. Often one or more loops will pop behind the iris while not touching the endothelium. Remaining loops are then positioned using the spatula and hook. Fig. 8-31 shows a sputnik lens in position for approximately 10 years.

There is nothing unique about the complications encountered with this lens when compared to other iris-clip lenses. The sphincter is impinged upon by the back loops at six points, so there are potentially more points for eccentric synechia formation and, in theory, more potential for dislocation with dilatation. This theoretical more than real potential is overcome by the fact that this lens has six areas of stabilizing support, making it probably the most stable of pupillary implants and the one with the least phakodonesis. Further, single loop or strut malpositions rarely need repair and should best be left alone (Fig. 8-32).

Secondary membrane formation may be a problem if miotics are utilized in the immediate postoperative period, particu-

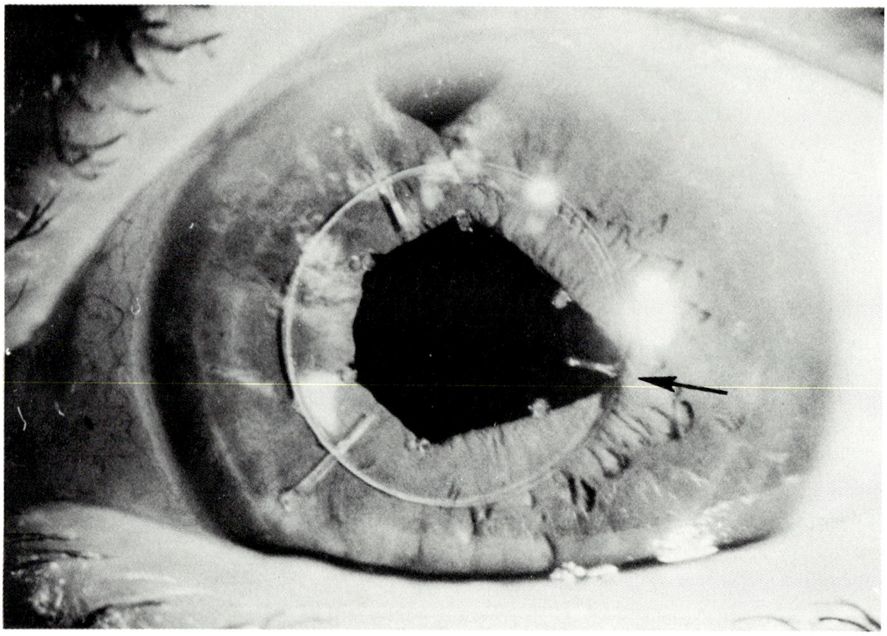

Fig. 8-32. Fyodorov sputnik lens with anterior strut posterior to iris *(arrow)*.

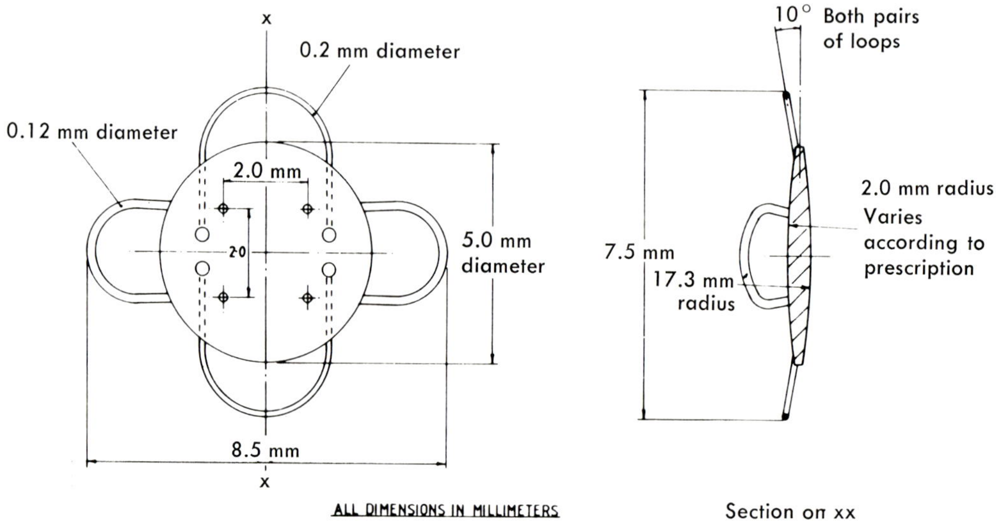

Fig. 8-33. Schema of Fyodorov-Binkhorst lens implant.

larly after extracapsular cataract extraction. After capsular fixation is achieved, prompt dilatation and steroids are essential. Mild dilating drops and steroids or steroids alone should be used after intracapsular extraction.

FYODOROV-BINKHORST LENS IMPLANT

Description

As with most implants, there are differences in design between manufacturers. Fig. 8-33 is Rayner's* model. There is a biconvex optic of polymethylmethacrylate 5 mm in diameter. The center optic thickness is approximately 0.66 mm, but this varies with dioptric power of the implant. Four nylon haptics originate from the optic, and each is angled posteriorly 10°. The anterior haptics are 0.12 mm in diameter and extend out from the plane of the optic. The total diameter from the tip of one anterior haptic to the other is 7.5 mm. The posterior haptics are 0.2 mm in diameter and arise from the back surface of the optic 0.50 to 0.75 mm posterior to the plane of the anterior loops. This is to avoid convolutions of the iris over the posterior haptics when the lens is in situ. Total diameter of the posterior haptics is 8 mm. The implant weighs 14.3 mg in air.

The implant has undergone some evolution. At various times the posterior haptics have been colored black or blue. This greatly helped identification of the haptics at surgery, but there were reports that the color leached out, and the loops were observed to become progressively paler. Currently Rayner manufactures this lens with all clear loops.

Surgical technique

This lens can be used following an intracapsular or extracapsular cataract extraction; the technique of insertion is

*Rayner & Keeler, Ltd., Chorleywood, Herts., England.

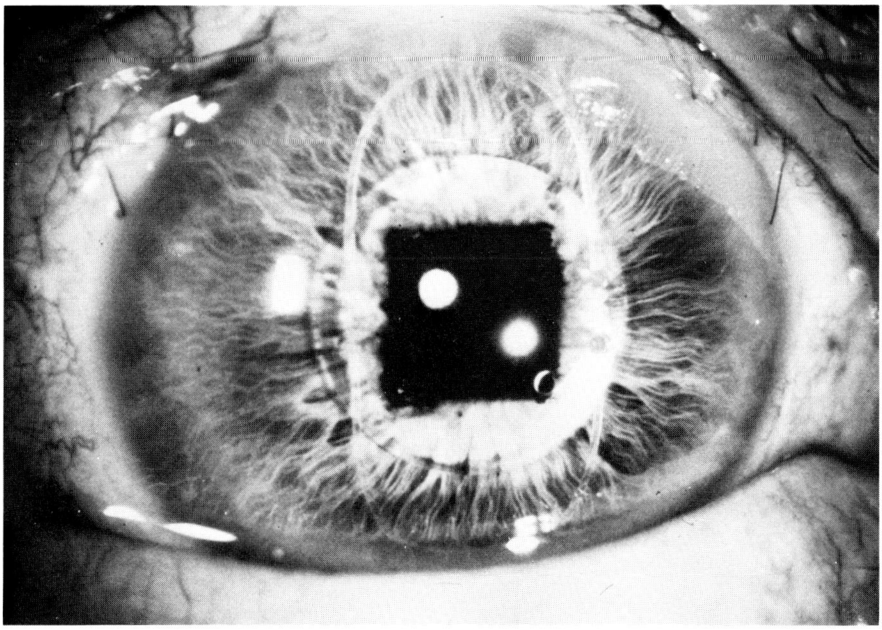

Fig. 8-34. Fyodorov-Binkhorst lens implant in situ with horizontal haptics posterior to iris. (From Jaffe, N. S.: Cataract surgery and its complications, ed. 2, St. Louis, 1976, The C. V. Mosby Co.)

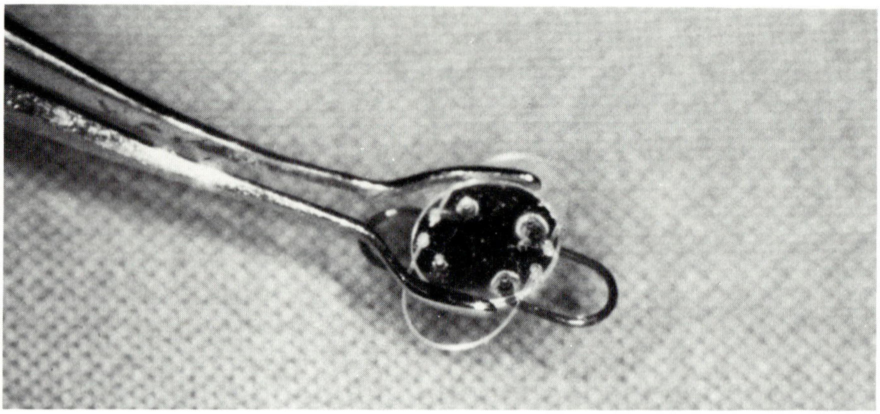

Fig. 8-35. Fyodorov-Binkhorst lens implant grasped with Binkhorst cross-action forceps. (From Jaffe, N. S.: Cataract surgery and its complications, ed. 2, St. Louis, 1976, The C. V. Mosby Co.)

the same. The implant's minimum horizontal diameter is that of the anterior haptics, namely 7.5 mm. Allowing for the thickness of the optic and clearance of haptics, it is improbable that the implant can be inserted through an incision smaller than 9 to 10 mm. As such, this implant does not lend itself to "mini-incision" techniques.

The lens can be inserted with the posterior haptics in a vertical position behind the iris, or conversely horizontally posterior to the iris (Fig. 8-34). There is no apparent optical advantage between these alternatives, but rather it is a matter of individual preference. In the first method the implant is grasped with the Binkhorst cross-action forceps (Fig. 8-35) so that the posterior inferior haptic may be slid under the iris at 6 o'clock. After this maneuver the cross-action forceps are released and withdrawn from the eye. The implant is steadied with a spatula held against the superior portion of the optic, while the superior iris is grasped with forceps and lifted over the posterior superior haptic. The implant is now in position. Alternately the implant can be grasped by the Binkhorst forceps with the posterior haptics in a horizontal plane. The right posterior haptic is inserted behind the iris at 9 o'clock. While one is still grasping the implant, the right lateral movement is continued until the left lateral posterior haptic clears the pupillary margin and the implant is moved to the left so that the left haptic falls behind the iris at 3 o'clock. The forceps are now released and the implant is in position. The implant can be inserted with other forceps, but the basic techniques are similar. An intracameral suture may be used to fixate the superior haptic to the superior iris, but is not essential.

The Fyodorov-Binkhorst implant is relatively easy to insert, yet the lens has not found wide popularity in the United States.

COPELAND LENS IMPLANT

Description

The Copeland lens is of one-piece design and made entirely of polymethylmethacrylate (Fig. 8-36). It is a modification of the earlier Epstein lens (Fig. 8-37) but lacks the fenestrations. The total diameter of the lens is 9 mm, comprising an optic zone of 4 mm and two haptics each 2.5 mm in length and 2.5 mm wide. The thickness is 0.14 mm at the haptics and 0.40 mm at the center of the optical portion (Fig. 8-38). The implant weighs

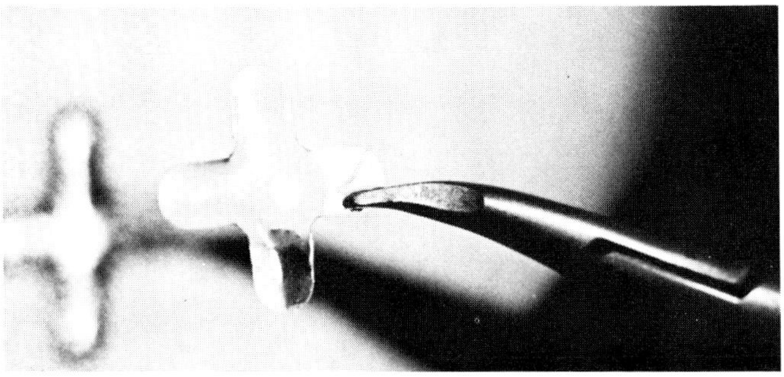

Fig. 8-36. Copeland lens implant. (From Jaffe, N. S.: Cataract surgery and its complications, ed. 2, St. Louis, 1976, The C. V. Mosby Co.)

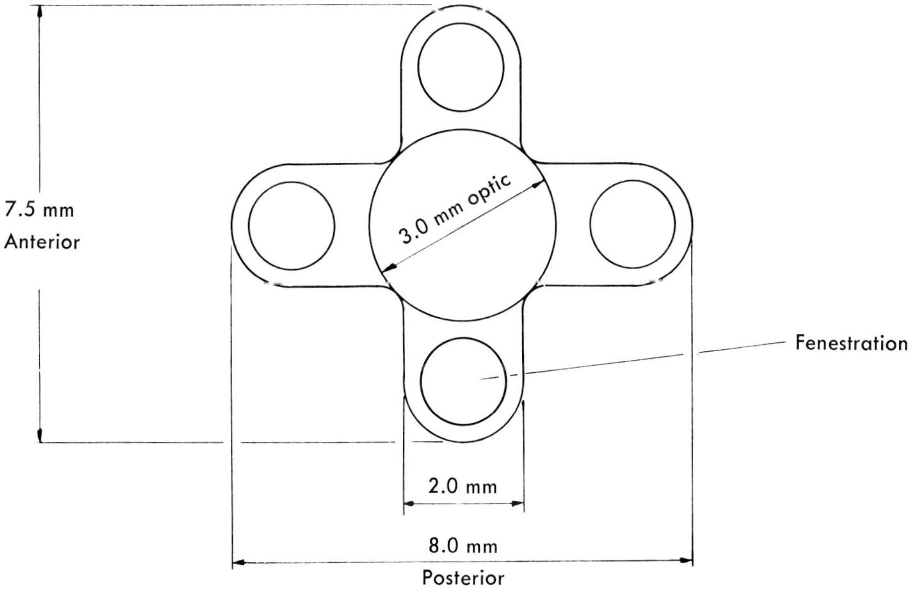

Fig. 8-37. Schema of Epstein lens implant.

7.2 mg in air. Copeland* will manufacture, on special order, a lens of 8 mm total diameter and can also supply thinner and narrower haptics. The lens was sterilized by the Ridley method and supplied in a single sterile vial of 0.5% sodium bicarbonate solution, but is now available in a dry sterile pack. Similar lenses from other manufacturers vary slightly in design and sterilization techniques. Though the optical portion of the Copeland lens implant protrudes slightly from the anterior surface of the implant, the implant is classified as iris-plane. This is in contradistinction to the Worst and Binkhorst implants in which the optic is clearly prepupillary. The Copeland lens has no loops and requires no iris suture, therefore the implant is relatively easy to insert.

*Copeland Intralenses, Inc., 129 E. 61st Street, New York, N.Y. 10021

Surgical technique with an intracapsular extraction

The implant is removed from its pack and irrigated with balanced salt solution.

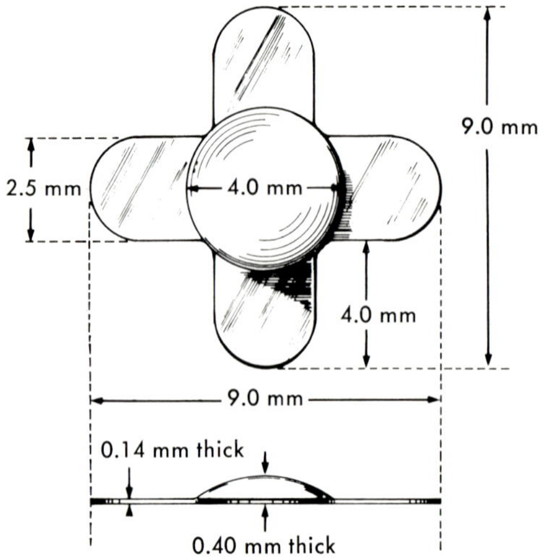

Fig. 8-38. Schema of Copeland lens implant.

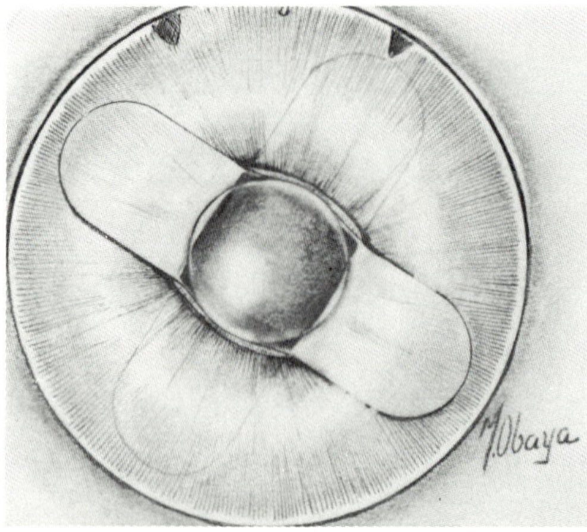

Fig. 8-40. Implant in situ in oblique axis (7-0 suture tied).

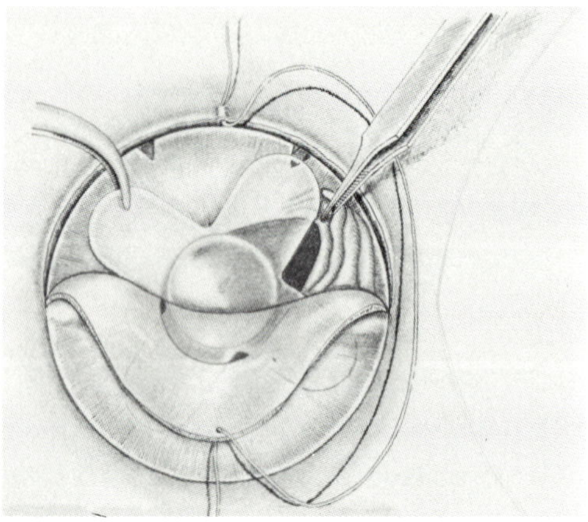

Fig. 8-39. Insertion of Copeland lens implant. Inferior arm is placed under iris at 7 o'clock. Grasp iris at 1 o'clock and pull over superior arm.

After an intracapsular cataract extraction the lens is inserted slightly obliquely. A right-handed surgeon would place the lens in the 1 to 7 o'clock axis through an adequate incision. The peripheral iridotomies or iridectomies are ideally 60° apart. Since the haptics of the implant are at a 90° angle, if the angle of the peripheral iridotomies coincided, it would be theoretically possible for both iridotomies to be obstructed by the implant, with an increased possibility of pupillary block. This is the rationale for suggesting 60°. After cataract extraction, acetylcholine (Miochol) or carbocholine (Miostat) is instilled into the anterior chamber to reconstrict the pupil. This important step is performed prior to implant insertion. The right, lateral haptic of the implant is grasped, and the inferior haptic is slid under the iris at 7 o'clock. Still holding the right haptic with the right hand, forceps held in the left hand grasp the iris at 1 o'clock and lift it over the superior haptic (Fig. 8-39). The implant is now in position (Fig. 8-40).

The lens does not have to be inserted obliquely. Lenses inserted horizontally and vertically are shown in Figs. 8-41 and 8-42, respectively. When the lens is inserted with the horizontal haptics posterior to the iris, the implant is grasped by the superior haptic. An intensely miotic pupil makes the insertion difficult, and a 4 to 5 mm pupillary diameter is ideal for this maneuver. The implant is inserted into the anterior chamber, and the right haptic is slid under the iris at 9 o'clock. The implant is further displaced to the right until the left haptic clears the pupillary margin, at which point the left haptic is slid under the iris at 3 o'clock.

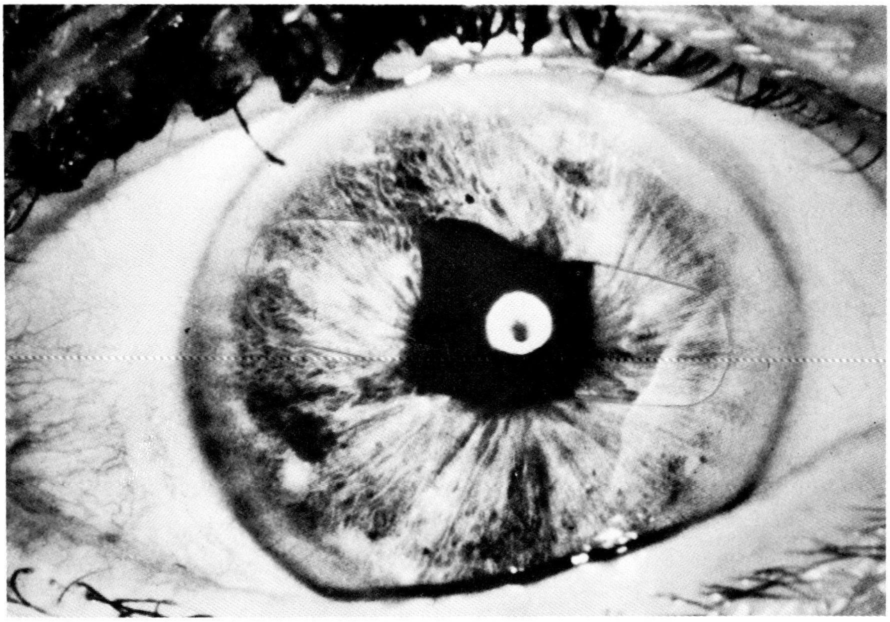

Fig. 8-41. Implant in situ in horizontal axis.

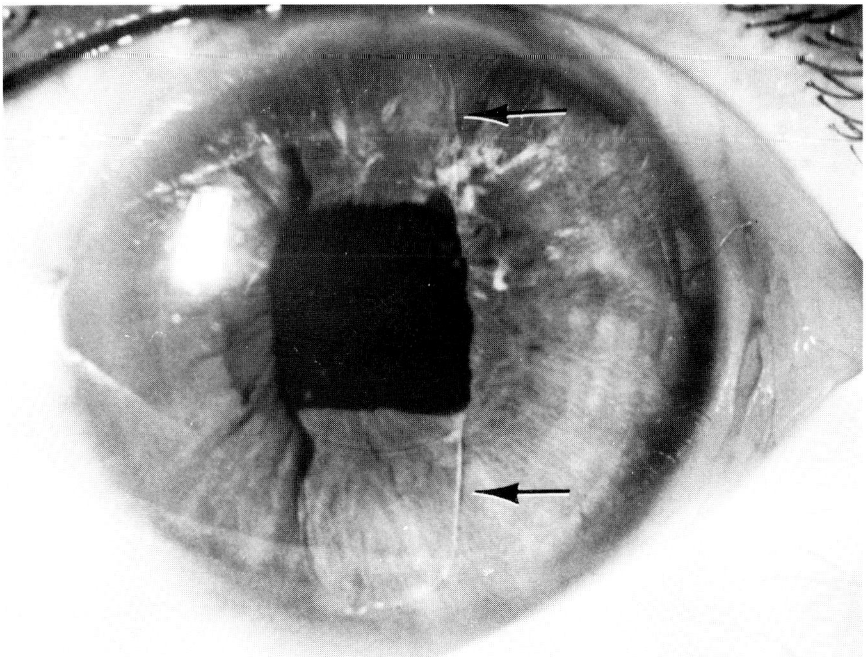

Fig. 8-42. Implant in situ in vertical axis. (From Jaffe, N. S.: Cataract surgery and its complications, ed. 2, St. Louis, 1976, The C. V. Mosby Co.)

The implant is in position, and acetylcholine is injected into the anterior chamber.

Surgical technique with an extracapsular extraction

Conventional and automated techniques are available for extracapsular cataract surgery, and the procedure of choice depends on the surgeon's preference. Thorough removal of lens cortex is advised inasmuch as it may be a catalyst for pupillary membrane formation, a complication possibly more frequent with the Copeland lens implant. The management of the posterior capsule is a matter of personal philosophy; however, a posterior capsulotomy is technically feasible after the implant is in situ and should not be performed prior to insertion, lest vitreous present.

The technique of insertion is the same as with the intracapsular technique, though the size of the incision may be smaller. It should be remembered that the diameter of the standard Copeland implant is 9 mm, and the surgeon will not err with a larger section.

Various instruments may be used for the Copeland implant technique. The implant may be held with either a nonlocking needle holder, Jaffe utility forceps, or Clayman or Shepard lens implant forceps. The iris is ideally grasped with Pierse No. 19 forceps.

After lens implantation the iris has a convoluted appearance because the haptics posterior to the iris indent the iris anteriorly, while the anterior haptics push the iris posteriorly. In effect the iris is draped over and around the implant, and this probably explains the implant's resistance to dislocation. Sometimes in the immediate postoperative period the lens is seen to be dislocated. Three haptics posterior to the iris is the usual situation, sometimes with vitreous anterior to the implant. The probable explanation is that the implant was malinserted at surgery and the true position of the haptics was not noticed at that time. It is important to be sure of the position of each haptic after implant insertion. If the position is incorrect, the lens should be repositioned. The management of dislocations is discussed on p. 174.

WORST MEDALLION LENS IMPLANT

Description

The Worst Medallion lens implant is one of the most widely used lens implants in the United States. In the 1975 survey conducted by the American Intra-Ocular Implant Society, it was ranked first in frequency among all lenses inserted. The model made by Medical Workshop of Holland* is a 2-loop lens with a lens body of polymethylmethacrylate, 6.2 mm in diameter (Fig. 8-43). The actual optic of the lens is 5 mm in diameter, and it sits eccentrically on the lens body. The rim of the lens body is 1 mm from the optic at its widest and narrows to 0.2 mm. The rim thickness is 0.15 mm, and the optic thickness varies with the dioptric power of the lens. A 20 D lens is 0.5 mm thick and weighs 11.3 mg in air. Two loops of nylon, 0.2 mm in diameter, originate from the back surface of the implant and pass posteriorly for 0.6 mm. They then angle horizontally, extending 0.5 mm beyond the lateral rim of the lens body. The total loop diameter is 7.6 mm. In the superior part of the lens body rim are two suture holes 2.5 mm apart and 0.6 mm in diameter. When the implant is in situ, the pupillary aperture at its smallest will be 2 mm square. Fig. 8-44 is a schema of the implant.

Implant design varies according to manufacturer. The loops may be nylon, polypropylene, platinum-iridium, or titanium. Sterilizing technique also varies. There are subtle differences in suture hole size between manufacturers, and this has technical ramifications in regard to passing the iris suture, as described below.

---

*Medical Workshop B. V., Heresingel 28, Groningen, Holland.

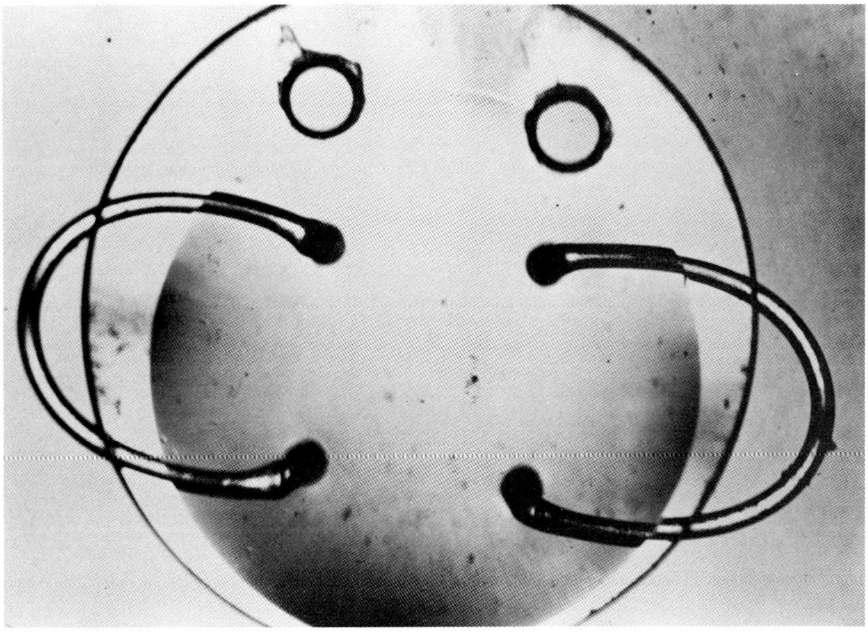

Fig. 8-43. Worst Medallion lens implant (Medical Workshop of Holland).

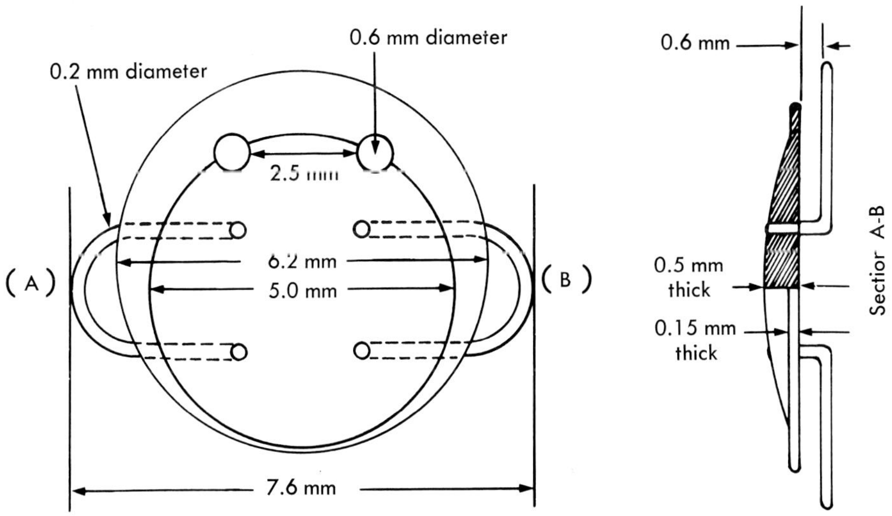

Fig. 8-44. Schema of Worst Medallion lens implant.

Surgical technique

The implant is removed from its container, washed, inspected, and set aside for further use. Some surgeons use a smaller incision with this implant, insert the loops vertically or obliquely, then rotate the lens to a horizontal position once it is centered in the pupillary aperture; this will be discussed later. Worst recommends a generous section, and this is advisable if the lens is inserted with loops horizontal.

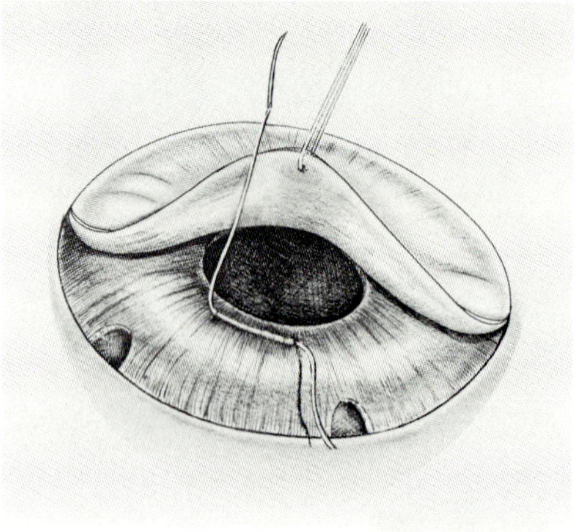

Fig. 8-45. Placement of iris suture in Worst Medallion implant technique.

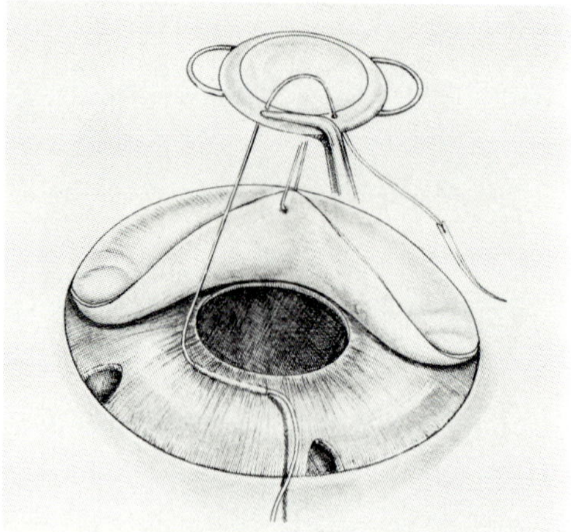

Fig. 8-46. Iris suture threaded through holes in Worst Medallion implant.

A 170° to 180° corneoscleral section is performed, and a 7-0 silk suture is placed at the 12 o'clock position for traction. Some surgeons perform two small superior iridectomies at this point, while others prefer to do this after the implant is inserted. The next step is crucial. A 9-0 or 10-0 nylon or polypropylene suture is placed through the iris stroma at the 12 o'clock position, 1 mm superior to the pupillary sphincter (Fig. 8-45). The bite should be approximately 2.5 mm in width, corresponding to the spacing of the suture holes in the implant. The passage of the iris suture is greatly facilitated by straightening the needle before the iris stroma is engaged. The iris is grasped with Hoskins No. 19 or similar forceps at 12 o'clock. The knuckle of iris is raised clear of the crystalline lens, and the needle is passed immediately below the tips of the forceps, through iris stroma, till the needle tip and shaft present at the other side of the bite. The needle is then regrasped and the bite is completed, always pulling the needle in a horizontal plane. Sufficient slack in the suture is required so that the needle may be placed in the canthus at the surgeon's left. Care should be taken that the long end of the suture remain on the surgeon's right, lest it inadvertently be snatched and result in iris damage. It is helpful to wet the suture so that it adheres to the drape. Cleaning of the suture by passing it through conjunctiva prior to iris placement has been advocated and this is optional. The cataract is then extracted.

A 4 to 5 mm pupil is ideal for insertion of the Worst Medallion lens implant. If the pupil is larger than this, acetylcholine solution is injected into the anterior chamber prior to insertion. Various forceps may be used to grasp the implant. The Clayman forceps are ideal. The implant is held with forceps in the right hand by the superior rim. Care should be taken that the jaws of the forceps do not occlude the suture holes. The needle of the iris suture, previously placed at the canthus to the surgeon's left, is picked up with fine forceps and placed through the left suture hole from back to front. The needle may be passed point or heel first. An assistant grasps the needle as it presents at the front of the left suture hole and passes it through the right suture hole front to back (Fig. 8-46). The rationale for this is that when the suture is ultimately tied, the knot will lie between the back surface of the implant and the iris and not pose a threat to the corneal endothelium.

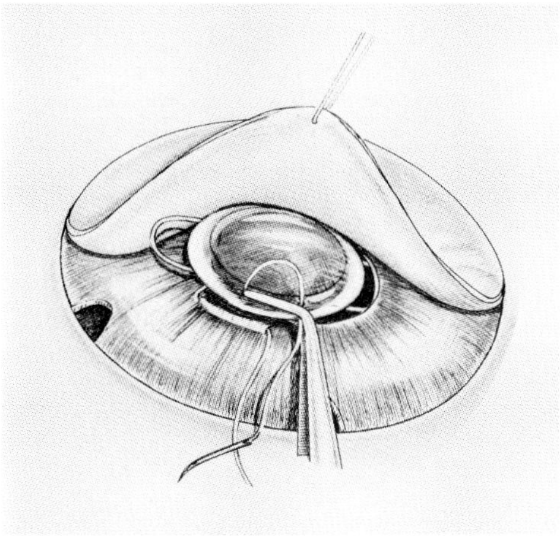

Fig. 8-47. Worst Medallion lens implant inserted with right loop under iris.

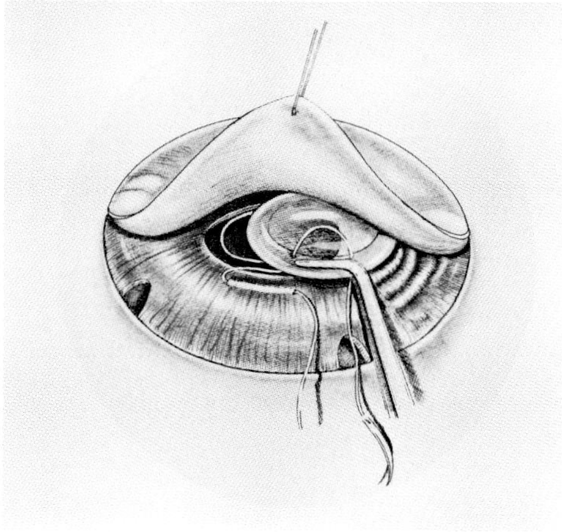

Fig. 8-48. Pupil is displaced slightly to right so left loop can clear pupillary margin.

With the assistant retracting the cornea, the implant is inserted into the pupillary aperture with a lateral motion to the right so that the right loop slides under the iris at 9 o'clock (Fig. 8-47). This motion is continued until the left loop clears the left pupillary margin (Fig. 8-48), at which point it is slid behind the iris at 3 o'clock. The reason for sliding the loop behind the iris at the surgeon's right (for a right-handed surgeon) first is that, if the left loop cannot be made to clear the margin of the pupil, the iris can be gently lifted with forceps held in the surgeon's left hand. One can see how awkward this maneuver would be if the order were reversed. The implant is now in position, and the pupil is constricted with acetylcholine solution. The next step is to tie the iris suture, which should be neither too tight nor too loose. We are reminded that the implant is referred to as the "medallion." A medallion is not tied to the neck but rather is suspended from it, and the same applies to the implant in regard to the iris.

The needle of the iris suture is layed on the closed cornea to the right of its midline. Any slack is taken up by pulling gently on the long end of the suture. The needle is cut off, and the long end is tied to the short end with a triple tie. The knot is tightened and slid under the implant with or without corneal retraction, according to the surgeon's preference. The knot is completed with two overhand ties, each individually tightened and slid under the implant as above. The suture is then cut flush with the edge of the implant (Fig. 8-49). It is not necessary to insinuate scissors under the implant to cut the suture directly on the knot; indeed this is hazardous.

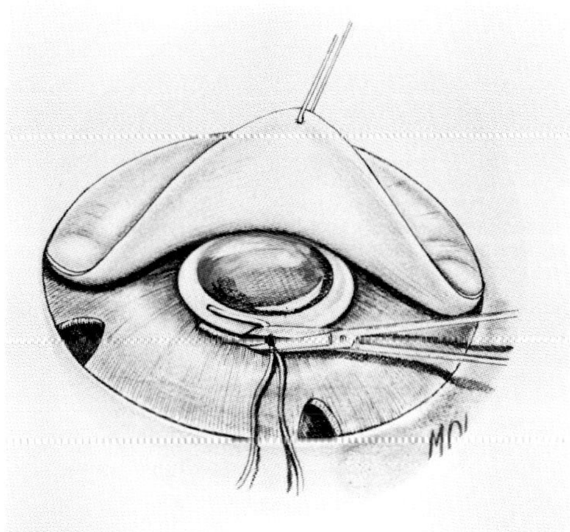

Fig. 8-49. Iris suture cut flush with edge of implant.

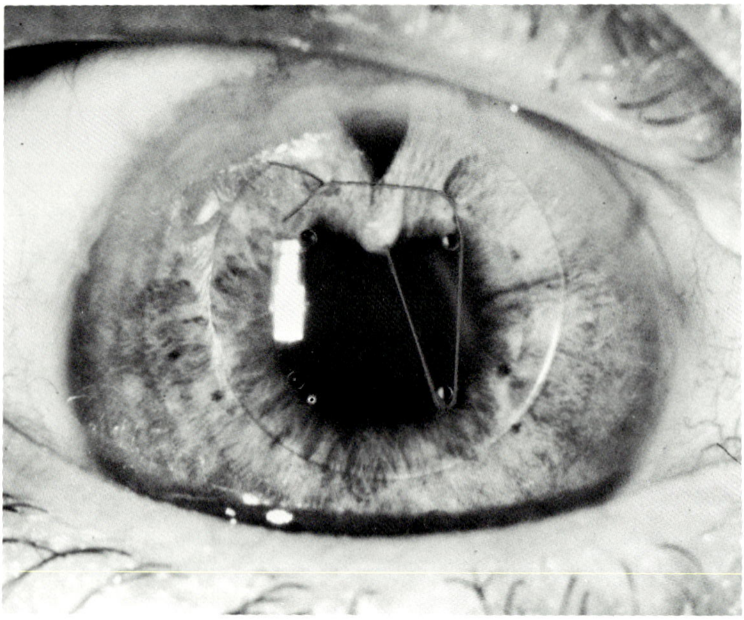

Fig. 8-50. Iris suture inadvertently tied around loop of implant. (Courtesy Dr. Robert Drews.)

Caution should be exercised as the implant is inserted so as not to drag the long arm of the iris suture into the anterior chamber with the right loop of the implant. Such a case is illustrated (Fig. 8-50).

If this is recognized after the implant is in position, but prior to tying the iris suture, the right loop of the implant should be dislocated anterior to the iris with a spatula and iris hook or forceps. The offending arm of the suture can then be withdrawn from the anterior chamber and the lens repositioned with a technique in reverse of the dislocating maneuver. A Jaffe spatula is used to move the implant laterally to the left, and the iris is engaged with a fine hook and lifted over the right haptic. The suture can now be tied. If this situation is recognized after the suture is tied, it is best left alone.

Hirschman advocates a different technique. A small corneoscleral incision of 120° to 130° is made. The iris suture is passed as described above, taking care to avoid injury to the pupillary sphincter and anterior lens capsule. The cataract is extracted with a cryoprobe, and acetylcholine is injected into the anterior chamber if the pupil is larger than 4 to 5 mm in diameter. The iris suture is threaded through the suture holes of the implant, and the implant is grasped by the haptic rim and brought into the anterior chamber with the right loop directed at the 6 o'clock position. Once in the anterior chamber, a clockwise and right lateral movement slides the right haptic under the iris at 8 o'clock. The lateral movement is continued to the right until the left haptic clears the pupillary margin, at which point the implant is moved to the left, sliding the left haptic under the iris at 2 o'clock. The implant is now rotated with forceps until the loops lay in a horizontal plane and the iris suture is tied. This technique also permits placement of the implant into the anterior chamber under an air bubble, since the narrower width of the implant passes through the incision.

Whichever method is used, it is pru-

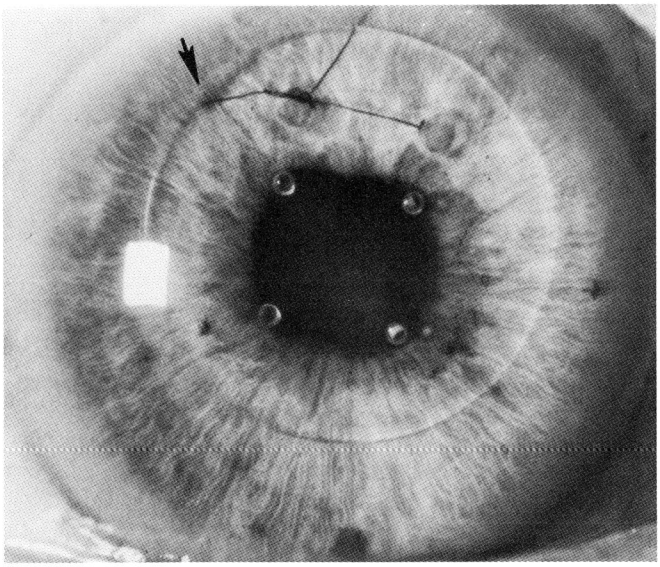

Fig. 8-51. Worst Medallion 2-loop lens implant in situ. Note iris suture *(arrow)*.

dent to inject an air bubble into the anterior chamber after implant insertion for two reasons. First, it reforms the chamber, and second, it serves as a cushion between the implant and the corneal endothelium while the corneoscleral incision is being sutured. Fig. 8-51 shows a patient with a Worst Medallion lens in situ. The iris suture is clearly visible *(arrow)*. When nylon has been used for the iris suture, suture failure has been noted after as little as 1 year of use, and in some cases this has proved to be troublesome to the patient and has required a second procedure for its removal. Polypropylene is now available and promises to be an improvement.

WORST PLATINUM-CLIP LENS IMPLANT

Description

The lens body and dimensions are identical with the Worst Medallion 2-loop lens, as manufactured by Medical Workshop of Holland. The nylon loops on the platinum-clip lens, however, are oriented vertically (Fig. 8-52). The inferior loop is longer than the superior, and

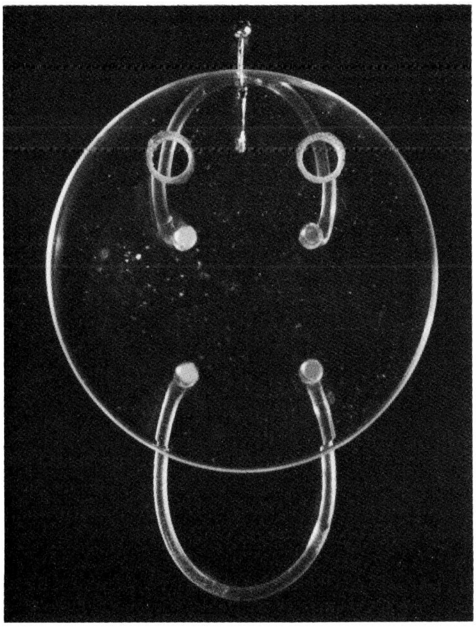

Fig. 8-52. Worst platinum-clip lens implant.

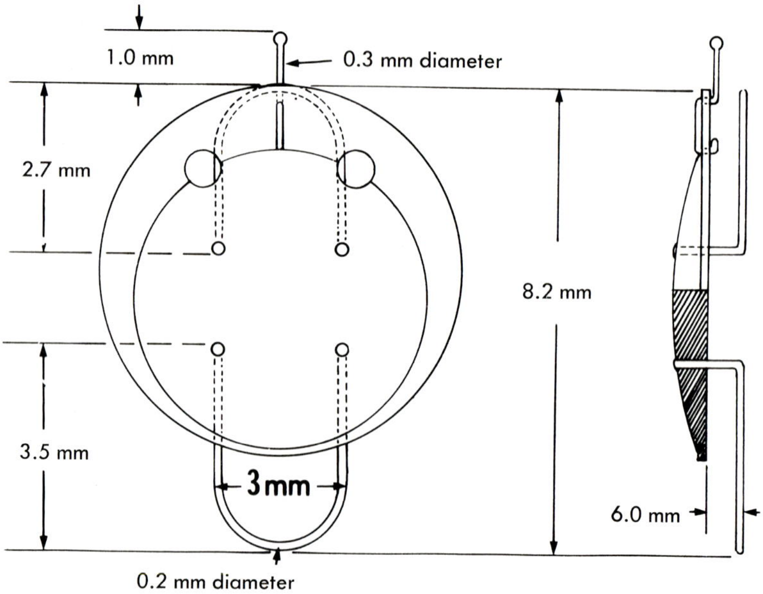

Fig. 8-53. Schema of Worst platinum-clip lens implant (approximate dimensions).

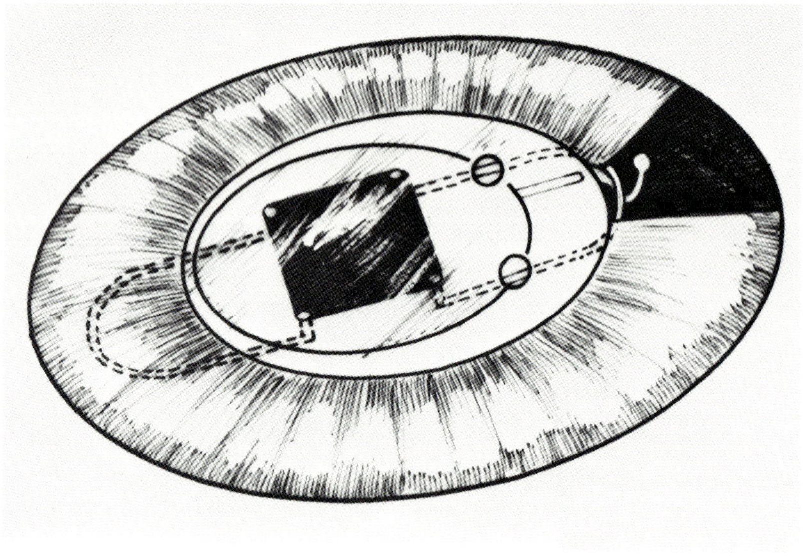

Fig. 8-54. Position of implant after insertion.

there is a small platinum wire 0.3 mm in diameter with a knob on its end imbedded in the haptic at the 12 o'clock position. The total loop diameter is 8.2 mm. Both loops originate from the back surface of the implant and pass posteriorly for approximately 0.6 mm before angling inferiorly and superiorly, respectively. The inferior loop is 3.5 mm long and the superior 2.7 mm long. The diameter of the loop is 0.2 mm. The platinum wire extends 1 to 2 mm and functions as a clip (Fig. 8-53). When the lens is in situ, the wire is bent posteriorly through the peripheral iridectomy to engage the apex of the superior loop, which is behind the

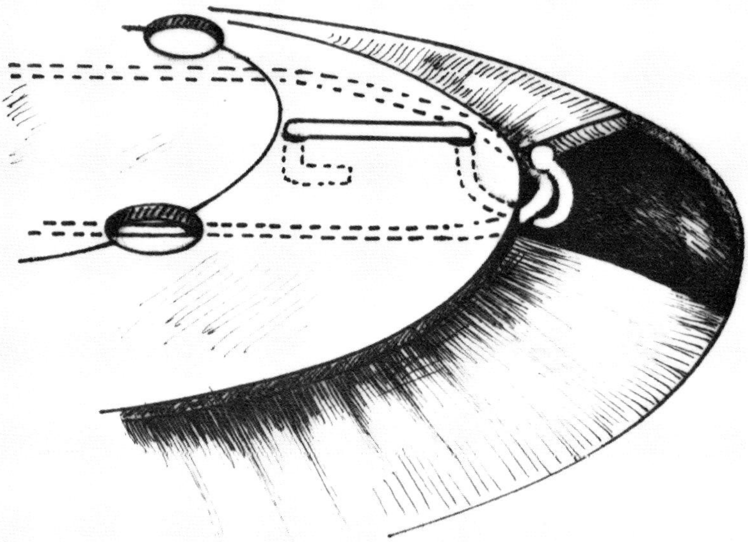

Fig. 8-55. Wire bent to form clip.

iris. Fig. 8-54 conceptualizes this implant after insertion. This lens was primarily designed for extracapsular cases, and is essentially similar to the Binkhorst 2-loop iridocapsular lens implant (p. 83). The platinum clip is an added feature that makes for reasonably secure fixation even if capsular fixation does not occur. The lens can also be used in conjunction with an intracapsular cataract extraction.

Surgical technique

The technique of insertion is similar in both extracapsular and intracapsular cataract extractions. The implant is grasped by the superior rim with Shepard or Clayman forceps. A 4 to 5 mm pupil is suitable for insertion. The inferior loop is placed behind the inferior iris at 6 o'clock (and in the inferior capsular bag in the case of extracapsular surgery). The inferior loop is longer than the superior in this implant, and in the initial maneuver the implant should not be decentered too far inferiorly lest the ciliary body be traumatized. Still holding the implant with the implant forceps, the superior iris is grasped with Pierse forceps or a fine hook, lifted over the superior loop, and placed between it and the platinum wire. Ideally, after an extracapsular cataract extraction the superior loop should be placed in the superior capsular bag, but this is not always easy to identify.

The peripheral iridectomy or iridotomy can be performed prior to cataract extraction, but with this lens implant it is advantageous to perform it after implant insertion so that the aperture may coincide with the exact position of the platinum wire. To clip the platinum wire to the superior loop the lens is lifted up to the 12 o'clock position and tilted slightly anteriorly. This brings the superior loop into the aperture of the peripheral iridectomy. The tip of the wire is held with forceps and brought down and through the iridectomy within the curve of the superior loop. The wire is released and regrasped from below the loop, and brought forward and around the superior extremity of the loop (Fig. 8-55). The platinum wire is extremely malleable and quite fragile. It may break off with repeated manipulation, and this should be avoided. The implant should be recentered with a fine

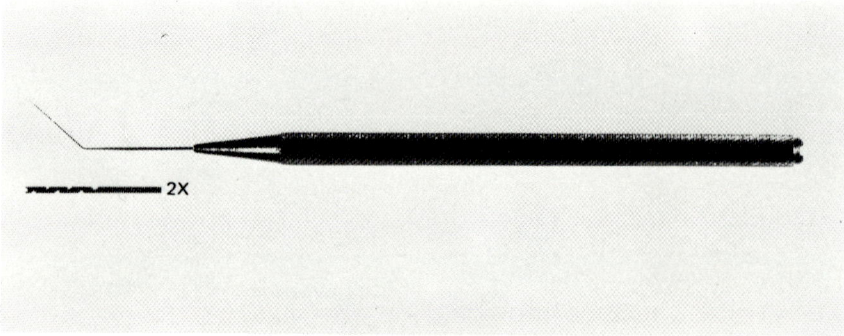

Fig. 8-56. Hirschman notched lens spatula.

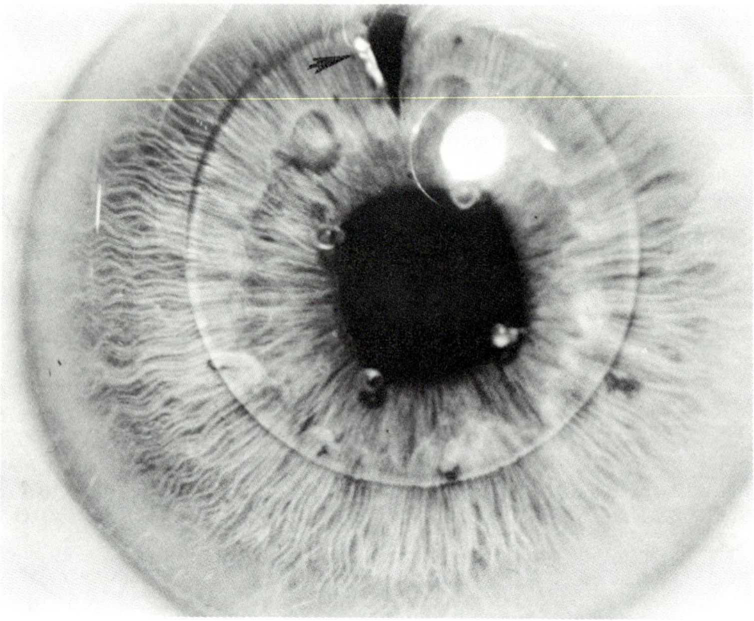

Fig. 8-57. Worst platinum-clip *(arrow)* lens implant in situ.

Jaffe or Hirschman spatula (Fig. 8-56). A bubble of air is instilled into the anterior chamber, and the incision is closed. Fig. 8-57 shows the lens in situ.

With this technique the peripheral iridectomy is of crucial importance. First, it must be positioned directly under the platinum wire and must be large enough to permit the clipping maneuvers. Furthermore, if the iridectomy is too peripheral, the inferior loop of the implant could dislocate with pupillary dilatation. On the other hand, if the iridectomy is too large, the lens may ride low and exhibit a pendular type of pseudophakodonesis as it hangs from the apex of the iridectomy.

The surgeon should be sure that the platinum wire correctly engages the superior loop. Occasionally the wire will be bent so that it protrudes anteriorly and could traumatize the endothelium. We have seen cortical remnants in the superior capsular cul-de-sac tilt the lens anteriorly and bring the clip into contact

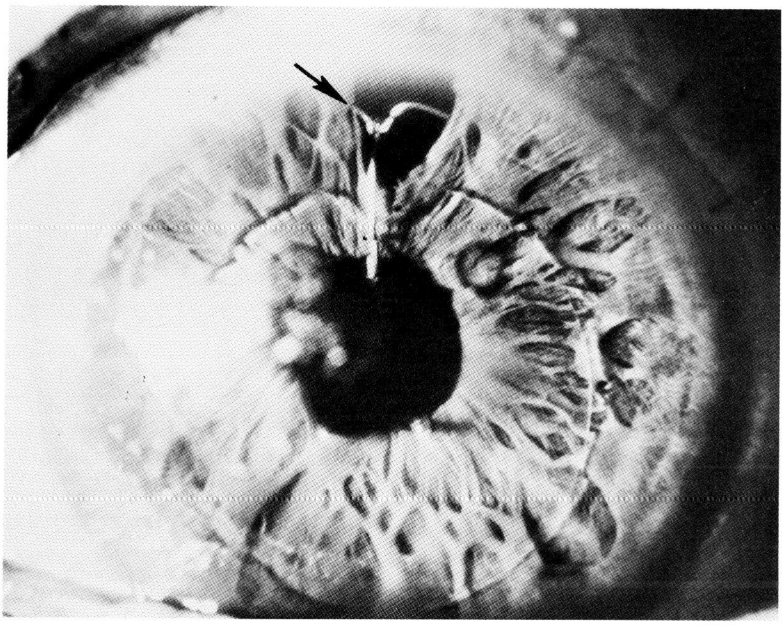

Fig. 8-58. Worst circular loop lens. Note platinum clip engaging a circular loop posterior to iris *(arrow)*.

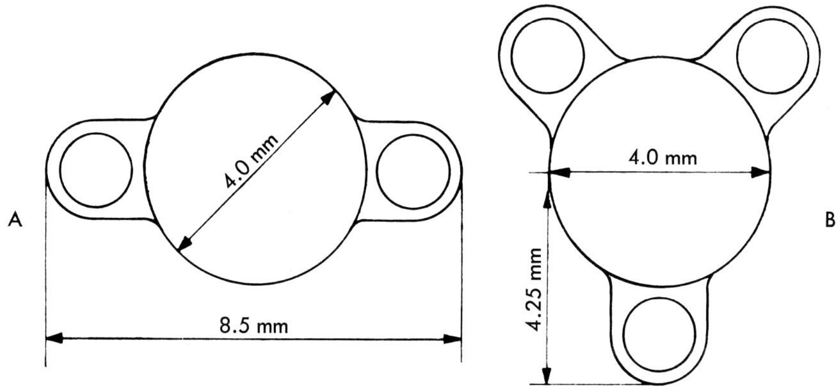

Fig. 8-59. Pearce posterior chamber implant. (From Pearce, J. L.: Trans. Ophthalmol. Soc. U.K. **96:**6, 1976.)

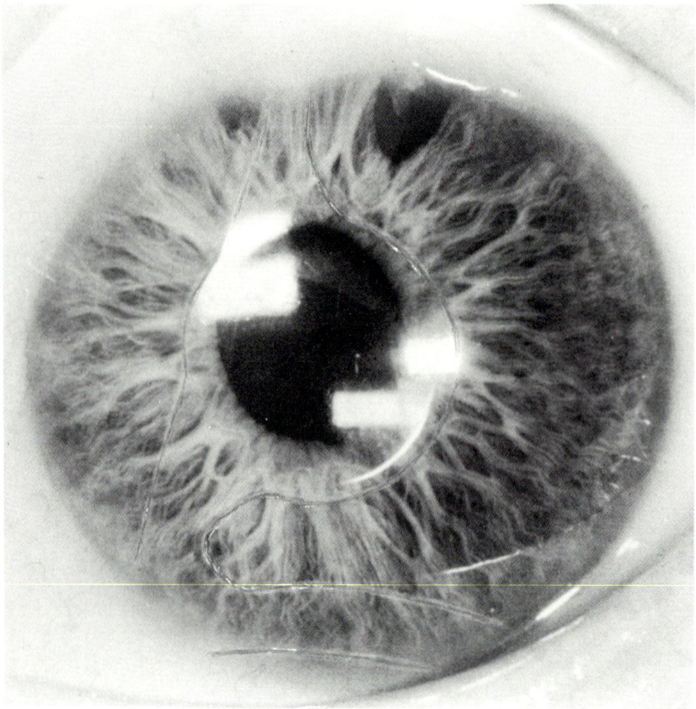

Fig. 8-60. Kelman anterior chamber lens. (Courtesy Dr. Charles Kelman.)

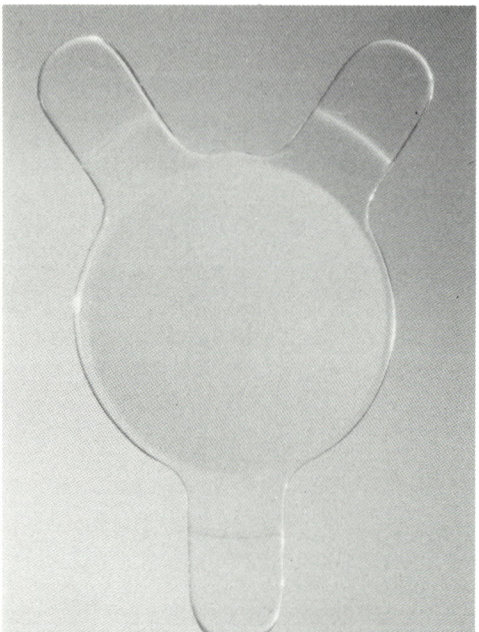

Fig. 8-61. Ridley anterior chamber lens implant.

with the back surface of the superior cornea.

OTHER LENSES

The Worst small incision, circular loop (Fig. 8-58), and "clover leaf" implants are not in wide clinical use. There are posterior chamber implants being designed (Fig. 8-59), but experience with these is limited to a few surgeons. The concept is, of course, predicated on extracapsular surgery. Anterior chamber lenses are currently of great interest. Kelman has designed an ingenious anterior chamber lens capable of being inserted through a 4.5 mm incision. This lens is approximately L-shaped, with a 4 mm optic originating from the vertical strut of the L (Fig. 8-60). The Ridley anterior chamber lens (Fig. 8-61) has not enjoyed the popularity of the Choyce Mark VIII implant, which is discussed in the next chapter.

CHAPTER 9

Choyce Mark VIII anterior chamber implant

D. P. CHOYCE, B.Sc., M.B., M.S. (London), F.R.C.S., D.O.M.S. (England)

HISTORY

Personal experience with the Ridley lens

From 1954 to 1955 I inserted a Ridley posterior chamber lens implant in eight cases of mature uniocular cataract, only two of which were satisfactory. What went wrong? First, Ridley stressed that the technical requirements of his posterior chamber lens implant operation would always be great, that extraction of the lens, leaving behind nothing but an intact posterior capsule, is not easy, and that small particles of residual lens cortex could give rise to phacoanaphylactic iridocyclitis. I think some of my failures were due to this latter phenomenon; others probably were due to the Cetavlon (cetrimide) sterilizing agent in which those early lens implants were sterilized. It was later established that even small amounts of this agent remaining on the surface of the lenticulus would set up a severe iridocyclitis.

Why early anterior chamber implants failed

The original Strampelli anterior chamber implant was used by him in November 1953 and was adopted enthusiastically in 1954 by Joaquin Barraquer. It is not generally realized that they treated not only aphakic patients but also phakic patients suffering from high myopia and high hypermetropia. In their publications they tended to merge their statistics with regard to these two widely different patient categories so that reading those papers today it is unclear how many aphakic cases developed complications as compared to the phakic cases. Clearly the two groups are not strictly comparable. Nor did they provide factual information as to the nature of the polymethylmethacrylate they used, nor the method of sterilization involved. All of these factors doubtless contributed to their heavy and much publicized complication rate. To some extent their early disappointments were duplicated in my first Mark I implant series (Table 9-1).

Table 9-1 clearly shows that the sequential modifications I introduced into the original Strampelli implant were associated with two related phenomena: (1) increased anterior depth, that is, the distance between the back surface of the cornea and the front surface of the implant optic; and (2) a decline in the incidence of endothelial corneal dystrophy, which was the main complication that discouraged their use by other ophthalmic surgeons. The mean anterior

□ President, International Intraocular Implant Club; Senior Consultant, Regional Eye Centre, Southend Group of Hospitals, Essex, England; Consultant Ophthalmologist, Hospital for Tropical Diseases, London.

chamber depth in phakic eyes is 2.85 mm,[1] so it is not surprising that the introduction of the Mark VIII implant reduced the incidence of endothelial corneal dystrophy to 1.5%. In contrast, 22% of the Mark I implants had developed corneal dystrophy by 1960, though it is possible that many of these were due to the cetrimide in which the first 30 implants had been sterilized. It is interesting that in the 17 years that have elapsed since, only six more have developed this dystrophy. In other words, those that were free of this complication 3 to 4 years after implantation have tended to remain free since, and those were the ones with deeper than average anterior chamber depths.

Details of Choyce modifications to the original Strampelli anterior chamber implant

In what respects does the Mark I (1955) implant differ from the Mark VIII (1963) model (Fig. 9-1)?

1. The thickness of the haptic portion

Table 9-1. Incidence of endothelial corneal dystrophy with Choyce anterior chamber implants

	No. eyes	Average follow-up in years	Average anterior chamber depths	Endothelial corneal dystrophy
Choyce Mark I	100	20	1.68 mm	28%
Choyce Mark II to VII	328	16	2.15 mm	7%
Choyce Mark VIII	850	7	2.85 mm	1.5%

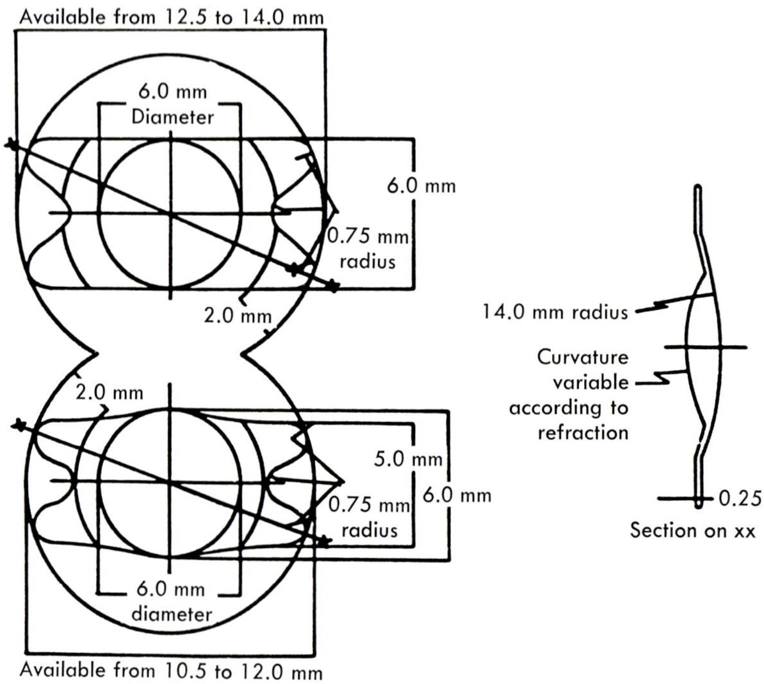

Fig. 9-1. Schema of Choyce Mark VIII anterior chamber lens implant (current model, as designed in 1963).

has been reduced from just under 1.0 mm to 0.25 mm, tapering to about 0.2 mm at the extremity of each foot.

2. It is a quadripedal implant instead of a tripod implant. The addition of the fourth foot makes it much more stable.

3. The four feet are flattened; that is, it is almost a one-plane horizontal implant. Each foot is flattened until it approaches the optic so that even in the shorter lengths (11.0 mm and 11.5 mm) not less than 2 mm of each foot is flat.

SECONDARY IMPLANTATION

Preoperative preparation

Because the anterior chamber implant was designed for secondary implantation, this will be considered first. The following preoperative procedures are essential:

1. Horizontal corneal diameter. This can be measured on the operating table. It saves time to measure it in the office using calipers read off on a metal ruler measured in half millimeters (Fig. 9-2).

2. Best corrected visual acuity with note of back vertex distance of major sphere.

3. Anterior chamber depth. Anything less than 3.0 mm will probably contraindicate implant insertion.

4. Examination of the corneal endothelium and anterior chamber with special reference to the absence of aqueous flare and cells and the presence or absence of vitreous in the anterior chamber. Its presence may not be a contraindication to secondary Mark VIII implantation, but obviously the surgeon will wish to know of its existence in the anterior chamber.

5. Gonioscopy. More than 30% occlusion of the angle would probably indicate the necessity for a preliminary operation to clear the angle if technically possible.

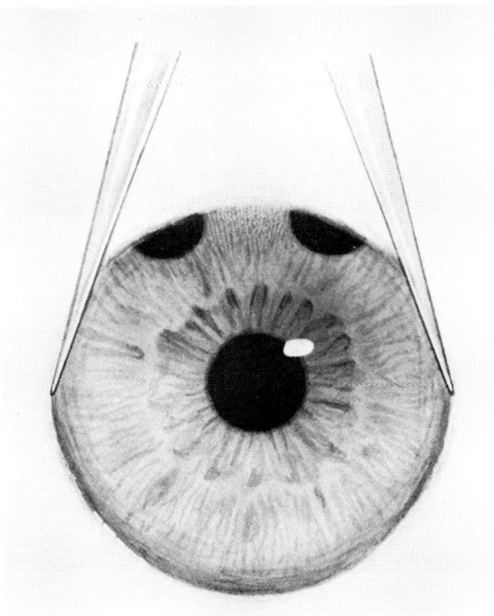

Fig. 9-2. Horizontal corneal diameter, limbal white to limbal white, measured with calipers.

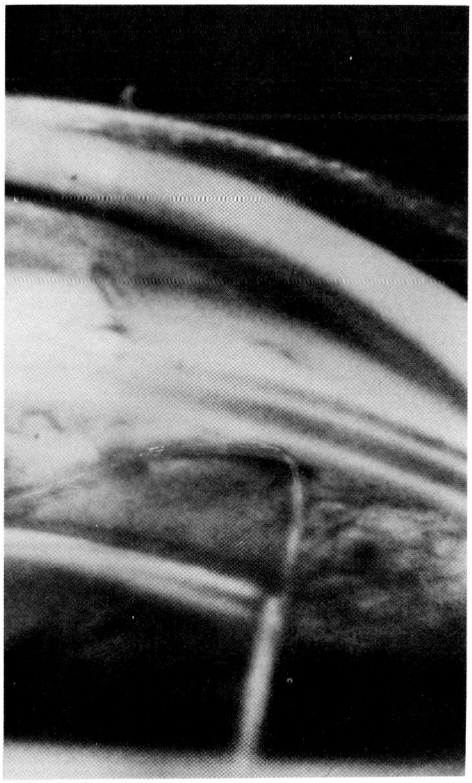

Fig. 9-3. Goniophotograph of foot of Mark VIII implant resting behind scleral spur. (Courtesy Dr. Jerald L. Tennant.)

These precautions are necessary because the four feet of the Mark VIII are designed to come to rest just behind the scleral spur (Fig. 9-3), and if access to this region is blocked by peripheral anterior synechiae, the adhesions must either be cleared by preliminary surgery or avoided by altering the axis of insertion.

6. Applanation tonometry, which should not exceed 20 mm Hg.

7. Funduscopy to identify any fundus pathology.

8. The eyelashes should be cut. Pilocarpine 4% (for miosis) and antibiotic drops should be instilled the night before and the morning of the operation.

9. Immediately prior to surgery, triamcinolone 40 mg is injected intramuscularly, and acetazolamide 500 mg is administered intravenously. General anesthesia is then induced. I do not give a retrobulbar injection, nor do I practice digital pressure.

Surgical technique

Secondary Mark VIII implantation is best performed temporally or from the upper temporal quadrant for the following reasons:

1. Ease of access, in that it should be possible to introduce the implant straight into the eye once the section has been made *without touching anything else on the way in*, whereas vertical insertion is more difficult because of the upper lid and the brow.

2. The astigmatism resulting from the conventional cataract incision from 3 to 9 o'clock usually leaves a degree of with-the-rule astigmatism, which will be canceled out in large degree by a temporal incision.

3. It is probably desirable to avoid reopening the previous cataract incision.

4. Gonioscopy should be repeated if this step was omitted in the preoperative preparation.

5. Exposure: a lid speculum with superior rectus bridle suture plus a small lateral canthotomy. One drop of 4% pilocarpine and one drop of 0.1% epinephrine (adrenaline) are instilled (to produce miosis and hemostasis, respectively).

6. The horizontal corneal diameter, white to white, is checked once more. This length plus 1 mm equals the probable length of implant necessary, but the surgeon must make sure that he has available additional implants of other lengths.

7. A light cautery barrage is layed down to seal off the limbal incision. I make the incision with a Graefe knife, a small Beaver blade being used. A good section is the basis for a successful anterior chamber implant operation. Many surgeons of the present generation have been trained to make the section with a razor-blade knife and scissors in preference to a Graefe knife. If a surgeon has more experience with the latter than with a Graefe knife, he should certainly use his preferred technique.

Cutting a temporal section of this nature is more difficult in a deep-set, small eye or if some blepharophimosis is present, hence the assistance provided by lateral canthotomy. It may also be expedient to make a smaller section than usual, enlarging it as necessary with Castroviejo's corneal scissors.

My usual method of cutting this section is as follows: The eye is fixed above by grasping and lifting the insertion of the superior rectus muscle with forceps. The knife enters at the 7 o'clock position in the right eye and at the 5 o'clock position in the left eye, exactly at the limbus, without raising a conjunctival flap. The knife is carried swiftly straight up to the 11 o'clock position on the right or to the 1 o'clock position on the left, where the counterpuncture is made again exactly at the limbus (Fig. 9-4). Care must be taken to avoid the pupil area so as not to pierce the hyaloid face. It will be appreciated at this stage how valuable preoperative constriction of the pupil is. The section is completed by cutting toward oneself,

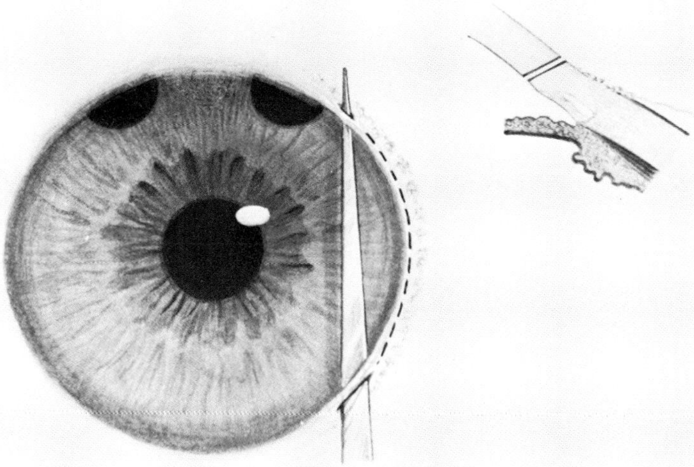

Fig. 9-4. Technique of cutting section for a secondary lens implantation (left eye illustrated).

very slowly and very gently, as in a slow-motion film, with the knife blade slightly rotated so as to cut a slightly corneal section that is avascular and has no conjunctival flap. The reason for this is that it is essential to leave a shelf or bevel of 1 mm of cornea so that the feet of the implant can be retained in the angle without dislocating from the eye before the suturing of the incision has been completed. To avoid dangerous pressure on the eye, the fixation forceps should be removed a few seconds before the section has been completed.

One of the most common mistakes made by those not used to this incision is making the section too small. Since the optic of the Mark VIII implant measures 6 mm across, the internal opening of the incision should be *not less than 8 mm.* Second, if the section is too scleral, it may bleed excessively. I do not make a conjunctival flap either limbal or fornix based. A surgeon who is experienced and skillful in cutting a right cataract section with the right hand and a left cataract section with the left hand should soon become expert in making the section used for the introduction of anterior chamber implant, though the procedure may feel initially somewhat strange.

Vitreous loss is most unlikely if the posterior capsule is intact or if the hyaloid face is intact, provided the operation is conducted in a gentle manner. If the hyaloid is broken and vitreous is already present in the anterior chamber opening, a certain amount will commonly escape on opening the eye. Some vitreous has been lost in about 10% of the aphakic cases in my series, but the amount was usually small and did not affect the ultimate result. I had considered using a Flieringa or similar ring in this type of case, but it has not been found necessary. If the patient is under general anesthesia, intravenous acetazolamide can keep vitreous loss within reasonable limits. Vitreous presenting on completion of the section should be cut off before the implant is inserted and again after implant insertion. After the corneal sutures have been tied, no vitreous should be present between the lips of the incision. In my opinion, vitreous loss should not deter the surgeon from completing the operation.

My most effective method of dealing with vitreous prolapse is by running a swab soaked in hyaluronidase along the incision; vitreous will adhere to this swab, enabling the surgeon to cut it off flush with the section using microscissors. The "vitreous" that escapes on reopening an aphakic eye is a mixture of aqueous and anterior vitreous and does not have the same jelly-like consistency of the formed vitreous, which may escape at the time of primary cataract extraction. Its escape from the eye in small quantities does not carry the same bad prognosis. It should not be followed back into the anterior chamber nor through the pupil.

8. The usual site of troublesome peripheral anterior synechiae is around the pillars of the superior iridectomy. Sometimes the iridectomy can scarcely be seen on gonioscopy because it is pushed up into the recesses of the angle by the vitreous without actually being included in the healed section. I have found that in most cases it is possible to separate these adhesions by releasing the peripheral iridectomy and centering the pupil with the use of a straight iris repositor or a synechia spatula. This is inserted in the superior part of the incision and runs along in the angle until it engages with the synechiae coming from the temporal pillar of the iridectomy. With this released, the tip of the repositor is engaged in the iridectomy, which is then delivered into the middle of the anterior chamber. This maneuver usually detaches any synechiae involving the nasal pillar of the iridectomy, but it is sometimes necessary to continue the process with the iris repositor. If carried out gently on a soft eye, this can usually be accomplished with little or no loss of vitreous.

When in doubt about the management of peripheral anterior synechiae, they should be left undisturbed. Efforts to free long-standing and dense adhesions often results in troublesome bleeding. The axis of implant insertion should be modified to avoid them, in preference to attempting to free them.

With a superior sector iridectomy or an eccentric pupil, the lower margin of the pupil may rise up behind the implant after its insertion and interfere with its optical function. This complication may be anticipated at this stage of the operation, before the implant is actually inserted, by carrying out a sphincterotomy at the 6 o'clock position.

9. Many surgeons inject air into the anterior chamber at this point to facilitate implant insertion. I prefer balanced salt solution at 30° C. Air is indicated to manage bleeding, and it acts as a tamponade. While the surgeon has been opening the eye and dealing with peripheral anterior synechiae, the operating room nurse will have taken the implant out of the container and will have washed it and placed it in a watchglass with balanced salt solution. The surgeon then picks up the implant across the optic portion with the Choyce 120° implant holding forceps. It is then transferred and placed right way up on the metal ruler for checking. The label on the container should match the surgeon's requirements in terms of length, power, and color (in the case of a colored haptic implant). The implant should be the right way up, and the length should be checked diagonally. Unfortunately there seems to be quite a bit of variation in the stated length, and if, for example, the implant labeled at 12.5 mm turns out to be 12.25 mm or 12.75 mm, the surgeon must use his judgment as to whether to go ahead and insert it into the eye or to open another package in the hope of finding an implant nearer to the stated length. On the whole I consider that 0.25 mm error is acceptable. All four feet should be in the horizontal plane, and this can be checked by observation and also by attempting to rock the implant by tapping the feet in rotation. No rocking means the feet are all in the horizontal plane and none of them are warped. The implant is examined carefully for flaws and foreign matter, the

optic in particular. The surgeon applies the 120° forceps to the optic once again, using his left hand if the implant is to be inserted into the right eye and the right hand if it is to be inserted into the left eye. With his other hand he grasps the feet with the 135° Choyce implant holding forceps and is now all set to slide the implant into the eye. The implant is rinsed one last time with balanced salt solution, and the distal feet are introduced through the section into the anterior chamber. Because the section is slightly beveled, it will be necessary to incline the feet down at an angle of about 30° until they are through the section into the anterior chamber. Then the implant is leveled off and slid if necessary with slight horizontal rocking movements across the anterior chamber. The surgeon is watching the distal feet during this process, making sure that they pass just in front of the constricted pupil, not touching the endothelium and not pushing the iris in front of it (Fig. 9-5).

Once those distal feet are safely across the pupil the surgeon's assistant should put a spatula in the temporal dovetail or crotch to steady the implant in that position, that is, nearly but not quite across the anterior chamber so that the surgeon can take off the 135° implant holding forceps without jerking the implant out of position.

The introduction of the distal feet into the section is sometimes helped by the insertion of a traction suture through the middle of the corneal lip of the section and gently lifting this up.

The surgeon then continues gently to push the implant across the anterior chamber with a spatula or needle holding forceps until the nasal feet rest snugly in the opposite angle. All that remains to be done then is to insert the temporal feet. This is accomplished by catching the outer (scleral) lip of the incision with fine-toothed forceps and retracting it *quite forcefully* out and slightly up while pressing gently on one foot of the implant with the tip of an iris repositor (Fig. 9-6). Usually the foot gives a little plop as it tips over the edge and takes up its position in the angle. The maneuver is re-

A

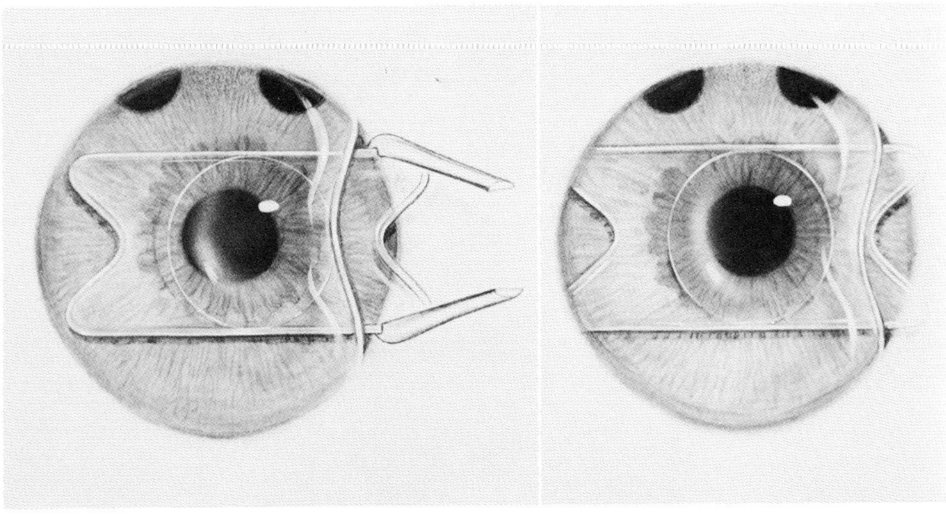

B

Fig. 9-5. Secondary lens implant technique (left eye illustrated). **A,** Implant held in Choyce 135° forceps, being slid across anterior chamber. **B,** Distal feet in situ and forceps now released. Note that less than 1.5 mm of temporal feet should extend beyond the incision.

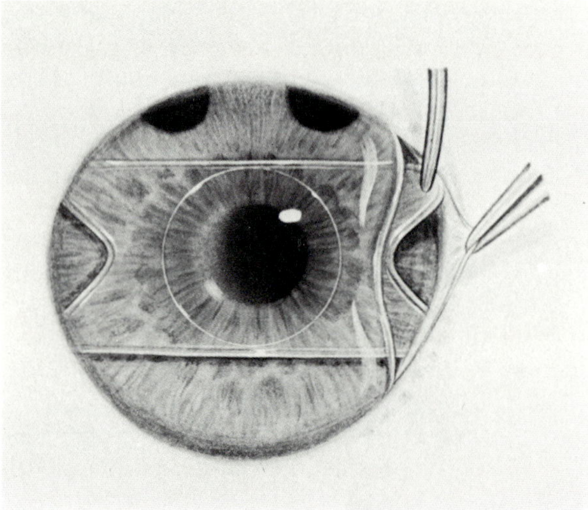

Fig. 9-6. Insertion of proximal feet.

peated for the other foot of the implant, and it is usually quite obvious when the feet are safely inside the anterior chamber and resting snugly in the angle. A fresh repositor is used to slide the length of the incision, making sure that the corneal part of the incision is not turned in.

A scleral hook or even a suture can be used to retract the outer lip of the incision during the placement of the feet. Which foot should be inserted first? Whichever foot looks as though it will go in with the greater ease; and having inserted it, it is easier to insert the remaining foot. How does the surgeon tell if the implant is the correct length? If the two proximal feet just drop into the angle without any effort being made to put them there, clearly the implant is too short. Conversely, if more than 1.5 mm sticks out across the section once the distal feet have taken up their proper position in the distal angle, it is probably too long. Either way the implant should be withdrawn from the eye and an implant half a millimeter longer or shorter, as required, should be used instead. It is very important not to push the proximal feet distally in order to get them over the bevel or ledge into the angle. Such movement would be transmitted to the distal feet, which might result in tearing of the distal iris root leading to hemorrhage, which may persist into the convalescent period and invalidate the functional result.

This insertion of the proximal feet is the crux of the operation; it is like so many other maneuvers in ophthalmic surgery which, when learned, are surprisingly simple. This is why I say that ideally a surgeon performing Mark VIII implantation for the first time should be assisted by a colleague who has done a number of these operations and knows exactly what is involved.

10. At this stage of the operation—after the implant has been inserted and before the incision has been closed—the surgeon may observe excessive bulging of the iris between the feet of the inserted implant, especially if the implant is a little on the long side, or if the anterior chamber was a little shallow, or if some goniosynechiae are still present. Bulging of the iris at this stage may precede anterior intraocular iris prolapse during convalescence, and it is desirable to perform a small additional peripheral iridectomy at this site. The apex of the bulging

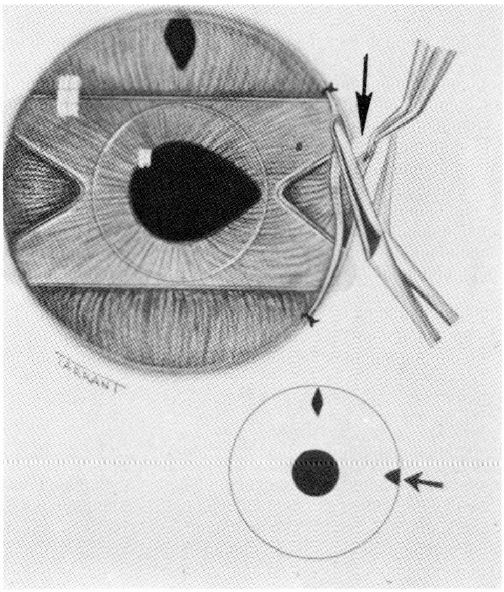

Fig. 9-7. Iridectomy *(arrows)* between proximal feet, if iris is bulging.

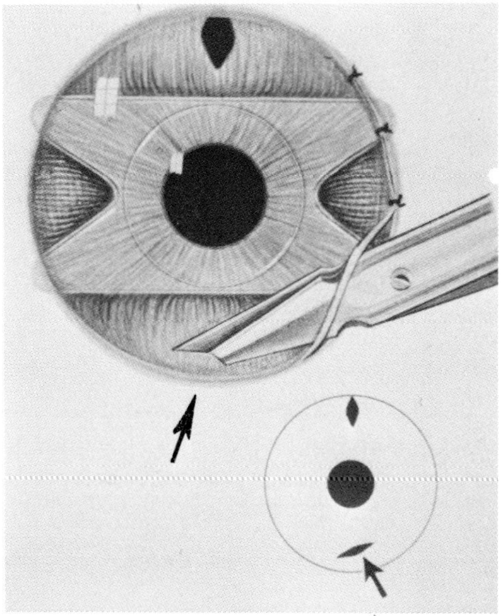

Fig. 9-8. Inferior iridotomy *(arrows)* performed with Vannas scissors.

iris is caught with iris forceps, and a small iridectomy is carried out leaving the sphincter intact (Fig. 9-7).

A further tendency for bulging of the iris in front of the lower margin of the implant should be relieved by inserting curved Vannas scissors through the lower part of the incision, pointing the lower blade slightly down, piercing the root of the iris around the 6 o'clock position with the single blade, and snipping through the iris stroma in the direction of its root (Fig. 9-8). This maneuver may be deferred until the top two sutures have been inserted and tied. It is most important that the surgeon remember that all these intracameral maneuvers must be carried out with great respect for the integrity of the corneal endothelium.

Six or seven interrupted sutures are usually required to close the incision. The needle should pass through the superficial layers only. This is sufficient for security purposes and avoids trauma to the endothelium. Any excess blood in the anterior chamber is irrigated and aspirated away during the suturing process;

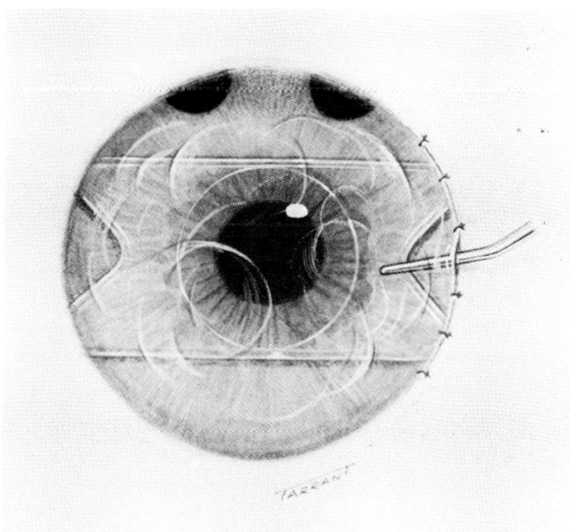

Fig. 9-9. Reinflation of anterior chamber with balanced saline solution.

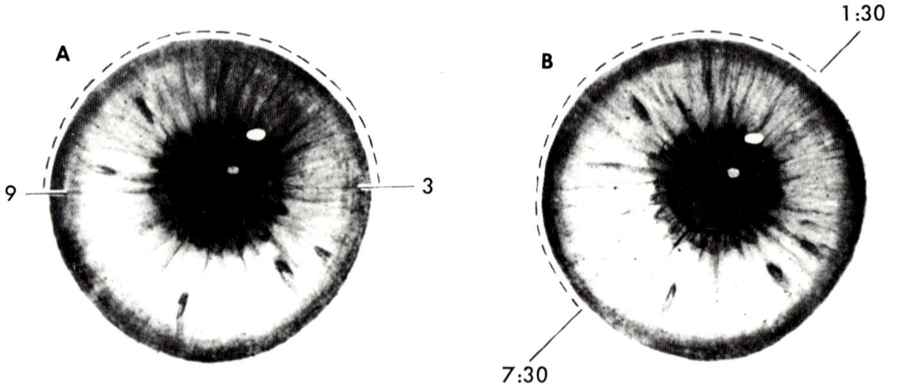

Fig. 9-10. Alteration of cataract incision axis if primary lens implantation planned (right eye illustrated). **A,** Routine cataract incision. **B,** Incision for primary lens implantation.

physiologic saline is used. When the suturing is finished, the implant should be very carefully centered by passing a synechia spatula between the sutures and exerting pressure on the upper or lower edge of the implant as necessary. Lastly, balanced salt solution is injected in sufficient quantities to reestablish the anterior chamber and push the iris behind the plane of the implant (Fig. 9-9). If the pupil is very constricted at the end of the operation, 2 drops of 1% cyclopentolate should be instilled to initiate postoperative mydriasis.

PRIMARY IMPLANTATION

My indications for primary anterior chamber implantation are (1) second eye, the first eye having been successfully implanted some time previously; and (2) poor general health and bad anesthetic risk for a two-stage procedure.

When confronted with the necessity for treating the second eye of a patient with a successful secondary implantation in the first eye, I insert an anterior chamber implant at the same time as the cataract is extracted. The experience gained with the first eye usually tells the surgeon both the length of implant required and the optical curve necessary.

Technically the operation is not difficult; convalescence is longer by several days than that following routine cataract surgery or secondary anterior chamber implant insertion. Primary insertion requires slight modification of my usual cataract extraction technique as follows: The 180° section should pass diagonally from the 10:30 to the 4:30 o'clock positions in the left eye, from the 7:30 to the 1:30 o'clock positions in the right eye (Fig. 9-10). I usually use a Graefe knife to make this incision; sometimes I have to enlarge it with corneal scissors. No conjunctival flap is cut. In an uncomplicated case, two basal peripheral iridectomies are made at the 11 and 1 o'clock positions. If circumstances require it, however, a sector iridectomy, with or without sphincterotomy, at the 6 o'clock position may be performed. Following appropriate treatment of the iris, two predelivery sutures are inserted at the 11 and 1 o'clock positions and the loops left long (Fig. 9-11).

Lens extraction is performed in the usual manner, either by the extracapsular method or the intracapsular method, according to the nature of the cataract. If the former procedure is used, it is very important that, so far as possible, all cortical remnants are irrigated from the eye before the implant is inserted.

Additional interrupted sutures are inserted to close off the nasal and superior part of the incision (Fig. 9-12). This will

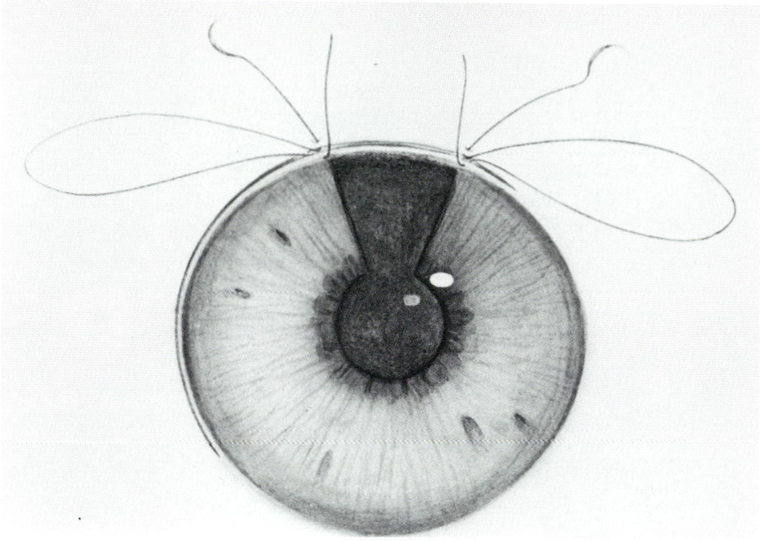

Fig. 9-11. Sector iridectomy and insertion of predelivery sutures.

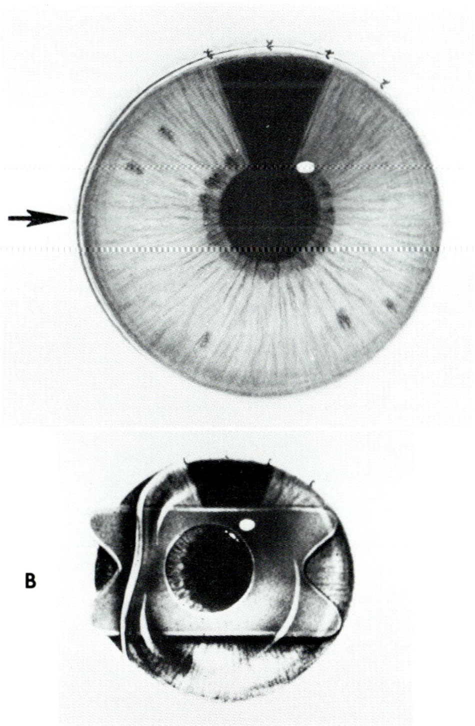

Fig. 9-12. A, Postextraction closure of upper and nasal parts of incision. Implant will be inserted temporally *(arrow)*. **B,** Insertion of implant.

leave a gap of about 8 mm temporally, which is adequate to permit introduction of the implant into the anterior chamber. If phacoemulsification has been performed, the incision must be enlarged to 8 mm to permit insertion of the implant. This is now done in the usual manner; a clear haptic implant will be used if a round pupil extraction has been performed, an implant with colored haptic being inserted if a sector iridectomy has been performed. Once all four feet of the implant are safely in the angle, the temporal part of the incision is closed with additional interrupted sutures (Fig. 9-13), the edges of the 180° incision are carefully probed with a fine spatula to ensure that no epithelium is in-turned, and balanced salt solution is injected through a fine cannula to reinflate the anterior chamber. Pilocarpine 4% drops are dropped on the cornea throughout this operation, after the cataract is extracted.

When I perform primary implantation I prefer to insert the implant either horizontally or diagonally. Tennant, however, has specialized in performing primary implantation vertically, that is, inserting the implant from 12 to 6 o'clock. Being a

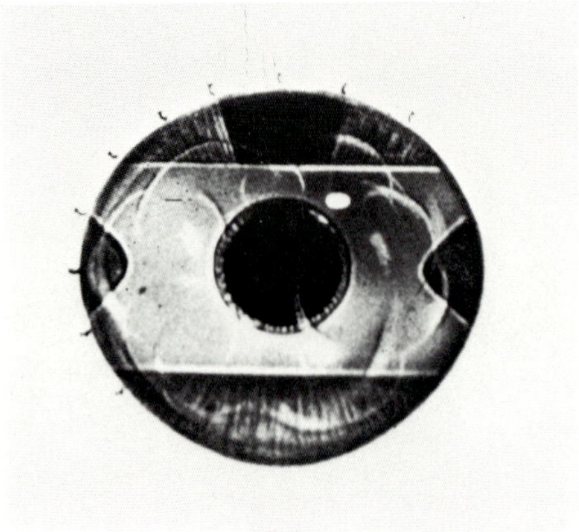

Fig. 9-13. Conclusion of primary implantation.

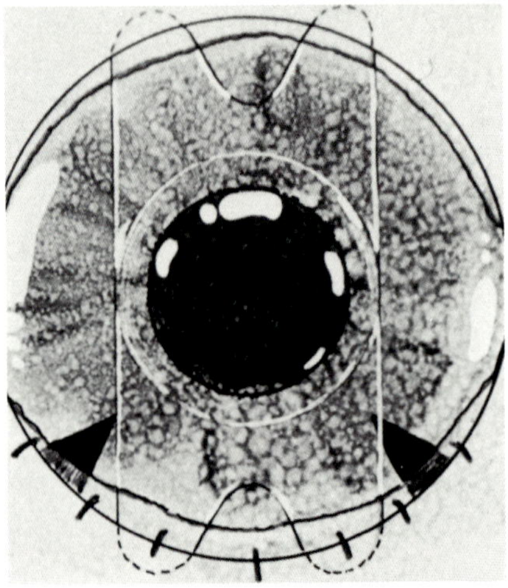

Fig. 9-14. Vertical insertion of Mark VIII implant. Implant length still equals *horizontal* corneal diameter + 1 mm. (Courtesy Dr. Jerald L. Tennant.)

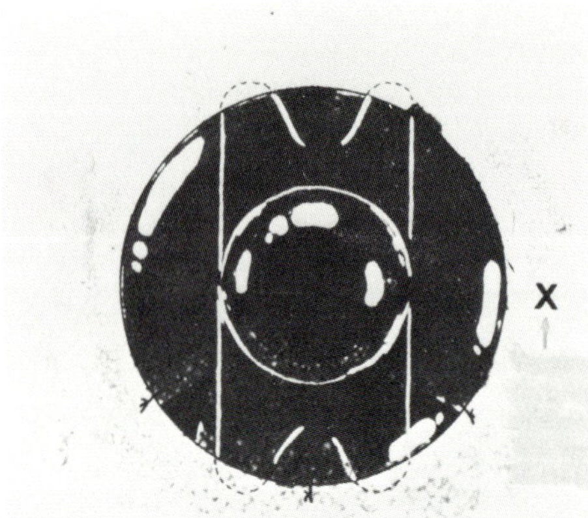

Fig. 9-15. Tap test to detect too short an implant at end of operation. Tap on sclera at *x*. Iris moves under lens, but lens itself is stable. (Courtesy Dr. Jerald L. Tennant.)

microsurgeon, he finds this approach easier. Two peripheral iridectomies are performed as far back as possible, that is, at 10 and 2 o'clock so that they are at least 8 mm apart, which is sufficient for the implant to be slid between them (Fig. 9-14).

The crux of the operation is the insertion of a fixed-length implant that is the right length for the individual eye. *How does the surgeon know this?* First, by adhering to the "horizontal corneal diameter plus 1 mm rule" regardless of the axis of insertion of the implant. Second, if the implant "falls" into the anterior chamber at the time of operation, it is very likely to be too short. Third, if the proximal feet stick out more than 1.5 mm over the scleral edge of a properly cut section, it is probably too long. Therefore, if in doubt, the surgeon should err on the side of too long rather than too short an implant. Clearly, experience is the best guide of all as to the correct length of implant to use. About one time in ten I find that the initial implant chosen is too long or too short and I have to go up or down 0.5 mm at the time of surgery before being satisfied.

Tennant has been responsible for devising two helpful tests for beginners in Mark VIII implantation—the "nudge" or "crotch" test after the implant has been inserted but before the incision has been sutured, and the "tap" test at the conclusion of the operation after reinflation of the anterior chamber—designed to detect that too short an implant has been inserted. In the nudge test, gentle downward movement with a spatula placed in the crotch should not bring the upper feet completely into view if the implant is the right length. If they are clearly seen then the implant is too short. The tap test, applied to the sclera in the region of the pars plana at right angles to the long axis of the inserted implant causes iridodonesis but not pseudophakodonesis, unless the implant is too short (Fig. 9-15).

INSERTION OF COLORED HAPTIC IMPLANTS

Colored haptic implants are used when there is a fairly substantial iris coloboma or a deformed pupil such as occurs after sphincterotomies have been performed. The insertion of a colored haptic implant is easier in one sense and more difficult in another. It is more difficult because, without a tight iris sphincter, extra care has to be taken not to roll up the iris or catch the pupil with the distal feet when the implant is slid across the anterior chamber. It is easier because it is easier to visualize the proximal feet when the time comes to guide them over the bevel or ledge into the angle beneath. With fairly substantial iris defects the question sometimes arises, Is it necessary for all four feet to have a backing of iris tissue? In practice it seems that iris tissue behind three of the four feet provides adequate support.

EXTERNAL-FIXATION IMPLANTS

It will be recalled that in 1960 I designed implants using a form of external fixation in aphakic patients with insufficient iris to prevent posterior dislocation of a standard anterior chamber implant, at that time the Choyce Mark V being the one in regular use. Since then the Mark VIII implant has been adapted for this purpose; implants for external fixation have loops at either one end or both ends and, on the whole, I think the 2-loop variety is the most successful (Fig. 9-16). However, the details of the use of these implants is outside the scope of this chapter, and readers are referred to Chapters 5, 11, and 25 in my monograph.[2]

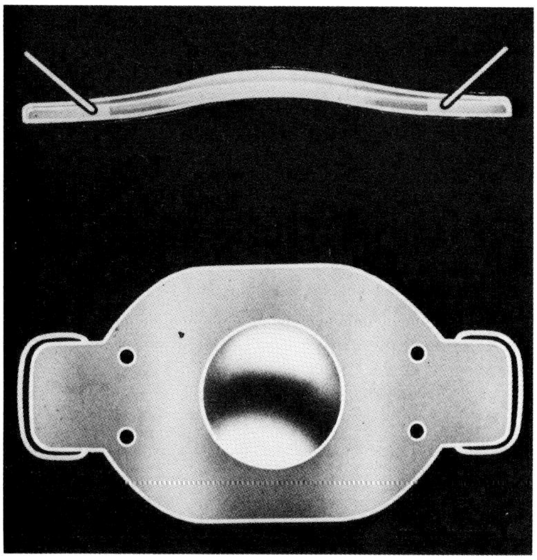

Fig. 9-16. Two-loop external-fixation Mark VIII implant.

COMPLICATIONS

1. Hyphema can be troublesome. The patient should be placed on bedrest, and I prescribe acetazolamide and mydriatics. The implant should not be disturbed unless the intraocular pressure is markedly raised for at least 2 to 3 weeks.

2. Bulging of the iris in front of the margins of the implant may occur, and if it does, it suggests that adequate apertures in the iris were not made or wound closure is imperfect so that some leakage of aqueous is occurring, and the section should be very closely examined with that possibility in mind. If the iris bulge persists for more than a few days and there is no leakage from the section, an additional ab externo peripheral iridectomy over the apex of the bulging iris should be performed and the anterior chamber reinflated with balanced salt solution. However, it is reassuring to know that even in this situation the implant cannot move forward to contact the endothelium.

3. Sometimes foreign body iridocy-

clitis is a little marked, in which case oral prednisolone is prescribed.

It is important to stress the vital importance of good mydriasis during the postoperative phase.

From hospital discharge up to 6 months

1. A low-grade iridocyclitis may persist and must be treated on the same lines as before.

2. The implant may reveal itself to be too short because it tends to revolve round the anterior chamber like a propeller. Pseudophakodonesis may also be present, which is not the case if the implant is a snug fit. Very often the implant that is a little too short eventually takes up a constant position and the eye gradually settles down and can be left alone, so there is no immediate urgency even if it is suspected that too short an implant has been inserted, but if after 3 to 6 months it is quite clear that this implant is manifestly too short and is acting as a loose foreign body in the anterior chamber, it must be removed and replaced with one at least 1 mm longer.

From 6 months to 14 years*

1. Slight deformation of the pupil sometimes occurs, usually becoming oval in the long axis of the implant. This suggests, however, that the implant used was a little on the long side or that, when it was inserted, a portion of peripheral iris was trapped by one of the feet. This is not a serious complication and does not interfere with the visual result.

2. Occasionally iridocyclitis occurs, particularly in eyes that were subject to this before surgery.

3. Rare cases of endothelial corneal dystrophy will be seen, but with the increasing use of a specular microscope for screening purposes before surgery, it is hoped that this occurrence will be infrequent.

An independent investigation of Choyce's cases by his colleague, John Pearce, disclosed an incidence of 1.5% of corneal dystrophy after an average follow-up period of 6 years.

INDICATIONS FOR REMOVAL OF AN IMPLANT

1. An implant that is too short and acting as a loose foreign body in the anterior chamber

2. Chronic iritis, most likely to be seen in those who suffer from chronic iritis before implantation

3. Subsequent trauma leading to hyphema with secondary glaucoma

If a Mark VIII implant has to be removed, it should be possible to remove it with comparative ease without seriously traumatizing the eye.

CONCLUSIONS

After a long latent interval—it was designed and used in 1963—the Mark VIII implant is now receiving a great deal of attention. It is likely to be more widely used in the future. What are the reasons for this?

1. Though designed as a secondary implant, for which purpose it is acknowledged to be the most suitable, contemporary studies by Choyce, Tennant, and many others show that it makes a very satisfactory primary implant.

2. It is the only pseudophakos that can be equipped with colored and opaque haptic portions.

3. It can be used following intracapsular or extracapsular extraction or following phacoemulsification.

4. The presence of vitreous in the anterior chamber is not a contraindication to its use.

5. Technically it is probably the easiest pseudophakos to insert and is certainly the easiest to remove.

6. No costly instrumentation is required; the use of an operating microscope is not essential. Loupes (4×) provide adequate magnification.

*This is the maximum time available for observation, since the Mark VIII implant was introduced in 1963.

7. A skillful and resourceful surgeon can perform Mark VIII implantation without a trained assistant.

8. There is so far no sign of a significantly raised incidence of endothelial corneal dystrophy.

For all of these reasons the Mark VIII anterior chamber implant has a wide appeal, particularly in those parts of the world where simplicity and speed of execution and the relative absence of complications are desired.

REFERENCES

1. Tornquist, R.: Shallow anterior chamber in acute glaucoma: a clinical and genetic study, Acta Ophthalmol. [Suppl.] (Kbh) vol. 39, 1953.
2. Choyce, D. P.: Intra-ocular lenses and implants, ed. 1, London, 1964, H. K. Lewis & Co.

CHAPTER 10

Surgery in special situations

This chapter will consider the propriety of lens implantation in special situations. It would be impossible to prognosticate every eventuality, but an attempt has been made to deal with some of the more frequently found clinical problems.

SECONDARY LENS IMPLANTATION

Secondary lens implantation is defined as the implantation of an intraocular lens in an eye that has previously been rendered aphakic. Primary lens implantation has evolved to the point of acceptance by a wide segment of the ophthalmic community. Secondary lens implantation, on the other hand, is currently one of the most controversial areas in the field of lens implant surgery.

Risk is inherent in any surgical procedure, and though cataract surgery enjoys a high success rate, it is not without complications. Responsible surgeons evaluate the patient's visual needs against the risk of surgery before deciding to operate, irrespective of whether an intraocular lens is used in the primary procedure.

When a patient is already aphakic, we have an eye capable of good vision with the appropriate optical correction. Yet there are monocular aphakic patients who, because of their inability to wear a contact lens, have achieved no benefit from cataract extraction and may indeed be worse visually. This class of patients could be considered candidates for a secondary lens implantation in their aphakic eye if they have some significant disability due to their monocular status. One could question the argument, however, that binocularity is essential for a normal life.

Most ophthalmologists have monocular patients who are gainfully employed and leading normal lives. If one considers only trauma and amblyopia as causes of monocular vision, there must be a considerable percentage of the population who only have one functioning eye and experience little visual difficulty.

In our combined experience we have resorted to secondary lens implantation in no more than 2% of our cases. There are, however, situations in which the risk of a secondary lens implant is justified. Before stating indications, it must be stressed that aphakia per se is *not* an indication, Second, if a patient is successfully wearing a contact lens, even though it is a nuisance and a bother to him, secondary lens implantation is *not* indicated. A bilaterally aphakic patient should not be subjected to a secondary lens implantation in both eyes because of the known complications of vitreous loss and the risk of corneal decompensation due to the endothelial cell population being depleted beyond viability.[1]

Indications

There are no specific indications; each case must be evaluated on its own merits. Reasonable indications include the following:

1. A child unilaterally aphakic due to trauma or congenital cataract, in the age range where amblyopia is expected. This is a contentious subject (discussed in Chapter 11), which comes down to

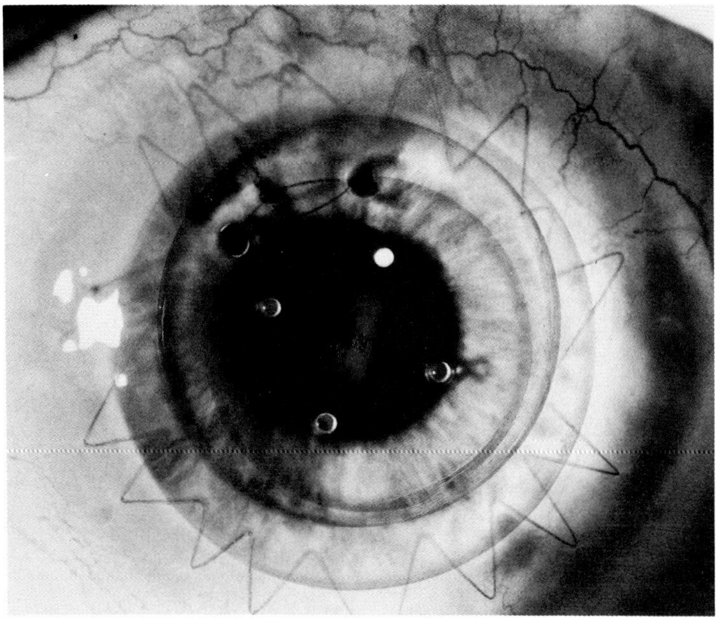

Fig. 10-1. Combined keratoplasty with secondary insertion of Worst Medallion lens implant.

whether the implant will last a lifetime without damage to the ocular structures versus the burden of irreversible amblyopia.

2. A monocular aphake, without any sign of cataract in the fellow eye, who is unable to wear a contact lens and absolutely requires binocular vision for occupational purposes.

3. A patient severely handicapped by monocular vision who is fully cognizant of the potential risks and knowingly undertakes them.

4. Special situations such as the monocular aphake who develops aphakic bullous keratopathy. After a successful keratoplasty, great difficulty will probably be experienced in fitting this patient with a contact lens. If the patient cannot wear a contact lens, no benefit will have been gained from the operation. If technically feasible, it is not illogical to insert a lens implant at the time of keratoplasty through the graft site. Fig. 10-1 shows a patient who had an opaque cornea after cataract surgery treated with an 8 mm penetrating keratoplasty combined with the secondary insertion of a Worst Medallion lens implant.

Unique circumstances can arise that challenge the surgeon, but should only be undertaken by surgeons of experience and substantial technical ability. Fig. 10-2, *A*, shows a patient operated on for cataract, who subsequently had an iris prolapse under a limbus-based flap. The patient was under the impression the eye was lost because it was never optically corrected, an understandable situation inasmuch as the patient had in excess of 16 D of astigmatism. The wound was explored, and prolapsed uvea was excised. The net result was a sufficiently viable iris to support a Binkhorst iris-clip lens implant inserted as a secondary implantation. The site of the excised iris prolapse was utilized as the peripheral iridectomy (Fig. 10-2, *B*).

At this point it should be stated that D. Peter Choyce has a completely different view of secondary lens implantation and considered lens implant surgery to be a

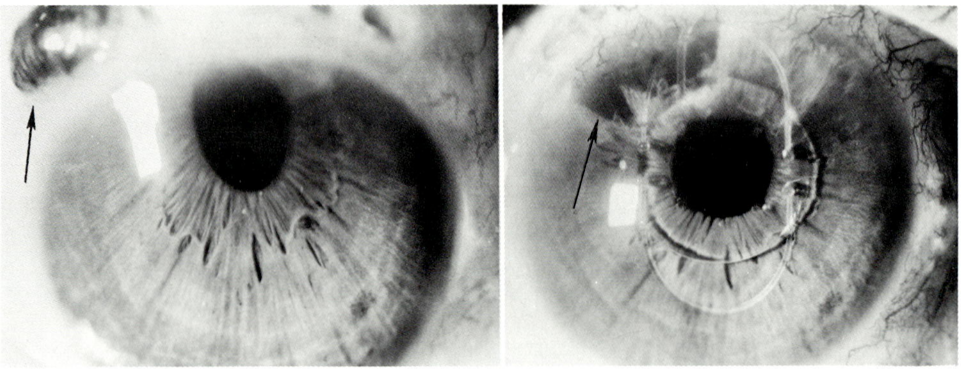

Fig. 10-2. A, Aphakic patient with iris prolapse *(arrow)* under conjunctival flap. **B,** Same patient after reconstruction of previous section and secondary insertion of Binkhorst iris-clip lens implant. Peripheral iridectomy *(arrow)* coincides with site of excised iris prolapse.

two-stage operation, with initial cataract extraction followed by lens implant insertion at a later date. Choyce discusses his views and techniques in Chapter 9, using the Choyce Mark VIII implant. *Other* techniques will be discussed here.

Techniques

Generally an intact posterior capsule makes secondary lens implantation easier, as the surgeon does not have to contend with the vitreous. Many implant surgeons prefer to avoid the initial incision because of possible bleb formation, wound leak, and unpredictable astigmatism. The alternatives would be a temporal section or a corneal incision. With a temporal section, care must be taken to avoid going to scleral. One can encounter serious and persistent bleeding from the long choroidal vessels with a posterior, temporal incision. Fig. 10-3 shows a Binkhorst iris-clip lens implant inserted as a secondary procedure through a small corneal incision.

Secondary lens implantation following an extracapsular cataract extraction. This applies only if the posterior capsule is intact. If a discission has been performed or the capsule has ruptured, the case should be managed as if it were an intracapsular extraction. Even though the posterior capsule is intact, in a secondary lens implantation the surgeon cannot be secure in expecting capsular fixation. Our choice would be to use a Binkhorst iridocapsular implant in this circumstance, with the proximal loop sutured to the iris stroma (p. 89). If peripheral iridectomies were performed at the initial procedure, it is not necessary to make additional openings. Alternatively, the Binkhorst iris-clip implant can be used. It offers better fixation, and with an intact posterior capsule a transiridectomy suture is not required. Posterior synechiae should be lysed as required to permit implant insertion, and care should be taken to avoid damage to the iris sphincter. Both model Binkhorst implants have the capability of being inserted through 7 mm incisions. The Worst platinum-clip implant can also be used, but may be troublesome if inserted in a horizontal position through a temporal section. The lens can pivot downward, and the clip could conceivably be displaced forward during horizontal eye movements, with resultant corneal touch.

Secondary lens implantation following a round pupil intracapsular cataract extraction. In this area of intraocular surgery the vitreous need not be feared, but it should be respected. Various types of automated equipment have been devised for the anterior segment to remove vitreous, yet

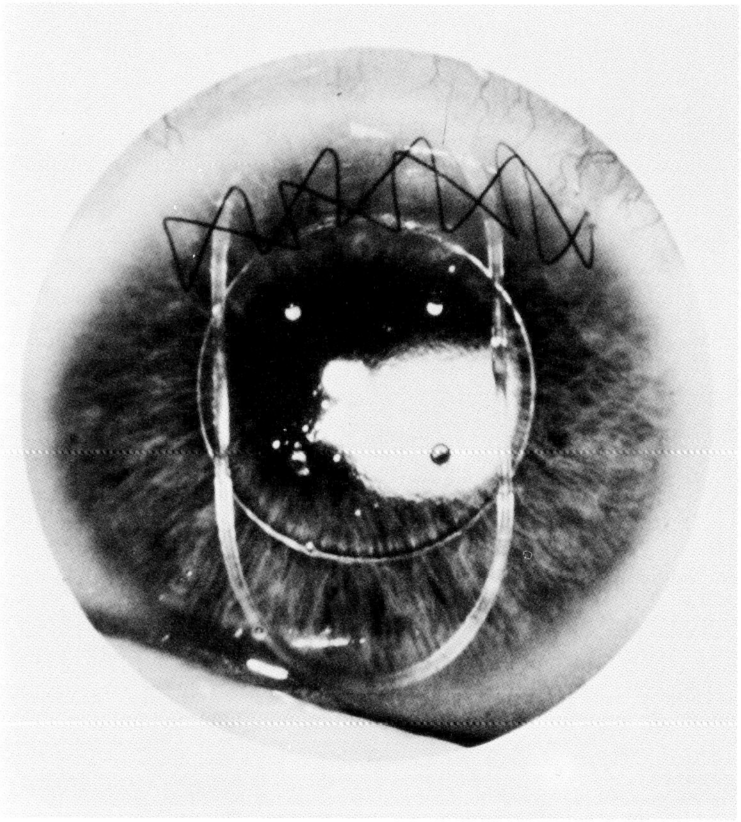

Fig. 10-3. Secondary implantation of Binkhorst iris-clip lens implant through a corneal incision.

vitreous is a living tissue. The surgeon should be mindful of the consequences of vitreous loss, such as the increased incidence of retinal detachment and cystoid macular edema, before undertaking a secondary lens implantation in an eye previously subjected to intracapsular cataract surgery. The preoperative exam is most important. If there is a substantial amount of free vitreous in the anterior chamber, we would not perform the procedure, a view not shared by Choyce. If the anterior hyaloid face is intact and posterior to the pupil, a secondary implant can be performed if care is taken to ensure that the anterior hyaloid face does not come forward. To this effect a Flieringa ring is desirable in conjunction with preoperative hyperosmotic agents. Judicious digital pressure is also helpful (p. 74). If the incision is large enough, any of the intracapsular lens implants could be used, but it seems prudent to use a small incision and to avoid the necessity of iris sutures because of the additional manipulation required over an exposed anterior hyaloid face. In this situation we would use a Binkhorst iris-clip lens implant without a transiridectomy suture. The Binkhorst forceps are difficult to use through a small incision, and Clayman or Shepard forceps (p. 77) are advantageous in this circumstance.

Transitional cases between an anterior chamber full of vitreous and an intact anterior hyaloid face well posterior must be individually evaluated as to the feasibility of implant insertion balanced against a critical appraisal of the patient's visual needs.

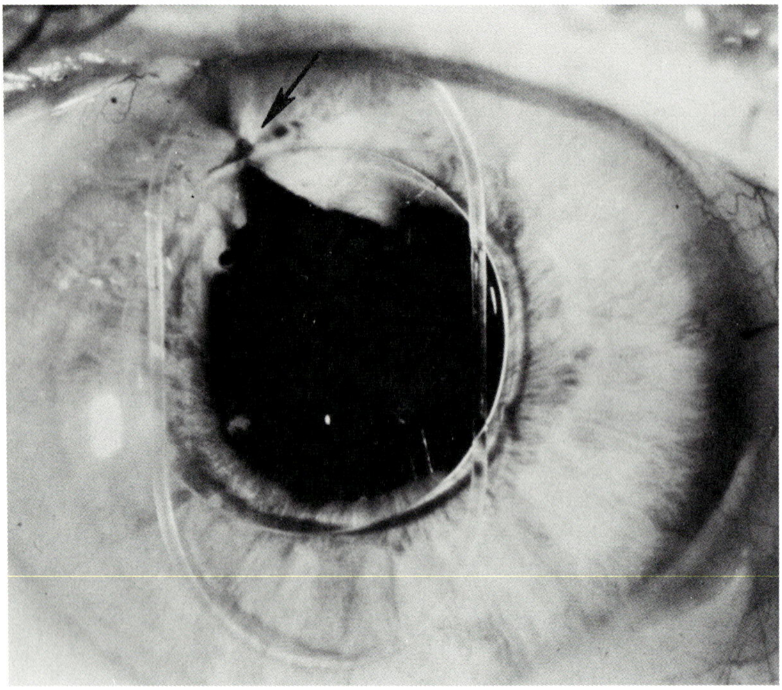

Fig. 10-4. Secondary implantation of Binkhorst iris-clip lens implant after surgical repair of iris coloboma *(arrow)*.

Secondary lens implantation following an intracapsular cataract extraction with a sector iridectomy. The iris coloboma has to be repaired prior to lens implant insertion for all currently available lens implants except the Choyce Mark VIII. If more than one-third of the iris is missing, the repair should not be undertaken. Furthermore, any vitreous bulge makes this a difficult operation that should not be performed unless the surgeon is prepared for vitreous loss and its consequences. The technique is discussed in Chapter 12. Briefly a 10-0 nylon or polypropylene suture is placed through the pillars of the iris coloboma approximately 2 mm distal to the sphincter. The reason for this is that if the pupil is too miotic, after the suture is tied it may pull out as the implant is being inserted. The suture is tightened, tied, and trimmed, thus reforming the pupil while maintaining an opening peripherally to function as a peripheral iridectomy. It is difficult to perform an iris repair through a small incision, and therefore the incision should be enlarged as the case dictates. We would again insert a Binkhorst iris-clip lens implant in this situation without a transiridectomy suture. Fig. 10-4 shows a Binkhorst iris-clip lens implant secondarily inserted after repair of an iris coloboma.

Summary

Secondary lens implantation should be undertaken only with great caution and conservatism. The surgeon is operating on an eye already capable of seeing well, and both the surgeon and the patient should realize that there is a possibility that the procedure may make the patient worse. Nevertheless there are patients who would benefit from secondary lens implantation, but in our experiences these patients have comprised a small fraction of the total number of implant insertions.

BILATERAL LENS IMPLANTATION

The situation faced here is whether an implant should be inserted in the second eye when the first is already pseudophakic. It is our opinion that an implant may be inserted in the second eye if the first eye fared well over a reasonable period of time, but prudence is advised. Clayman analyzed 730 cases with well-documented follow-up.[2] This data included current Binkhorst and Worst implant series together with Jaffe's previously published experiences with the Copeland lens implant.[3] Forty-four (6%) of the 730 patients had bilateral implants, and of these, 88% of the patients had consecutive surgery more than 1 year apart and 50% more than 2 years apart. Table 10-1 shows the final visual acuities with follow up ranging from 6 months to 8 years. Eighty-six percent of the bilateral implant patients obtained a visual acuity of 20/40 or better in the first eye, and 83% had 20/40 or better in the second eye. The predominant cause of visual acuity less than 20/40 was senile macular choroidal degeneration (Table 10-2). Figs. 10-5 and 10-6 show representative bilateral implant cases.

Table 10-1. Final visual acuity following bilateral implants in 44 of 730 patients*

Visual acuity	First eye	Second eye
20/20 to 20/40	86%	83%
20/50 to 20/400	10%	10%
<20/400	4%	7%

*From Clayman, H., Jaffe, N., Light, D., and Eichenbaum, D.: Lens implantation in surgery in the second eye, Ophthalmic Surg. 8:45-48, 1977.

Table 10-2. Visual acuity of <20/40 in 14 eyes following bilateral implants in 44 of 730 patients*

Cause	No. eyes
Senile macular choroidal degeneration	7
Cystoid macular edema	4
Diabetic retinopathy	1
Ischemic optic neuropathy	1
Keratopathy	1

*From Clayman, H., Jaffe, N., Light, D., and Eichenbaum, D.: Lens implantation in surgery in the second eye, Ophthalmic Surg. 8:45-48, 1977.

A

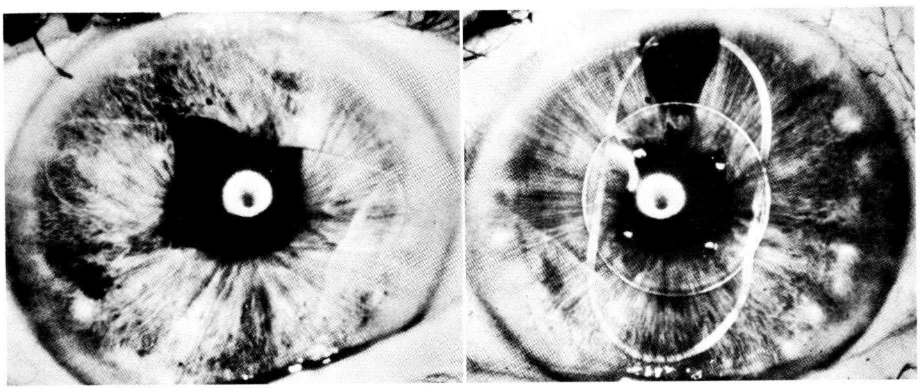

B

Fig. 10-5. Patient with bilateral lens implant. **A,** Copeland lens in right eye. **B,** Binkhorst iris-clip lens implant in left eye. (From Clayman, H. M., Jaffe, N. S., Light, D. S., and Eichenbaum, D. M.: Ophthalmic Surg. 8:45, 1977.)

A 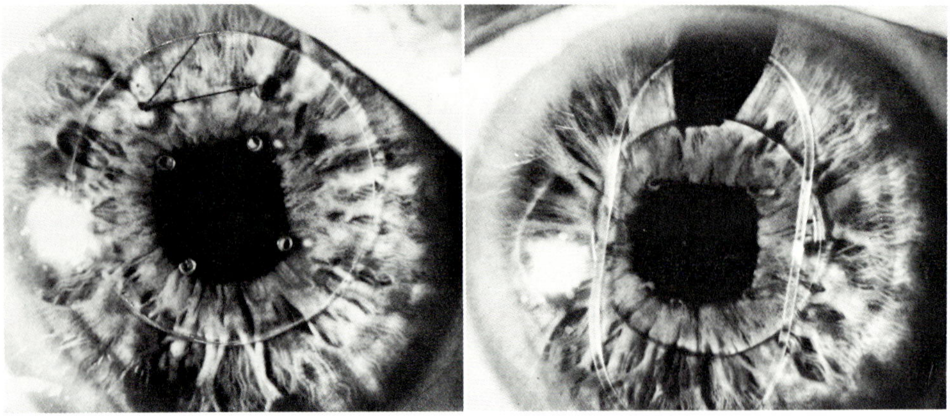 B

Fig. 10-6. Patient with bilateral implants. **A,** Worst Medallion lens implant in right eye. **B,** Binkhorst iris-clip lens implant in left eye. (From Clayman, H. M., Jaffe, N. S., Light, D. S., and Eichenbaum, D. M.: Ophthalmic Surg. **8**:45, 1977.)

Table 10-3. Indications and contraindications for lens implant in second eye*

Indications	Contraindications
Young patient (60 to 67 yr)	Elderly patient managing well with one eye
Patient troubled by cataract in second eye	Any patient satisfied with current status
Active patient	Poor result in first eye
Occupational	

*From Clayman, H., Jaffe, N., Light, D., and Eichenbaum, D.: Lens implantation in surgery in the second eye, Ophthalmic Surg. **8**:45-48, 1977.

Indications and contraindications for bilateral lens implant insertion are given in Table 10-3. Admittedly these are nonspecific and rather general because ultimately the decision to operate on the second eye must rest with the surgeon and the individual patient's visual needs. A conservative approach is advised whereby the interval between operating on the first and second eyes is of sufficient length that the outcome of the first operation may be reasonably ascertained.

COMBINED CATARACT EXTRACTION AND KERATOPLASTY WITH IMPLANT INSERTION

The patient with *unilaterally* significant corneal disease and a cataract poses a problem when visual rehabilitation is required. There is a substantial length of time following combined keratoplasty and cataract extraction to ultimate visual recovery. This is even longer if a two-stage procedure is performed, with an interval of several months between operations. If the patient cannot be fitted with a contact lens postoperatively, then the operation would have been to no avail. Since astigmatism postkeratoplasty can be excessive, there is a definite probability that a contact lens will not be tolerated.

It is reasonable to consider lens implant insertion in conjunction with the cataract extraction and keratoplasty, assuming no other ocular contraindications. The presence of an implant in such cases can be beneficial, inasmuch as the vitreous is held back behind the iris-pseudophakos diaphragm, precluding vitreous touch to the endothelial surface of the graft. Calculation of lens implant power is often difficult because presumably the condition of the cornea makes accurate keratometry difficult (p. 60). A history of previous refraction is helpful here.

Another consideration is what model lens implant should be used. Since the technique described below utilizes an intracapsular cataract extraction through the keratoplasty site, the implant must be

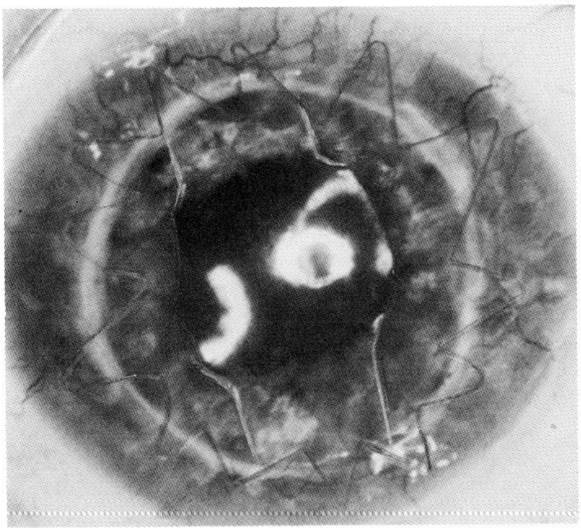

Fig. 10-7. Postoperative appearance of patient who had combined cataract extraction and keratoplasty with insertion of Copeland lens implant.

amenable to this technique, and the Binkhorst iridocapsular lens implant would not be suitable. Furthermore, the length of the Choyce Mark VIII implant makes it unwieldy to insert through the keratoplasty opening. The Binkhorst iris-clip, the Fyodorov sputnik, the Fyodorov-Binkhorst, the Copeland, the Worst Medallion, and the Worst platinum-clip implants all can be inserted in conjunction with a cataract extraction and keratoplasty.[4,5] Difficulty may be experienced with the platinum-clip implant in manipulating the clip under the shelf of the host cornea at the keratoplasty site. Our experience has shown that the Copeland implant (Fig. 10-7) or the Binkhorst iris-clip implant are technically the easiest under these circumstances. The latter is inserted without a transiridectomy suture; however, an iris stromal suture may be used to anchor either the superior or inferior anterior loops to the iris stroma.

Technique

A soft eye is essential, and adequate digital pressure should be applied. Hyperosmotic agents may be administered if the patient's general medical condition permits. We routinely perform a lateral canthotomy and use a 19 mm Flieringa ring sutured to each scleral quadrant with an interrupted 7-0 black silk suture. The intraocular pressure is monitored with a Schiøtz tonometer, and the eye is not entered until a scale reading of at least 15 with a 5.5 g weight is attained. These cases are difficult technically, and great care should be exercised with these preliminaries. The first question is what size graft to use. The patient's corneal bed must be of sufficient size to permit both cataract extraction and implant insertion. We do not advise less than an 8.5 mm graft. After the donor corneal button is trephined, the trephine is placed on the patient's cornea in the desired position. No attempt is made to trephine a full thickness button of host cornea, but rather a mark is made with the trephine, which is then slightly tipped in one quadrant to enter the anterior chamber. Conversely, the chamber can be entered with a razor knife in the line of the trephine. The dissection of the corneal button is completed with right- and left-handed curved corneal section scissors. Peripheral iridotomies are performed by reaching under the superior shelf of the host cornea and snipping the iris with microscissors. The cataract is then extracted with a cryoprobe through a dilated pupil, and acetylcholine is instilled into the anterior chamber to reconstrict the pupil. The implant is inserted.

If the Binkhorst iris-clip lens implant is used, Jaffe's technique (p. 78) is advantageous with one modification. Instead of holding the implant with Binkhorst cross-action forceps, an anterior loop, either upper or lower, is grasped with utility forceps. The contralateral set of loops is clipped onto the iris at whichever position is most convenient, and the implant is then released. The other set of loops is maneuvered into position by displacing the implant with a Jaffe spatula until the posterior loop clears the pupillary margin, at which point the iris is allowed to pass between the two loops as the implant springs back from its displaced position. Forceps may be used to facilitate this.

The donor corneal button is then placed in the recipient corneal bed and approximated with eight interrupted 10-0 nylon sutures. A running 10-0 nylon suture is placed in a purse-string fashion, taking a sufficient number of bites to ensure wound closure. Infra-Tenon's corticosteroid is injected at the conclusion of the procedure,[6] and topical corticosteroid drops are prescribed postoperatively. In the subsequent months the interrupted sutures may gradually be removed, but the running suture can be left indefinitely unless its presence excites corneal vascularization.

Related situations

The patient with a previous keratoplasty and a cataract is another type of case in which the surgeon may consider implant insertion, although the prognosis is less favorable. With a routine cataract extraction a previous corneal graft may deteriorate from the trauma of surgery. Decompensation can also occur from subsequent vitreocorneal endothelial touch. The surgeon does not have to contend with this or aphakia after an implant is inserted. On the other hand, lens implant surgery requires more manipulation than routine cataract surgery, and its effect on the corneal endothelium has been documented (p. 186). Implant insertion

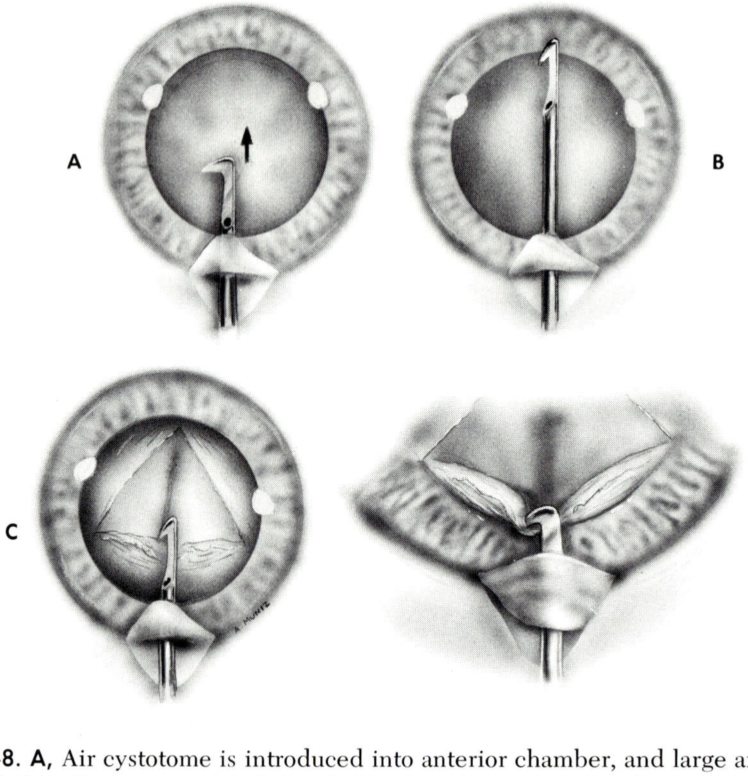

Fig. 10-8. A, Air cystotome is introduced into anterior chamber, and large air bubble is instilled. **B,** Cystotome extended to 6 o'clock position. **C,** Point of cystotome engages anterior capsule and is withdrawn superiorly, forming a Christmas tree–shaped wedge of capsule. **D,** Apex of torn capsule being withdrawn to limbal wound. (From Jaffe, N. S.: Cataract surgery and its complications, ed. 2, St. Louis, 1976, The C. V. Mosby Co.)

can cause decompensation of a previous corneal graft.

Some authors[4] have reported relatively good results with implant insertion in the presence of a previous keratoplasty; however, the series has been small with a relatively short follow-up. A definitive statement cannot be made as to whether an implant is indicated in this circumstance. The surgeon's own judgment and experience should be the guide.

PHACOEMULSIFICATION AND LENS IMPLANTS

The first decision in cataract surgery is whether an intracapsular or extracapsular cataract extraction should be performed. If the surgeon chooses the extracapsular procedure, then the technique of extracapsular extraction is the next decision. The standard extracapsular extraction with implant insertion has been described in Chapter 8 (p. 83) and elsewhere.[7] Does phacoemulsification offer the *implant* surgeon any advantages?

The technique of phacoemulsification requires a 3 mm incision into the anterior chamber at the surgical limbus. An irrigating cystotome is introduced through this opening, and an anterior capsulectomy is performed (Fig. 10-8). The nucleus is then engaged with the cystotome and prolapsed into the anterior chamber (Fig. 10-9), whereupon the cystotome is

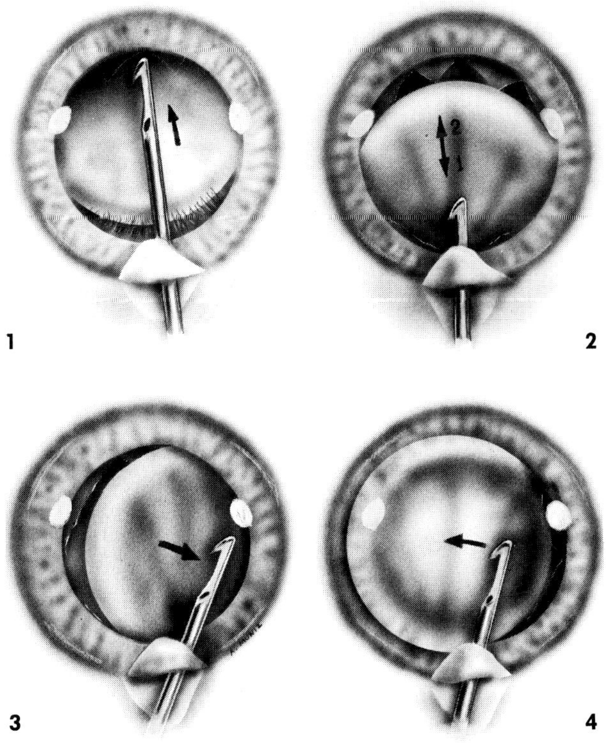

Fig. 10-9. Point of cystotome engages nucleus, and through a vertical seesaw maneuver (or, if necessary, a lateral seesaw), nucleus is prolapsed into anterior chamber. (From Jaffe, N. S.: Cataract surgery and its complications, ed. 2, St. Louis, 1976, The C. V. Mosby Co.)

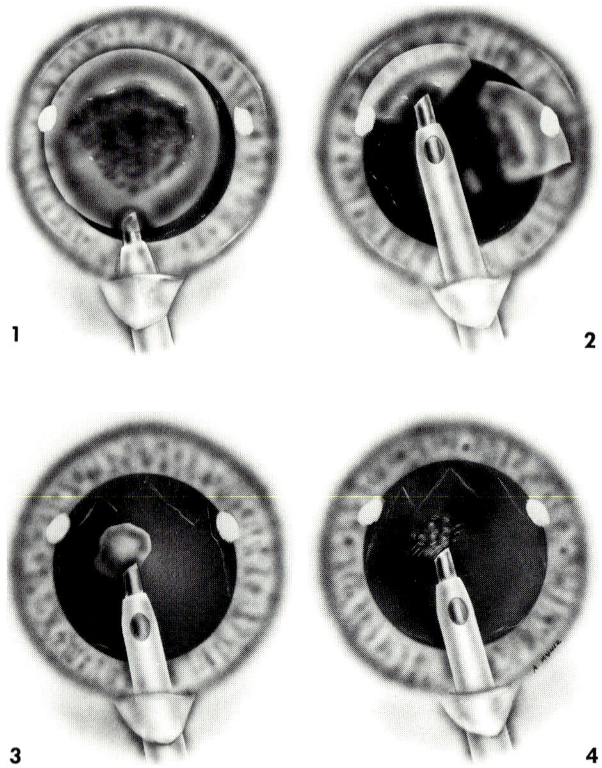

Fig. 10-10. Ultrasonic tip performing emulsification and aspiration. (From Jaffe, N. S.: Cataract surgery and its complications, ed. 2, St. Louis, 1976, The C. V. Mosby Co.)

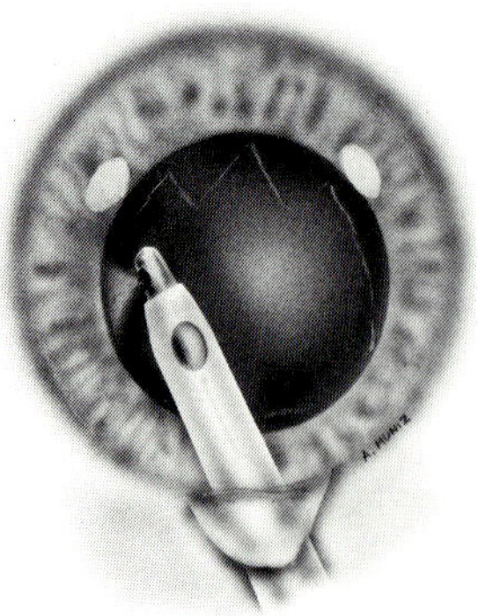

Fig. 10-11. The nonultrasonic tip is used with only irrigation and aspiration to clear out cortical remnants. (From Jaffe, N. S.: Cataract surgery and its complications, ed. 2, St. Louis, 1976, The C. V. Mosby Co.)

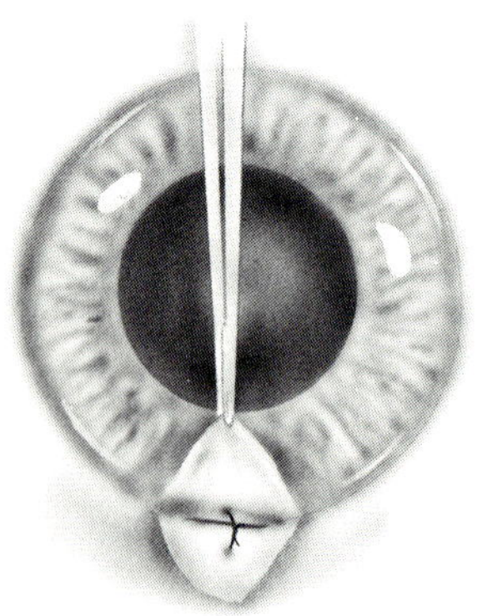

Fig. 10-12. Incision closed with one suture. (From Jaffe, N. S.: Cataract surgery and its complications, ed. 2, St. Louis, 1976, The C. V. Mosby Co.)

withdrawn from the eye. The ultrasonic tip of the Cavitron/Kelman phacoemulsifier is passed through the 3 mm incision, and the nucleus is emulsified and aspirated (Fig. 10-10). Cortical remnants are removed with an irrigating, aspirating tip (Fig. 10-11). A peripheral iridectomy is made through the original incision, which is then closed with a single suture (Fig. 10-12).

When this procedure is performed satisfactorily, the postoperative care and convalescence are minimal. The aphakic correction can be prescribed as early as 3 weeks after surgery. We feel that the rapid physical and visual rehabilitation is due to the 3 mm incision rather than the extracapsular technique or an intact posterior capsule. Kelman and others are routinely performing a posterior capsulotomy or capsulectomy at the initial procedure in a large percentage of their cases because of late posterior capsule opacification in many patients.[8]

Phacoemulsification is not easy, and the main advantage is lost when the 3 mm incision has to be enlarged to at least 6 to 7 mm to permit insertion of a lens implant into the anterior chamber. Additionally, one has to contend with corneal endo-

A B C D

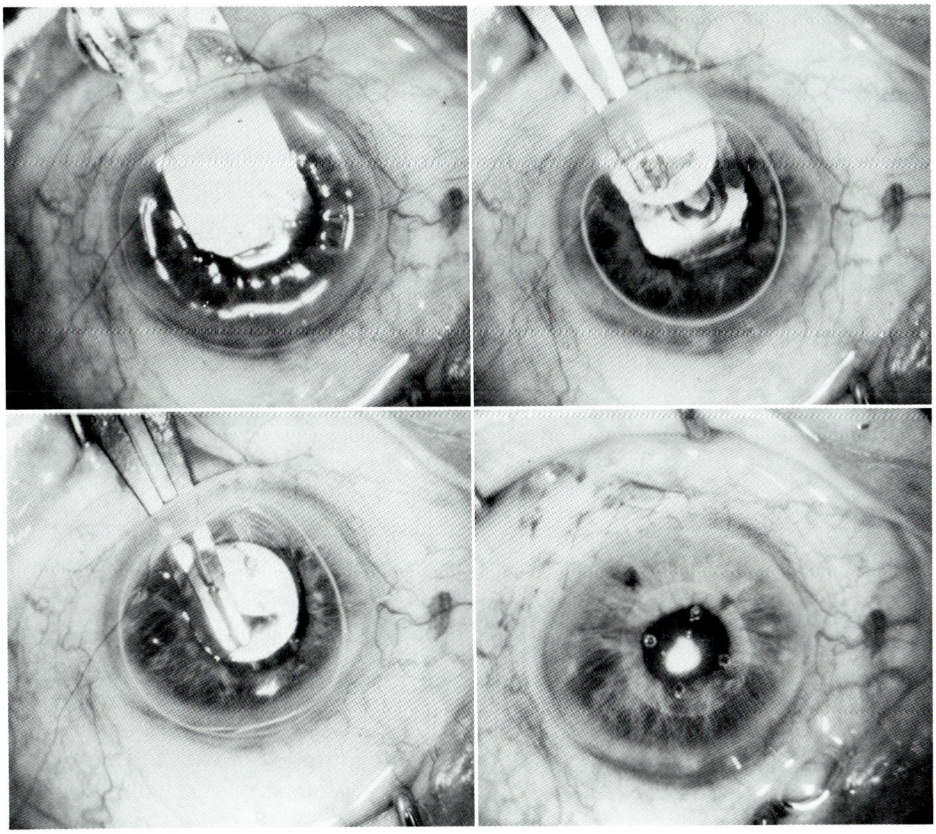

Fig. 10-13. Lens implantation after phacoemulsification. **A,** Sheets glide in situ. Binkhorst iridocapsular lens implant being introduced into the anterior chamber through a small incision after phacoemulsification. **B,** Implant within anterior chamber. Sheets glide still in situ. **C,** Inferior loop of implant under iris guided into position along plane of Sheets glide. **D,** Lens in situ with sutures placed in "triple X" wound closure. (Courtesy Dr. John H. Sheets.)

thelial trauma from both lens implantation[1,9] and increased instrumentation and irrigation.[10] Hirschman combined phacoemulsification with several hundred cases of lens implantation. He continues to use phacoemulsification, within its indications, for cataract extraction without lens implantation. However, when an implant is to be inserted, he prefers a microsurgical adaptation of the standard extracapsular technique, which he feels gives more consistent results and is technically easier.

In the hands of several outstanding surgeons phacoemulsification with lens implantation enjoys results that compare favorably with any other surgical technique (Fig. 10-13), but for the colleague of average ability and surgical load, who does neither phacoemulsification or lens implantation regularly, the combination could be hazardous. Since both techniques are still controversial, additional pressures are placed upon the surgeon.

GLAUCOMA AND LENS IMPLANTATION

Two questions arise when a glaucoma patient is considered for lens implant surgery. Does preexisting glaucoma contraindicate lens implant surgery? If not, should the surgery be modified?

First, we would *not* insert an implant in a case where the patient is on maximum topical and systemic therapy and still has an unacceptable intraocular pressure. It would be naive to expect the cataract surgery with lens implantation will have a beneficial effect on uncontrolled glaucoma, assuming that the angle is open. Any subsequent iritis may compound the underlying disease and place the surgeon in a therapeutic dilemma. The traditional treatment for iritis, mydriatics and cortisone derivatives, has significant drawbacks in this situation. Mydriatics may cause the implant to dislocate, and cortisone or its analogs can increase the intraocular pressure in susceptible patients.[11]

In uncontrolled glaucoma a combined cataract extraction and filtering procedure in conjunction with lens implantation is dangerous. First, the patient may have a flat or shallow anterior chamber in the postoperative period. Combined cataract surgery and trabeculectomy has been described[12] and supposedly has a low incidence of anterior chamber shallowing, but a flat or shallow anterior chamber after trabeculectomy can occur. This would be a significant problem with a lens implant in situ because the implant would be in contact with the corneal endothelium. The deleterious effects of physical contact between polymethylmethacrylate and corneal endothelium has been studied.[9] The usual treatment for a flat chamber, pressure patching and maximal dilatation, is often unsatisfactory. The former will push the corneal endothelium further against the implant, and the latter can cause the implant to dislocate.

The second point against combined glaucoma, cataract, and lens implant surgery is that the glaucoma phase of the operation may not succeed. The net result is a patient with an implant and uncontrolled glaucoma. All the currently available glaucoma medications have some disadvantages. It is our clinical impression that implant patients on chronic miotic therapy have a higher incidence of retrolenticular membranes (p. 177) and synechiae. Topical epinephrine compounds may cause maculopathy,[13,14] and echothiophate iodide has been suspected of precipitating retinal detachment[15] and iris cysts.[16] Retinal detachment would be difficult to repair if synechiae or chronic miosis prevented adequate pupillary dilatation. When the intraocular pressures are uncontrolled and the patient has a significant cataract, we generally operate the glaucoma first and perform a trabeculectomy in the superior nasal quadrant. This leaves the temporal limbus available for cataract extraction at a later date, with or without implant insertion.

With a filtering bleb present superior nasally, the cataract may be extracted

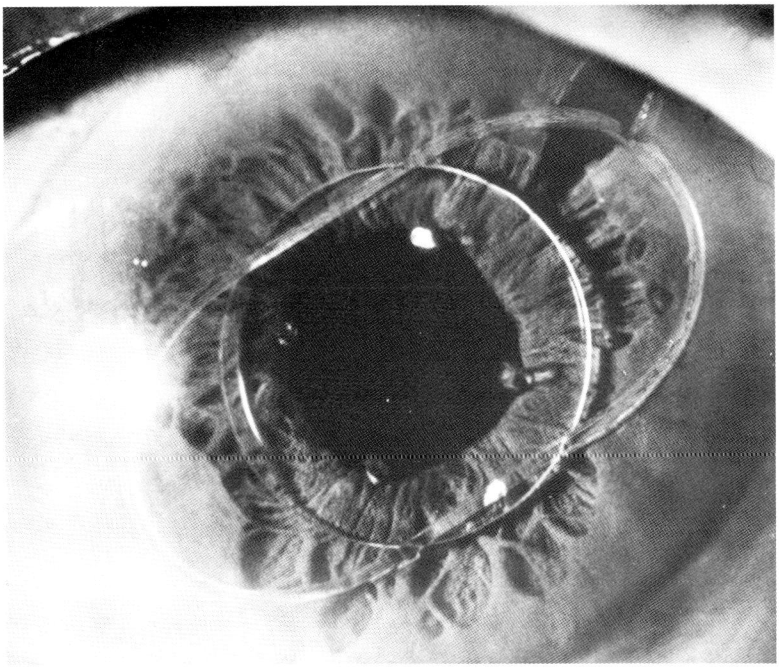

Fig. 10-14. Binkhorst iris-clip lens implant inserted obliquely through temporal section.

through a temporal section. A superior bleb or superior temporal bleb requires a corneal or inferior section. An inferior section is very cumbersome, especially for a microsurgeon, and care should be taken to avoid inadvertent external pressure on the inferior lid speculum. We prefer the Binkhorst iris-clip lens implant when an implant is to be inserted through an atypical cataract section. The implant may be inserted horizontally or obliquely (Fig. 10-14). A transiridectomy or iris-fixation suture is optional in this situation.

Implant surgery is probably *not* contraindicated in chronic open-angle glaucoma, provided that the intraocular pressure has been satisfactorily controlled on a modest glaucoma regimen. A retrospective study[17] of 623 patients in the Miami Collaborative Intraocular Lens Implant Survey[18] produced 17 patients with preoperative glaucoma who had a Copeland implant inserted and 7 additional glaucoma patients with Binkhorst implants inserted between 1974 and 1975. In the Copeland group, one patient developed a central retinal artery occlusion 18 months postoperatively, and another patient had the implant removed because of iritis and uncontrolled glaucoma (Fig. 10-15). Fig. 10-16 shows the Binkhorst series. The study concluded that intraocular lens implantation does not adversely affect intraocular pressure or its control in those patients with preexisting glaucoma or ocular hypertension.

Lens implant surgery would not be contraindicated in narrow-angle glaucoma, provided the pressures are in reasonable control. Patients with the less frequent types of glaucoma must be individually evaluated before they can be considered candidates for lens implantation.

The surgical technique frequently has to be modified when chronic miosis or posterior synechiae preclude adequate dilatation, and this is discussed in Chapter 12. When one is performing an irido-

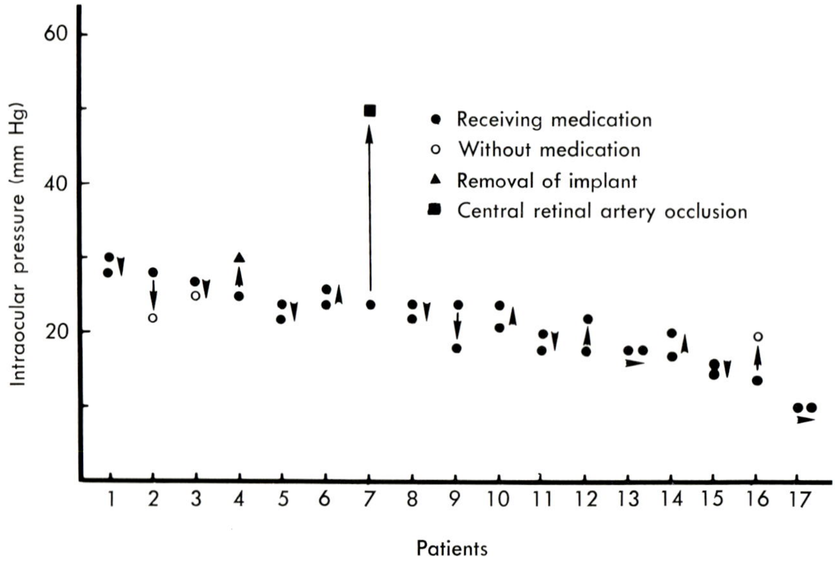

Fig. 10-15. Patients with Copeland lens implants and preexisting glaucoma. (From Smith, J. A., and Anderson, D. R.: Arch. Ophthalmol. **94**:1292, 1976.)

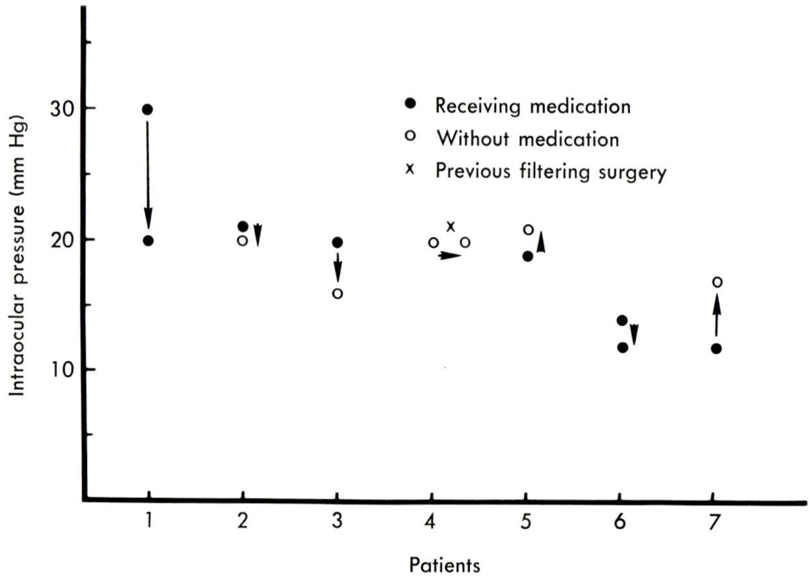

Fig. 10-16. Patients with Binkhorst implants and preexisting glaucoma. (From Smith, J. A., and Anderson, D. R.: Arch. Ophthalmol. **94**:1292, 1976.)

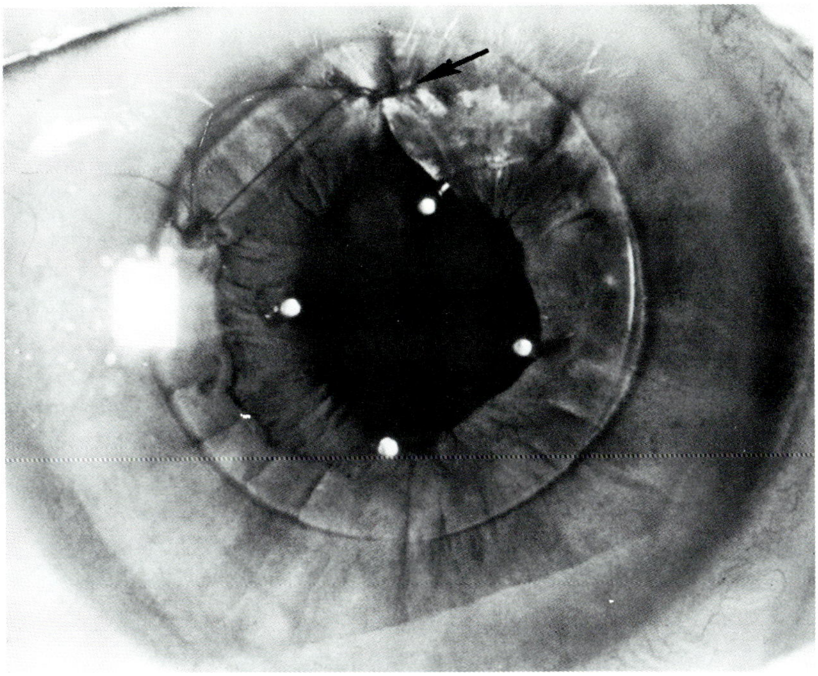

Fig. 10-17. Superior pupillary notch after iridoplasty *(arrow)* and insertion of Worst Medallion lens implant.

plasty for miosis, the pupil should not be reconstructed back to its preoperative size, as great difficulty will be encountered inserting the implant without sphincter rupture. The iridoplasty suture is inserted slightly distal to the sphincter, producing a small pupillary notch superiorly (Fig. 10-17). Significant cataracts and chronic miosis are particularly disabling. Patients who have had successful cataract extraction with lens implantation and relief of their miosis are generally most grateful to their surgeon.

CONCLUSIONS

Undoubtedly situations will arise that have not been covered here. The surgeon is reminded that often an operation is technically feasible, but its subsequent effects on the eye may be less than satisfactory. Caution is advised in selecting cases for lens implantation where concurrent disease or technical demands place the patient at an unwarranted risk.

Lens implantation in children is a subject of sufficient magnitude and complexity to merit a separate chapter, which follows.

REFERENCES

1. Forstot, S. L., Blackwell, W. L., Jaffe, N. S., and Kaufman, H. E.: Effect of intraocular lens implantation on corneal endothelium, Trans. Am. Acad. Ophthalmol. Otolaryngol. **83:**OP195-203, 1977.
2. Clayman, H., Jaffe, N., Light, D., and Eichenbaum, D.: Lens implantation surgery in the second eye, Ophthalmic Surg. **8:**45-48, 1977.
3. Jaffe, N. S., and Duffner, L. R.: The iris-plane (Copeland) pseudophakos, Arch. Ophthalmol. **94:**420-424, 1976.
4. Taylor, D. M., and Khaliq, A.: Keratoplasty and intraocular lenses: follow-up study, Ophthalmic Surg. **8:**49-57, 1977.
5. Lee, J. R., and Dohlman, C. H.: Intraocular lens implantation in combination with keratoplasty, Ann. Ophthalmol. **9:**513-518, 1977.
6. Smith, J. L., McCrary, J. A., Bird, A. C., et al.: Sub-Tenon steroid injection for optic neuritis, Trans. Am. Acad. Ophthalmol. Otolaryngol. **74:**1249-1253, 1970.

7. Binkhorst, C. D.: Lenses in pseudophakia, Trans. Am. Acad. Ophthalmol. Otolaryngol. **77**:OP589-617, 1973.
8. Jaffe, N. S.: Cataract surgery and its complications. 2, St. Louis, 1976, The C. V. Mosby Co., p. 142.
9. Katz, J., Kaufman, H. E., Goldberg, E. P., and Sheets, J. W.: Prevention of endothelial damage from intraocular lens insertion, Trans. Am. Acad. Ophthalmol. Otolaryngol. **83**:204-211, 1977.
10. Edelhauser, H. F., Van Horn, D. L., Hyndiuk, R. A., and Schultz, R. O.: Intraocular irrigating solutions, Arch. Ophthalmol. **93**:648-657, 1975.
11. Becker, B.: Intraocular pressure response to topical corticosteroids, Invest. Ophthalmol. **4**:198-205, 1965.
12. Clayman, H.: Combined trabeculectomy and cataract extraction. In Emery, J., and Paton, D., editors: Current concepts in cataract surgery: proceedings of the Fourth Biennial Cataract Surgery Conference, St. Louis, 1976, The C. V. Mosby Co., pp. 147-150.
13. Kolker, A. E., and Becker, B.: Epinephrine maculopathy, Arch. Ophthalmol. **79**:552-562, 1968.
14. Mackool, R. J., Muldoon, T., Fortier, A., and Nelson, D.: Epinephrine-induced cystoid macula edema in aphakic eyes, Arch. Ophthalmol. **95**:791-793, 1977.
15. Heimann, K., and Kyrielis, E.: Netzhautablösung bei miotischer therapie, Klin. Monatsbl. Augenheilkd. **156**:98-104, 1970.
16. Chin, N. B., Gold, A. A., and Breinin, G. M.: Iris cysts and miotics, Arch. Ophthalmol. **71**:611-616, 1964.
17. Smith, J. A., and Anderson, D. R.: Effect of the intraocular lens on intraocular pressure, Arch. Ophthalmol. **94**:1291-1294, 1976.
18. Duffner, L. R., Wallace, W. K., and Stiles, W. R.: The Miami Cooperative Community Study on the Copeland intraocular lens (pseudophakos), Am. J. Ophthalmol. **82**:590-593, 1976.

CHAPTER 11

Intraocular lens in the pediatric patient

DAVID A. HILES, M.D.

The insertion of an intraocular lens following senile cataract extraction has been followed with great interest by pediatric ophthalmic surgeons for many years. The surgical difficulties and the complications encountered following intraocular lens insertion in aphakic adults have kept these same pediatric eye surgeons wary of the intraocular lens as a technique that may be safely applied to children.[1] Binkhorst and his associates in Europe, however, have developed intraocular lens and implantation techniques that have been successfully applied to children since 1959.[2]

Infantile cataract surgery has been performed with greater ease and fewer complications since the advent of Scheie's small limbal incision aspiration procedure and its many modifications, including phacoemulsification.[3,4] The main obstacle in performing infantile cataract surgery is not always the surgery itself, but is the rehabilitation of these often traumatized or congenitally malformed eyes. Amblyopia produced by high anisometropic refractive errors and aniseikonia, strabismus, organic defects, and deprivation commonly coexist. Spectacle, contact lens, and amblyopia patch failures are also common in children and add to the difficulties of rehabilitation.[2,5-7] The intraocular lens appears to offer an additional method to reduce some of the rehabilitative complications in eyes that would otherwise achieve little visual success.[2]

□ Clinical Associate Professor, Department of Ophthalmology, University of Pittsburgh School of Medicine, Pittsburgh, Pennsylvania.

INDICATIONS

Visual acuity

There are several indications for intraocular lens implantations in children. The first and most important is to preserve vision and prevent amblyopia.[1,2] Anterior segment trauma producing corneal scars often precludes successful contact lens wear in these patients. Increasing suppression and amblyopia may occur following traumatic cataract and its surgery in young children. This factor is related to the young ages of the patients at the time of the occlusion of the visual axis and the interval before rehabilitation of the eye. The longer this time interval exists, the greater the possibility of irreversible amblyopia.[6,8,9]

Children with unilateral congenital cataract often have severe deprivation amblyopia that may not be able to be reversed, and some surgeons have advised against any surgery for these patients.[2,9-14] However, Binkhorst and Gobin[15] in 1970 reported an improvement in vision in all cases of unilateral infantile cataract. While the acuity remained less than normal, the patients accepted occlusion of the sound eye more readily and the nystagmoid ocular movements were improved.

The research of Wiesel and Hubel[16-19]

and von Noorden et al.[20,21] has demonstrated that in both cats and monkeys, irreversible anatomic changes occur in the lateral geniculate body as the result of visual deprivation. In addition, there is a diminution of the cortical driving following visual deprivation within the first few months of life. These findings have prompted ophthalmic surgeons to perform cataract surgery within the first few weeks or months of life and to undertake more vigorous and rapid rehabilitation methods for these patients.[7,22] These methods have included optical correction with contact lens, amblyopia occlusion therapy, strabismus surgery, and secondary membrane capsulotomy.[8]

Spectacle correction accompanied by occlusion seldom preserves visual function in aphakic eyes.[23] Poor spectacle centering and marked retinal image disparities lead to active suppression and amblyopia.[2] Contact lens, while reducing the retinal image disparity considerably, still does not reduce the problem of low-riding lens with decentration, induced vertical diplopia, and the resultant suppression.[2,5] Ocular movements and blinking also affect contact lens centration. Strabismus is commonly associated with infantile cataracts and frequently requires corrective surgery.[2,24] Variations in the strabismic angles have been reported in patients wearing aphakic contact lens. Diplopia or suppression were constant findings in these patients.[1,15,24] The absence of accommodation is present in all aphakic corrections and places additional barriers upon the maintenance of clear form-vision over the total viewing range.[1]

All of the above factors contribute to the presence of amblyopia, a lack of binocular function, and the ultimate production of strabismus in some patients.[2,24] The presence of an intraocular lens, however, does not preclude the necessity for amblyopia occlusion therapy. Binkhorst and Gobin have reported a regression of visual acuity in patients neglecting such therapy. They also report long-term improvement with its continuation.[15,24]

Fusion

A second major consideration for intraocular lens implantation in children is the preservation of some form of fusion.[2] If the eyes maintain relatively equal acuities (isometropia), equal retinal image sizes (iseikonia), and a normal alignment, the possibility of the development of peripheral fusion increases.[25] This effect helps to maintain a stable ocular alignment without the later tendency to develop heterotropia. In some patients a preexisting deviation may even be alleviated.[24]

Specific indications

My specific indications for intraocular lens implantation in children have been tempered by the existing conservative climate surrounding this type of surgery in the United States. Two separate groups of patients were considered. The first group was composed of children who had traumatic, irregular corneal scars and cataracts. A lens extraction and intraocular lens implantation at the same operation (primary) was performed when the visual axis became occluded. Those children who had sustained a traumatic cataract with or without corneal scarring and who had had an unsuccessful aphakic contact lens trial were also candidates for implantation (secondary). Some of these patients had had a previous discission of their posterior lens capsule. This finding complicates, but does not negate, the possibility of intraocular lens insertion, providing that vitreous is not present in the anterior chamber at the time of intraocular lens implantation.

The second group of children consisted of those with unilateral infantile cataracts who were 8 months of age or older but usually less than 8 years of age.[2,15] Intraocular lens implantation in eyes less than 8 months of age has not been attempted because of the caution by Binkhorst of the "surgical misbehavior" accompanying such surgery.[15,25,26] The complications have included hemorrhage, prolapse of ocular contents, iris incarceration, anterior synechiae formation, iris bombé, iritis, and intractable pupillary fibrotic membranes.[10,26] However, it just may be these eyes that will most benefit from such a procedure in the future. Very early intraocular lens implantation may yet prove as surgically and visually successful as is the very early removal of the congenital cataract. No intraocular lenses were implanted in eyes with chronic ocular inflammatory diseases, rubella, marked microphthalmos, or infantile glaucoma.

Since the long-term effects of the intraocular lens in children are unknown,[9] no binocular lenses were inserted. The intraocular lens has been used by others in binocular aphakes to prevent or relieve strabismus or in mentally retarded children.[25,26] Unilateral implantation in the eye with the worst vision may improve its acuity and thus prevent fusional disruption and strabismus. If the acuity then fails in the fellow eye or strabismus does occur, an intraocular lens implantation has been suggested for this eye also.[9,10,25]

Prior to the decision to implant an intraocular lens, the parents of each patient are informed of the alleged advantages and disadvantages of the procedure as well as the current information derived from the lay press and television. They are also well prepared for any eventuality that may occur such as infection, lens dislocation, secondary membrane or post-pseudophakos membrane surgery, strabismus surgery, macular changes, retinal detachment, and possible late intraocular lens removal. The final decision is jointly made by the ophthalmologist and the child's properly informed parents.

INTRAOCULAR LENS

The Worst Medallion implant is the intraocular lens model most frequently implanted in children. Its selection depends upon the need for fixation due to the age of the patients or to the condition of the anterior segment related to previous surgery or trauma.

The intraocular lens should permit adequate pupillary activity for the examination of the fundus, avoidance of pupillary block, and easy access for secondary membrane surgery.[26] The intraocular lens loops have been composed of inert metals of either platinum-iridium alloy or titanium rather than of potentially degradable and absorbable synthetic materials such as Supramid (nylon 6).[1,26,27] The heavier metallic loops have been adequately supported by the iris and capsular membrane and by synechiae formation.[25,27] Recently, polypropylene loops have supplanted these other materials. These loops are lighter in weight, are not considered to be biodegradable over a long period of time, and do not produce iris sphincter erosion.

The Binkhorst 2-loop iridocapsular intraocular lens had been used for young children who formed synechiae readily.[27] Most children do, however, require an ancillary method of intraocular lens fixation. Iris fixation consists of a suture placed through the iris and the haptic holes of the Worst Medallion implant. Other methods employed occasionally consist of a suture passed through the iris and around a loop of the Binkhorst 2-loop intraocular lens or that of the Worst trans-iridectomy fixation clip.

Intraocular lens powers

The intraocular lens powers are either estimated by the method of Binkhorst[28] or are calculated from keratometer readings, A-scan axial lengths, anterior chamber depths, and known preoperative or aphakic refractive errors (Chapter 6).[26,29] If the intraocular lens strength has not been precalculated, a lens in the 19 to 20 D range is selected.[1] Postoperatively, a spectacle correction is placed in instances where the sphere or cylinder or both are significant for visual improvement. Children over the age of 4 to 5 years are also given a bifocal addition for near work.

TECHNIQUE

The technique of insertion of the intraocular lens is divided into three major categories: (1) simultaneous extracapsular cataract extraction and intraocular lens implantation performed at the same operation; (2) extracapsular cataract extraction followed by an intraocular lens implantation at a later date; and (3) extracapsular cataract extraction and capsulotomy followed by intraocular lens insertion at a later date. The techniques of the three procedures are described.

Simultaneous extracapsular cataract extraction and intraocular lens implantation

The patient is admitted to the hospital the day prior to surgery. The pupil is dilated with 1 drop each of 10% phenylephrine and 2% cyclopentolate administered upon admission. These drops are repeated at bedtime along with 1 drop of 1% atropine. The drops are repeated at 7 AM the morning of surgery and again 45 minutes preoperatively. Topical or systemic antibiotics have not been used routinely.[30]

The patient is placed under general endotracheal anesthesia. A mannitol "push" of 0.2 g/kg of body weight of a 25% solution is given as an intravenous injection after the endotracheal tube has been inserted. This is considered to be the test dose for adults but is in the therapeutic range for children and significantly lowers the intraocular pressure. Ocular massage also aids in the further reduction of the intraocular pressure. Schiøtz tonometry is performed prior to the initial incision, and the pressure desired is 15 mm Hg or less. The surgical microscope is used for all procedures. Continuous external drop irrigation on the corneal surface assures clear visibility throughout the procedure.

A suitable size Flieringa ring is eccentrically superiorly placed around the cornea and the anterior segment of the eye. This ring supplies the needed support to the collapsible infantile sclera when the larger incision necessary for intraocular lens implantation is made. A 2 to 3 mm wide and 8 to 10 mm long limbus-based flap is fashioned and reflected over the cornea. Care is taken to cleanly dissect the entire exposed surgical limbus with a round-bladed knife. Wet-field cautery is applied to the area to shrink the prominent episcleral vasculature.

An 8 mm grooved ab externo incision is made with a razor blade or other knife. The incision is made in the surgical limbus at the junction of its anterior two-thirds with the posterior one-third and is carried down to the level of the posterior corneal stroma and Descemet's membrane. The incision must be long enough to allow an easy insertion of the intraocular lens without trauma to the intraocular structures. No preplaced corneoscleral sutures are used. A 2 mm keratome incision enters the anterior chamber through the groove at the 12 o'clock position. The keratome is rotated slightly to the right and to the left to enlarge the internal aspect of the wound by 0.5 mm on each side (Fig. 11-1).

An anterior capsulotomy is performed with a sharp irrigating cystotome. The capsulotomy opening forms an H-shaped figure that prepares the capsular cul-de-sacs for the placement of the posterior intraocular lens loops (Fig. 11-2). No capsule is removed. The phacoemulsifier or other aspiration instrument is passed into the lens capsular sac, and the lens cortex and nucleus are emulsified and aspirated. At the conclusion of aspiration the pupil is rendered miotic with acetylcholine solution (1:100) to protect the fragile posterior capsule from rupture while the intraocular lens is being inserted.

The corneoscleral wound is carefully enlarged by cutting the few remaining posterior stromal fibers and Descemet's membrane with right and left microcorneal scissors.

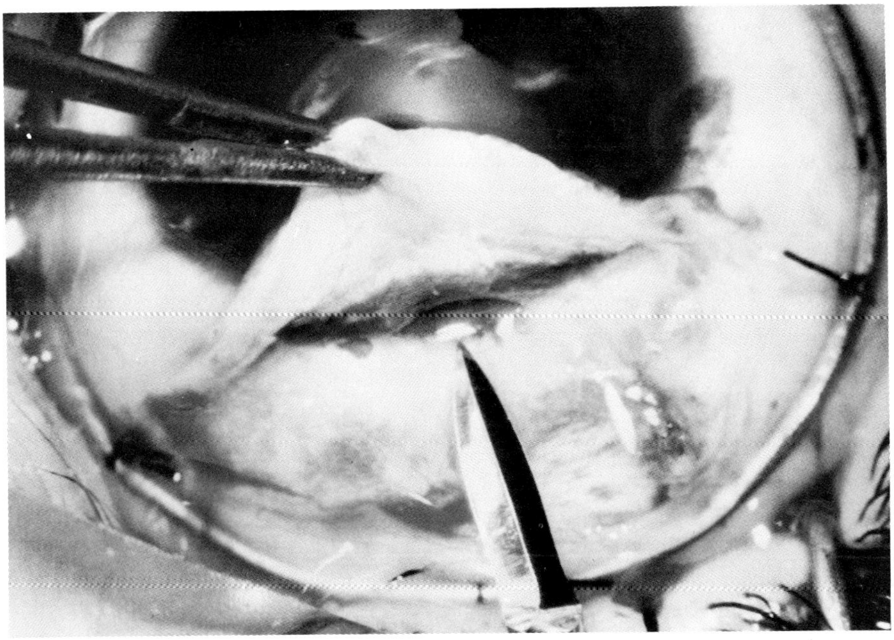

Fig. 11-1. Flieringa ring surrounds cornea. Corneoscleral incision is prepared and keratome is placed for initial incision.

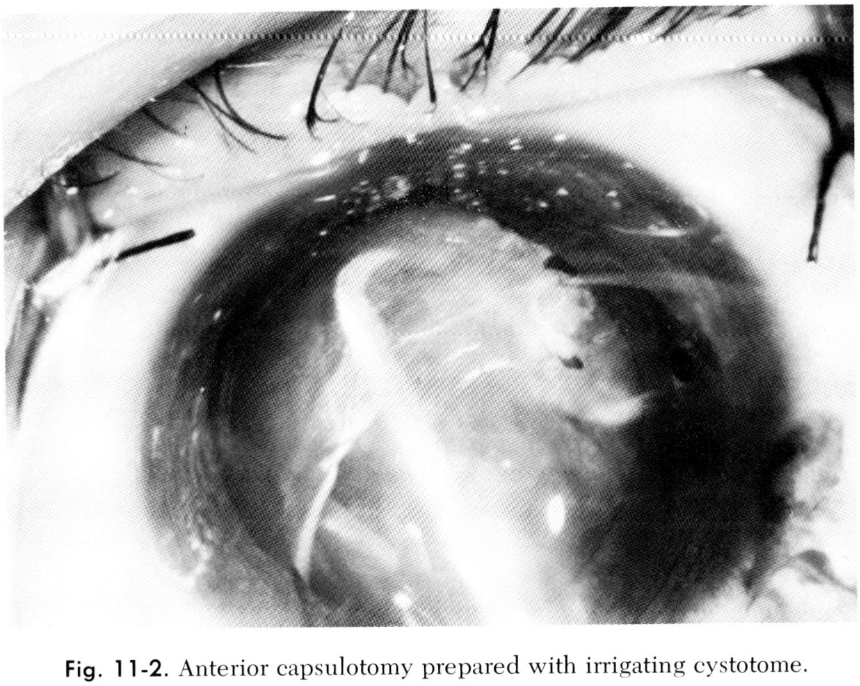

Fig. 11-2. Anterior capsulotomy prepared with irrigating cystotome.

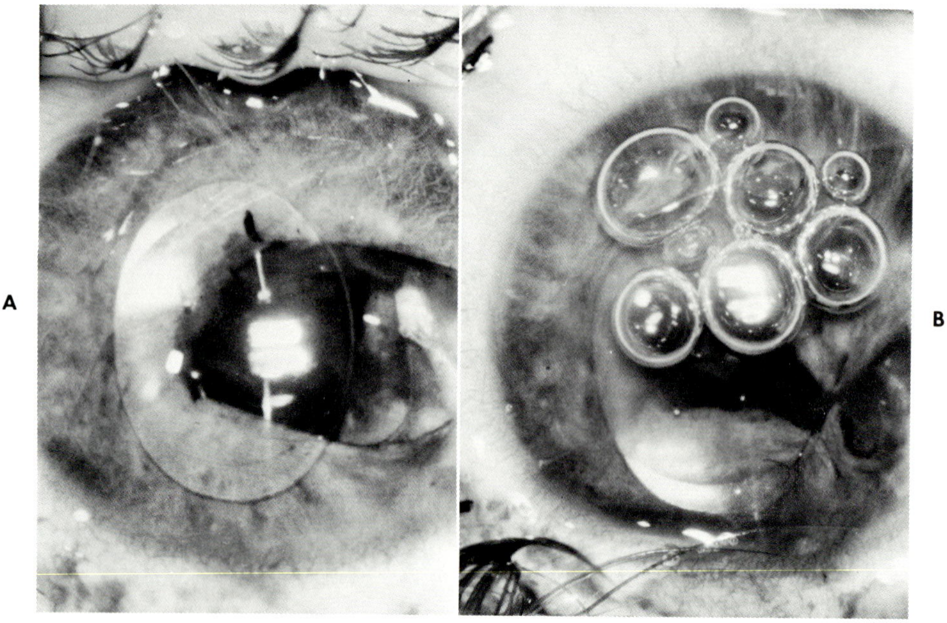

Fig. 11-3. A, Intraocular lens in pupillary space. A traumatic iris coloboma is present. **B,** Iris suture closes coloboma and secures intraocular lens in pupillary space.

Traumatic adherent iridocorneal synechiae must by lysed before an intraocular lens may be inserted. Adhesions between the iris and cornea that do not involve the angle are cut with scissors, and the presence of the intraocular lens in the anterior chamber prevents the readhesion of the two structures. Adhesions extending into the angle are released by performing radial iridotomies on each side of the adhesion down to, but short of, the angle (Fig. 11-3, *A*). This step is necessary to prevent late intraocular lens tilt or corneal touch. The iris coloboma created may then be closed or bridged with an iris suture later in the operation (Fig. 11-3, *B*). However, some patients have such wide sector iridectomies that they are unable to be closed. The intraocular lens loops are placed within the capsular cul-de-sacs, and adhesions readily form to hold the loops in place.[1] An iris-fixation suture or a transiridectomy clip is also utilized to assure stable intraocular lens fixation (Fig. 11-4).

The intraocular lens is transferred from its storage container or dry pack into a neutralizing fluid or saline rinse and is inspected for defects. It may be implanted by a variety of forceps, but the optimum seems to be one in which an irrigation tip precedes the intraocular lens or its loops into the anterior chamber. The infusion of fluid or air aids in the maintenance of anterior chamber depth and in the separation of the iris, cornea, and lens capsular flaps. An elongated, bent McPherson or irrigating Nevyas forceps that grasps the vertical portion of two of the intraocular lens loops is very useful for inserting most intraocular lenses. The intraocular lens is carefully slipped over the iris surface and into the anterior chamber.[27] Care is taken to avoid contact with the corneal endothelium. This task is greatly complicated in children, however, by the collapsible sclera and the forward pressure of the iris-lens capsular diaphragm.

A Sheets intraocular lens glide (p. 168) is a useful adjunct to the insertion of the intraocular lens. The glide is inserted

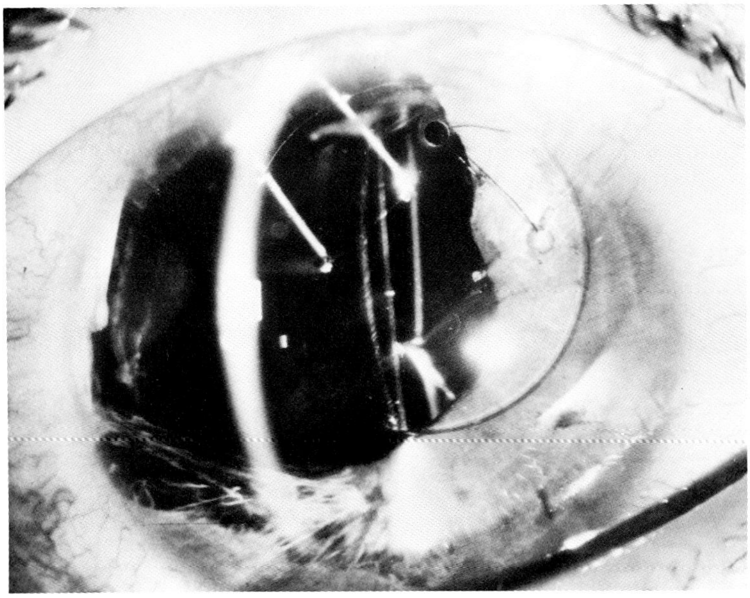

Fig. 11-4. A large, traumatic iridectomy existed prior to cataract extraction and intraocular lens implantation. Superior lens loops were placed into capsular cul-de-sac and became adherent to it (slit-lamp view).

through the incision and over the iris surface to completely cover the pupil. The intraocular lens is placed over the pupillary aperture, and the glide is removed. One horizontal intraocular lens loop is inserted under the iris and into the capsular cul-de-sac. The opposite intraocular lens loop is carefully placed into the opposite cul-de-sac by teasing the iris and lens capsule over the superior loop with a small iris spatula. The final placement of the intraocular lens is undertaken with a Hirschman serrated lens spatula. Acetylcholine solution (1:100) is injected into the anterior chamber to further center the intraocular lens in the pupil. Either one or two peripheral iridectomies are performed.

It is highly suggested that the intraocular lens be fixed to the ocular structures even though synechiae formation is prevalent in children. The Worst Medallion implant is secured to the iris by passing a 3 mm bite of a single 9-0 polypropylene suture (Ethicon, Inc., Somerville, N.J.) through the iris just above the sphincter. The Worst platinum-clip intraocular lens is fixed by passing the iris transfixation hook over the anterior surface of the iris superiorly and clipping it through the iridectomy to the superior intraocular lens loop that lies posterior to the iris. An elliptically performed iridectomy aids in this maneuver. The Choyce Mark VIII intraocular lens is supported by the sclera, and no additional fixation is needed.

When the intraocular lens is properly positioned, air is injected into the anterior chamber to separate the intraocular lens from the corneal endothelium.[1] The incision is closed to air-tight consistency with multiple interrupted 8-0 polygalactin sutures. The anterior chamber is partially filled with balanced salt or acetylcholine solution (1:100), and the remainder is filled with a small air bubble. The optical portion of the intraocular lens remains at the level of the flat iris plane at the conclusion of the procedure. The conjunctiva may be closed with several interrupted sutures or by appositional adhesions produced by the wet-field cautery.

Pilocarpine 2% and antibiotic-steroid combination drops are placed onto the cornea.[1,26] The eye is not patched, but is covered with a perforated shield. Intravenous dexamethasone is given at the conclusion of the operation to reduce the operative iridocyclitis. The patient is discharged from the hospital on the first postoperative day and reexamined in the office at 2- to 3-day intervals. Since operative iridocyclitis and striate keratitis occur commonly, systemic prednisone (20 to 40 mg, based upon body weight and administered every morning with breakfast) is used in decreasing dosages for 8 to 10 days to reduce the inflammatory reaction. Acetazolamide maintains a soft eye for the first 2 to 3 postoperative days.[26] Topical pilocarpine is used four times per day for several days or until firm capsular adhesions have occurred. Mydriatic medications may then be used. Topical antibiotic-corticosteroid drops are instilled four times a day for 4 to 6 weeks.

A discission under the intraocular lens may be performed at the conclusion of the lens insertion. The preferred technique, a discission performed at a second operation following the intraocular lens implantation surgery, prevents lens displacement or vitreous prolapse into the anterior chamber.[2,27]

Extracapsular cataract extraction followed by intraocular lens implantation at a later date

Secondary intraocular lens implantation is undertaken in the same manner as primary implantation except that the crystalline lens is absent, and synechiae have often formed between the anterior and posterior capsular layers and the iris. Preoperative dilatation is necessary only to identify the areas of synechiae formation.[3,26] The conjunctival flap and a deeply grooved corneoscleral ab externo incision are prepared. The incision into

A

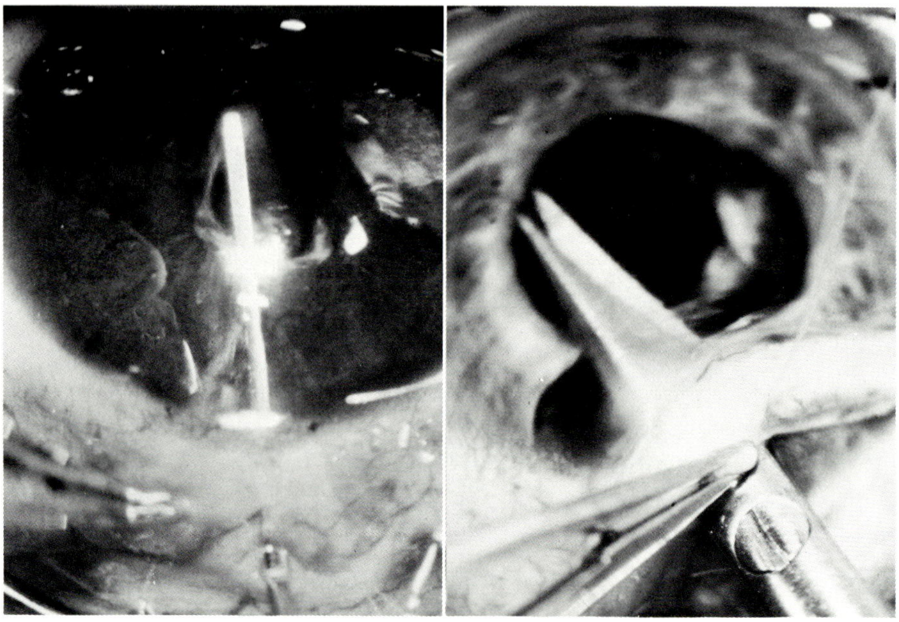

B

Fig. 11-5. A, Formation of capsular cul-de-sacs with thin spatula. **B,** Dissection of cul-de-sacs with Vannas scissors.

the anterior chamber is opened with a razor blade or keratome at its extreme right for the right-handed surgeon. The incision is completed to the left with microcorneal scissors. Great care is taken not to inadvertently rupture the posterior capsule. If the capsule is ruptured early in the procedure and vitreous is lost, an anterior vitrectomy is performed to remove all formed vitreous from the anterior chamber prior to intraocular lens insertion. If a capsular rupture occurs after the intraocular lens is in place, the wound and the anterior chamber must be cleared of vitreous before the final closure is completed.

Careful dissection with a spatula, discission knife, or Vannas scissors frees the adhesions between the iris and lens capsule and produces cul-de-sacs for the placement of the intraocular lens loops (Fig. 11-5, *A* and *B*). The intraocular lens is inserted into the pupillary space, and the loops are placed in the newly created cul-de-sacs.[1,26,27] Synechiae formation usually occurs rapidly, and firm fixation of the intraocular lens takes place in young patients within a few days. However, additional intraocular lens fixation methods are routinely employed. An additional peripheral iridectomy may also be necessary if there is question as to the patency of the original iridectomy opening.

Extracapsular cataract extraction and capsulotomy followed by intraocular lens implantation at a later date

The obvious complication arising from this technique is that of vitreous involvement.[26,27] If vitreous is present in the anterior chamber preoperatively, an anterior vitrectomy is performed.[1,26] Synechiae exist between the capsule, the iris, and the vitreous face, and careful dissection is required to create the cul-de-sacs for the placement of the intraocular lens loops. Very careful manipulation places the intraocular lens loops within the clefts. Intraocular lens fixation is then accomplished as described above.

COMPLICATIONS OF INTRAOCULAR LENS IMPLANTATION

There are numerous operative and postoperative complications of intraocular lens implantation in children that must be anticipated. The operative complications consist of scleral collapse with a flattening of the anterior chamber, posterior capsular rupture with vitreous loss, and hyphema. The more common pediatric postoperative complications consist of striate keratitis, iridocyclitis, secondary and postpseudophakos membrane formation, lenticular precipitates, and intraocular lens dislocations. The uncommon complications are corneal dystrophy, glaucoma, cystoid macular degeneration, and retinal detachment.

Operative complications

Scleral collapse. Reduced scleral rigidity in children predisposes to scleral collapse with the possibility of extrusion of the intraocular contents. The probability of the occurrence of these events is increased with the creation of the larger corneoscleral incision necessary for intraocular lens implantation. The iris-lens-capsular diaphragm presses forward to the corneal endothelial surface even with the use of the Flieringa ring and intravenous mannitol. During intraocular lens insertion, care is taken not to unduly traumatize the corneal endothelium or to rupture the fragile posterior capsule. The insufflation of air or fluid into the anterior chamber during intraocular lens insertion aids in preserving this space, but the maintenance of a deep anterior chamber remains difficult.

Vitreous loss. Posterior capsular rupture and vitreous loss were strong contraindications to the lens implantation in children.[26] Vitreous loss may lead to corneal dystrophy, uveitis, pupillary block glaucoma, distorted or updrawn pupils, intraocular lens tilt and displacement, secondary glaucoma, cyclitic membranes, and detached retinas.[1] If vitreous loss occurs, standard vitreous management techniques, including anterior chamber vitrectomy with mechanical vitrectors, are instituted to clear the anterior chamber, iris surface, and incision before further intraocular lens surgery is completed.

Hyphema. Small hyphemas absorb without sequelae. Larger collections of blood should be irrigated from the anterior chamber prior to wound closure. The site of bleeding is usually in the corneoscleral wound, the iridectomy site, or at a vascularized anterior synechia. Local cautery or anterior chamber air tamponade controls bleeding.

Postoperative complications

Striate keratitis. Transient striate keratitis commonly occurs in children following intraocular lens insertion and is due to the scleral collapse that flattens the anterior chamber when the eye is widely opened. The endothelial surface is often rubbed when the intraocular lens is inserted. The cornea clears again, without sequelae, in 48 to 72 hours. Permanent corneal edema is rare in children because of the presence of an otherwise healthy corneal endothelium.[30]

Iridocyclitis. Operative iridocyclitis occurs in most pediatric patients, and topical and systemic corticosteroids are used to control it.[26] No complications have ensued from the iridocyclitis, and, in fact, its presence is beneficial to assure adequate synechiae formation between the intraocular lens loops and the ocular tissues. The anterior chamber flare and cells usually do not persist longer than the third postoperative week. The systemic corticosteroids used to control the iridocyclitis are rapidly reduced over a 9-day period. The topical corticosteroids are gradually reduced and discontinued when the anterior chamber remains clear of inflammatory activity.

Secondary membrane. Most pediatric patients develop an opaque secondary membrane over a period of time and require a capsulotomy.[2,26] This surgery may be accomplished at the time of the intraocular lens implantation or as a secondary procedure.[1,2,30] The secondary discission is preferred because it has been noted that the posterior capsule becomes taut or rigid over the first few weeks following the cataract aspiration. It also separates from the underlying anterior vitreous face. These factors present the surgeon with the opportunity to perform a controlled discission through a tight membranous posterior capsule without disturbing the vitreous face, introducing vitreous into the anterior chamber or displacing the intraocular lens.

The capsulotomy is performed by passing a very sharp 2 to 2.5 mm Haab discission knife through a limbal incision, under the edge of the intraocular lens, and into the pupillary space between the intraocular lens loops. An opening in the posterior capsule is created without disturbing the intraocular lens (Fig. 11-6). An air bubble is introduced into the anterior chamber to maintain the chamber depth, to keep the intraocular lens in its centered position, and to force the vitreous face posterior to the capsulotomy cleft. Postoperatively, 2% pilocarpine is used for 2 to 3 days. It is accompanied by an antibiotic-corticosteroid drop instilled four times a day until the anterior chamber inflammatory reaction has totally subsided. This usually requires 7 to 10 days. All but four patients in this series have had a posterior capsulotomy.

Postpseudophakos membrane. Kulvin et al.[31] have described a postpseudophakos intraocular lens membrane occurring in as many as 15% of patients. It may arise any time from 6 weeks to 3 years after intraocular lens implantation. The dense or filamentous membrane may adhere to the surfaces of the intraocular lens or lie behind it. The membrane is easily separated from the intraocular lens with a discission knife, and a visual opening may thus be created through it. Six (7.5%) of my patients have developed postpseudo-

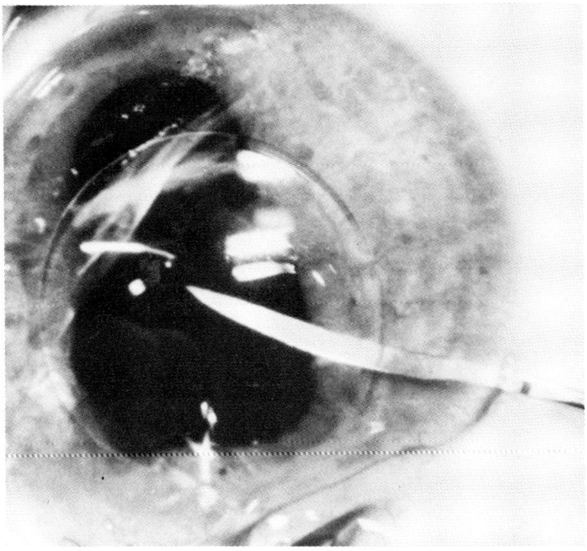

Fig. 11-6. Discission knife passes between intraocular lens loops to create posterior capsular opening in visual axis.

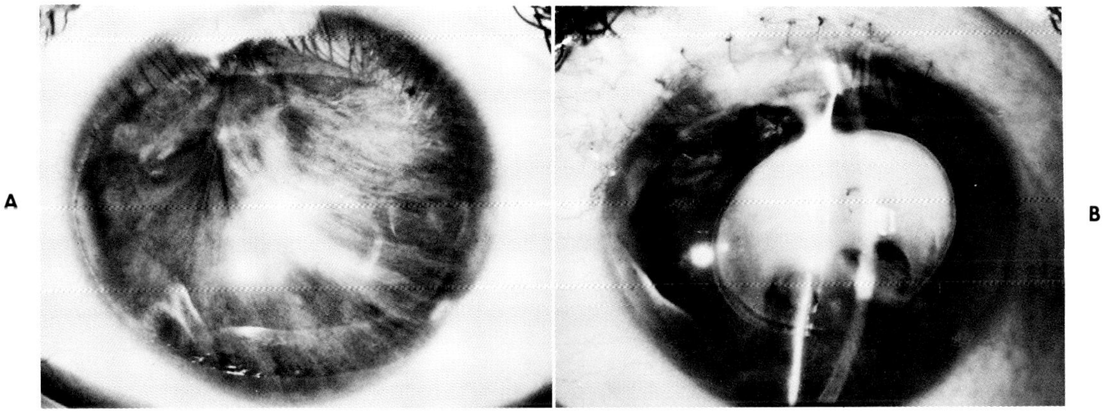

Fig. 11-7. A, Traumatic corneal scar and updrawn pupil. **B,** Stable dense white membrane covering anterior and posterior surface of intraocular lens.

phakos membranes behind their intraocular lenses, and they have required repeat discissions to clear their visual axes.

One of my patients developed a dense postpseudophakos membrane surrounding the intraocular lens in an otherwise quiet eye. Four years prior to the implantation this patient had had a traumatic central corneal perforation with penetration through the lens and into the vitreous body. Surgery had been performed previously to remove the cataract, but the pupil has subsequently become totally updrawn (Fig. 11-7, *A*). Repeated surgical efforts at creating a pupillary aperture were unsuccessful. An intraocular lens was inserted to form and maintain a pupillary opening. Several weeks following the intraocular lens insertion a dense white membrane covered a large part of the intraocular lens surfaces, and then as suddenly as it started, the membrane

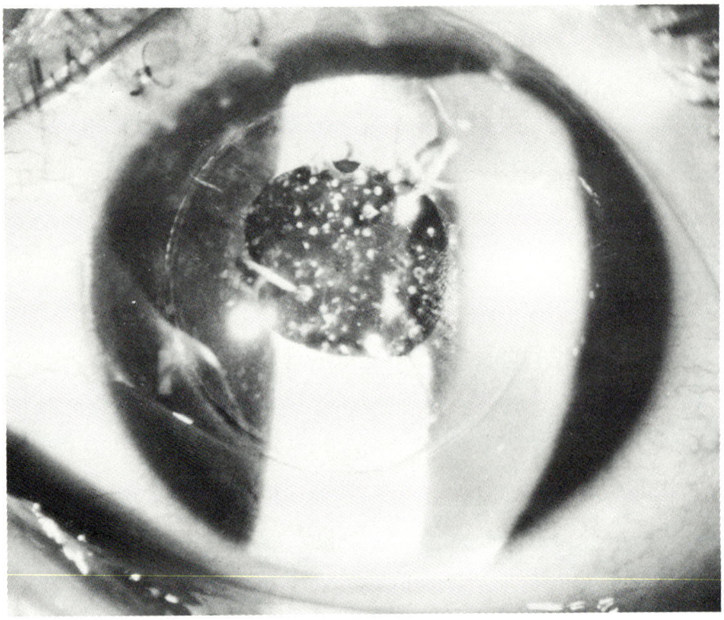

Fig. 11-8. Multiple pigmented precipitates over intraocular lens surface and on surface of posterior lens capsule.

ceased growing and remained stationary (Fig. 11-7, *B*).

Lenticular precipitates. Lenticular precipitates are often noted in the postoperative period. They may have a greasy consistency and are usually pigmented, or they may be gray-white in color and composed of lens elements or inflammatory cellular debris (Fig. 11-8). These precipitates may be cleared with the use of topical corticosteroids, but they do tend to disappear spontaneously over several months.[26]

Intraocular lens dislocation. Intraocular lens dislocations do occur in children despite their very rapid ability to form synechiae. Two dislocations have occurred in my experience, and both were with unfixed intraocular lenses. One 4-year-old child dislocated an unfixed Binkhorst iridocapsular 2-loop lens into the anterior chamber following a lens extraction for traumatic cataract. The surgery was complicated by the presence of a large vascular corneal scar and adherent leukoma. The lens was surgically repositioned, and the loops were sutured to the iris. The second patient, a 16-year-old male, dislocated an unsecured Binkhorst 2-loop iridocapsular intraocular lens. Conservative methods of repositioning the lens were tried without success. The lens was easily surgically replaced into its proper position, and it was also sutured to the iris. Following these incidents, it became my preference to fix *each* intraocular lens implanted in children by a suture.

Uncommon postoperative complications

There are many uncommon postoperative complications that may also occur following pediatric intraocular lens implantation but are not peculiar to children. These consist of intraocular infection, detached retinas,[9,26,32] secondary glaucoma,[26] cystoid macular edema,[32] and endothelial corneal dystrophy.[26] Their management is discussed elsewhere in this text.

RESULTS

Eighty pediatric patients have undergone intraocular lens implantation over a 36-month period. Fifty patients were male and 30 were females. This trend reflects the increased amount of trauma or the poorer contact lens wear noted in boys. The average age at implantation was 6.7 years and ranged from 8 months to 24 years. However, only 11 of the patients were 12 years of age or older. Thirty-seven patients had implantations following ocular trauma, and 43 intraocular lenses were implanted in children with a variety of unilateral infantile cataracts. Fifty patients had cataract aspirations (phacoemulsification) combined with an intraocular lens implantation. Thirty patients had secondary implantations, and 22 of these were implanted in eyes following both cataract aspirations and discissions of their secondary membranes. All of the secondary implantations were in children who were contact lens failures. In several instances implantation was offered as a last resort to salvage an eye that otherwise was relegated to intractable deprivation amblyopia.

Visual acuity

The evaluation of the visual acuity of pediatric aphakic patients is complicated by the preoperative and postoperative presence of other ocular anatomical defects and sensory and motor anomalies peculiar to children.[10] In a review of my series, 25 patients have 20/20 to 20/40 and 15 patients have 20/50 to 20/100 corrected visual acuities. Ten patients have 20/200 and 12 have less than 20/200 visual acuities. Eighteen patients are too young or too uncooperative to determine accurate visual measurements (Tables 11-1 to 11-4). The final visual acuity was usually better in the uncomplicated traumatic cataract group than in the infantile cataract group. This is probably related to the higher incidence of abnormalities associated with infantile cataracts. However, organic, strabismic, refractive, and deprivation amblyopia are the major causes of visual defects in both groups. Amblyopia is also related to the age of the patient at the time of visual obstruction

Table 11-1. Patient age at intraocular lens surgery and postoperative visual acuity versus cataract type

Trauma (37 patients)		Infantile (43 patients)	
Age	Visual acuity	Age	Visual acuity
12	400	5	40
11	LP	7	200
6	80	8	20
9	40	8	30
8	20	9	200
11	20	6	70
6	20	2	200
11	30	2	70
16	20	5	50
14	25	2	Ecc
17	20	5	200
24	20	2	50
2	200	2	70
1	Ecc	7	40
9	30	6	50
4	800	7	100
4	30	9	400
5	30	2	800
7	25	10	400
18	40	3	?
3	?	3	?
6	25	1	?
15	30	5	4/200
8	?	1	?
21	20	1	?
5	30	4	?
16	400	5	200
4	800	4	100
9	?	4	70
8	30	4	80
20	50	1	?
5	50	2	?
4	30	2	?
6	200	5	80
5	50	5	200
8	30	1	?
6	200	3	?
		5	?
		5	?
		1	?
		7	200
		14	400
		2	?

Table 11-2. Visual acuity following intraocular lens implantation (number of eyes)

	20/20 to 20/40	20/50 to 20/100	20/200	<20/200	Unknown	Total
Traumatic	21	4	3	6	3	37
Infantile	4	11	7	6	15	43
TOTAL	25	15	10	12	18	80

Table 11-3. Traumatic cataracts

Patient no.	Age		Interval (in years)		Best corrected visual acuity
	At injury	At IOL surgery	From trauma to cataract surgery	From cataract surgery to IOL implant	
1	4	12	8	=* 0	20/400
2	7	11	0	4	LP
3	5	6	5 mo	= 0	20/80
6	8	9	1	= 0	20/40
7	7	8	1	= 0	20/20
8	11	11	2 mo	= 0	20/20
11	6	6	2 mo	= 0	20/20
12	6 mo	11	10	= 0	20/30
15	7	16	8	1	20/20
18	8	14	6	= 0	20/25
19	11	17	0	6	20/20
21	11	24	8	13	20/20
22	1	2	1	= 0	20/200
24	1	1	8 mo	= 0	Ecc?
27	8	9	7 mo	= 0	20/30
33	4	4	4 mo	= 0	20/800
34	4	4	2 mo	= 0	20/30
36	5	5	1 mo	= 0	20/30
37	7	7	1 mo	= 0	20/25
39	15	18	3	= 0	20/40
40	3	3	2 mo	= 0	?
41	4	6	2	= 0	20/25
47	9	15	2	4	20/30
48	8	8	2 mo	= 0	?
50	7	21	7	7	20/20
53	5	5	3 mo	= 0	20/30
65	4	16	12	= 0	20/400
66	3	4	1	= 0	20/800
68	5	9	1 mo	4	?
69	5	8	1 mo	3	20/30
70	14	20	6	= 0	20/50
73	5	5	1 mo	= 0	20/50
74	4	4	1 mo	= 0	20/30
75	5	6	1	= 0	20/200
76	3	5	2	= 0	20/50
77	8	8	1 mo	= 0	20/30
80	4	6	1 mo	2	20/200

*=Denotes simultaneous cataract aspiration and intraocular lens implantation.

Table 11-4. Visual acuity with traumatic cataracts (number of eyes)

Age at IOL implantation	20/20 to 20/40	20/50 to 20/100	20/200	<20/200	Unknown	Total
6 yr or less	6	3	3	3	1	16
Over 6 yr	15	1	0	3	2	21
TOTAL	21	4	3	6	3	37

by the cataract, the length of time prior to cataract surgery and optical correction, the success of the amblyopia therapy, the associated anatomical anomalies of the eye, and the presence of strabismus[1] (Table 11-3).

Occlusion therapy has been instituted in all patients under 8 years of age manifesting poor fixation responses or linear visual acuity differences of two lines or more.

Residual refractive errors

The postoperative spherical equivalent refractive errors ranged from −3 to +2.5 D in all but 10 patients. The cylinders ranged up to 3 D in all but three patients. A spectacle has been prescribed for all patients in whom the sphere or cylinder was significant for visual improvement. Most patients were also given a bifocal correction for their near work.

Strabismus

I found that strabismus complicated infantile cataract surgery and intraocular lens implantation in 51% of these patients (Table 11-5). Strabismus may exist prior to the cataract surgery or it may arise after the crystalline lens is removed and the intraocular lens is implanted. It may arise in children of all ages who did not have strabismus before their fusion was disrupted by the occurrence of the cataract and aphakia.

The treatment of aphakic strabismic children consists of occlusion for the amblyopia if it is felt that the amblyopia is remediable. Spectacles are prescribed for the residual sphere or cylinder encountered, and a bifocal addition is used for near work. When the strabismic angle has become stable for several months, strabismus surgery is performed. The amount of surgical correction corresponds to that undertaken for other children with strabismus. Long-term deviations require surgery more frequently and in larger amounts than do deviations of recent onset.[2,24]

Fusion

Fusional responses vary according to the depth of the amblyopia, the placement of the optimum correction, and the absence of strabismus. Other authors have reported fusional successes in children following cataract surgery and intraocular lens implantation for traumatic cataract.[1,2,24] Fusional responses were obtained in 23 (29%) patients.

SUMMARY

The intraocular lens offers an additional experimental parameter to be considered for the visual rehabilitation of children with traumatic or unilateral infantile cataracts. The disadvantages of aphakic spectacles or contact lens and amblyopia have committed many of these eyes to the status of visual cripples. In this series of 81 patients, with a maximum of 36 months follow-up, it has been concluded that the intraocular lens may be successfully implanted.

I wish to reemphasize that vitreous involvement does not preclude intraocular lens implantation, providing all the vitreous is removed from the anterior chamber before the conclusion of the operation. Discission of secondary membranes should be performed if there is any doubt

Table 11-5. Fusion and strabismus results related to intraocular lens implantation

Patient no.	Strabismus present before IOL	Strabismus surgery	Strabismus amblyopia	Persistent strabismus before IOL	Strabismus after IOL	Strabismus surgery after IOL	Final alignment	Fusion +/0	Type of cataract	Best visual acuity
1	0				0		EX	0	T	400
2	ET	R&R	+		0		ME	0	T	LP
3	0		+		XT	Needed	XT=40	0	T	80
4	HT	LIO	+		XT		MX	0	C	40
5	0				0		EX	0	C	200
6	0				0		EX	+	T	40
7	0				0		EX	+	T	20
8	0				0		EX	+	T	20
9	0				0		EX	+	C	20
10	0				0		EX	+	C	30
11	0				XT	R&R	EX	+	T	20
12	0				0		EX	+	T	30
13	ET	Nystagmus Surg.	+	+	ET		ME	0	C	200
14	ET		+	+	ET	R&R	ME	0	C	70
15	0		+	+	0		EX	+	T	20
16	ET	R&R	+	+	ET	MM, RR	ME	0	C	200
17	ET	R&R	+	+	ET	MM, RR	ET=25	0	C	70
18	0				0		EX	+	T	25
19	0				0		EX	+	T	20
20	XT		+	+	XT	Needed	XT=20	0	C	50
21	XT	R&R	0	+	XT	MM, RR	EX	+	T	25
22	0				0		EX	0	T	200
23	0				X(T)	Needed	XT=30 DVD	0	C	Ecc
24	0				XT	R&R	MX	0	T	Ecc
25	0				ET		ME	0	C	200
26	ET		+	+	ET		ME	0	C	50
27	0				0		EX	0	T	30
28	ET	R&R	+	+	ET	Needed	ET=25	0	C	70
29	0				0		EX	+	C	40
30	0				0		EX	+	C	50
31	0				0		EX	+	C	100
32	0				0		EX	0	C	400
33	0				0		EX	0	T	800
34	0				0		EX	+	T	30
35	ET	R&R	+	+	0		ME	0	C	800
36	0				0		EX	+	T	30
37	0				0		EX	+	T	25
38	XT		+	+	XT	R&R	EX	0	C	400
39	0				0		EX	+	T	40
40	0				XT	R&R	MX	?	T	?
41	0				0		EX	+	T	25
42	ET	R&R (simultaneous IOL)		+	ME		ME	0	C	?

Abbreviations: EX, orthophoria; ME, monofixational esophoria; MX, monofixational exophoria; DVD, dissociated vertical deviation; MM, marginal myotomy; RR, reresection; Ecc, eccentric fixation; C, congenital; T, traumatic.

Table 11-5. Fusion and strabismus results related to intraocular lens implantation—cont'd

Patient no.	Strabismus present before IOL	Strabismus surgery	Strabismus amblyopia	Persistent strabismus before IOL	Strabismus after IOL	Strabismus surgery after IOL	Final alignment	Fusion +/0	Type of cataract	Best visual acuity
43	ET		+	+	ET	Needed	ET=30	0	C	?
44	ET		+	+	ET	Needed	ET=20	0	C	?
45	0				XT	Needed	X(T)=20	0	C	4/200
46	ET, LHT		+	+	ET		ME	0	C	?
47	ET-XT	R&R Reverse R&R		+	X		ME	+	T	30
48	0				0		EX	?	T	?
49	XT	Simultaneous R&R	+	+	MX		MX	0	C	?
50	XT	0	0	+	XT	—	EX	0	T	20
51	XT		+	+	XT		XT	0	C	?
52	ET	Simultaneous R&R	+	+	XT		XT	0	C	200
53	0				0		MX	+	T	30
54	ET		+	+	ET		ME	0	C	100
55	XT		+	+	XT		XT−18	0	C	70
56	XT	R&R	+	0	EX		EX	0	C	80
57	ET		+	+	ET	R&R	ME	0	C	?
58	XT		+	+	X		MX	0	C	?
59	0				0		EX	0	C	?
60	0				0		XT=16	+	C	80
61	ET		+	+	ME		ME	0	C	200
62	0				0		EX	?	C	?
63	XT	0	+	+	X		MX	0	C	?
64	0				0		EX	?	C	?
65	XT		+	+	XT	R&R	MX	0	T	400
66	0				0		EX	0	T	800
67	X		+	X	XT		XT	0	C	?
68	0				0		EX	?	T	?
69	0				0		EX	+	T	30
70	XT			+	XT, HT	R&R, IO	MX	0	T	50
71	0				ET	Needed	ET	0	C	?
72	Nystagmus	Kestenbaum			0		ME	0	C	200
73	0				0		EX	?	T	50
74	0				0		EX	?	T	30
75	0				0		EX	?	T	200
76	0				0		EX	0	T	50
77	XT	Rec. IOOU Rec. LROU			0		ME	0	T	30
78	ET				0		ME	0	C	400
79	0				0		EX	0	C	?
80	XT			+	XT		XT	0	T	200

as to the clarity of the membrane. All patients should be repeatedly refracted and the overrefraction prescribed to assure that the child is obtaining the best possible form vision to the aphakic eye. Bifocals are prescribed for near work. Vigorous occlusion therapy is undertaken in all patients exhibiting amblyopia.

REFERENCES

1. Binkhorst, C. D., Gobin, M. H., and Leonard, P. A. M.: Post-traumatic artificial lens implants (pseudophakoi) in children, Br. J. Ophthalmol. **53**:518, 1969.
2. Binkhorst, C. D., and Gobin, M. H.: Injuries to the eye with lens opacity in young children, Ophthalmologica **148**:169, 1964.
3. Kelman, C. D.: Phacoemulsification and aspiration: a new technique of cataract removal, Am. J. Ophthalmol. **64**:23, 1967.
4. Scheie, H. G.: Aspiration of congenital or soft cataracts: a new technique, Am. J. Ophthalmol. **50**:1048, 1960.
5. Rubinstein, K.: Management of unilateral aphakia, Br. Orthopt. J. **17**:82, 1960.
6. Van Balen, A. T.: Binkhorst's method of implantation of pseudophakoi in unilateral traumatic cataract, Ophthalmologica **165**:490, 1972.
7. von Noorden, G. K., Ryan, S. J., and Maumenee, A. E.: Management of congenital cataracts, Trans. Am. Acad. Ophthalmol. Otolaryngol. **74**:352, 1970.
8. Parks, M. M., and Hiles, D. A.: Management of infantile cataracts, Am. J. Ophthalmol. **63**:10, 1967.
9. Van Balen, A. T.: Four years' experience with Binkhorst lens implantation, Am. J. Ophthalmol. **75**:755, 1973.
10. Binkhorst, C. D., and Gobin, M. H.: Congenital cataract and lens implantation, Ophthalmologica **164**:392, 1972.
11. Costenbader, F. D., and Albert, D. G.: Conservatism in the management of congenital cataract, Arch. Ophthalmol. **58**:426, 1957.
12. François, J.: Treatment of congenital cataracts, Ann. Ophthalmol. **2**:131, 1970.
13. Frey, T., Friendly, D., and Wyatt, D.: Re-evaluation of monocular cataracts in children, Am. J. Ophthalmol. **76**:381, 1973.
14. Nordlohne, M. E.: The intraocular implant lens: development and results with special reference to the Binkhorst lens, The Hague, 1975, Dr. W. Funk, B. V.
15. Binkhorst, C. D., and Gobin, M. H.: Treatment of congenital and juvenile cataract with intraocular lens implants (pseudophakoi), Br. J. Ophthalmol. **54**:759, 1970.
16. Wiesel, T. N., and Hubel, D. H.: Effects of visual deprivation on morphology and physiology of cells in the cats lateral geniculate body, J. Neurophysiol. **26**:978, 1963.
17. Wiesel, T. N., and Hubel, D. H.: Single-cell responses in striate cortex of kittens deprived of vision in one eye, J. Neurophysiol. **26**:1003, 1963.
18. Wiesel, T. N., and Hubel, D. H.: Comparison of the effects of unilateral and bilateral eye closure on cortical unit responses in kittens, J. Neurophysiol. **28**:1029, 1965.
19. Wiesel, T. N., and Hubel, D. H.: Extent of recovery from the affects of visual deprivation in kittens, J. Neurophysiol. **28**:1060, 1965.
20. Baker, F. H., Grigg, P., and von Noorden, G. K.: Effects of visual deprivation and strabismus on the responses of neurons in the visual cortex of the monkey, including studies on the striate and pre-striate cortex in the normal animal, Brain Res. **66**:185, 1974.
21. von Noorden, G. K.: Experimental amblyopia in monkeys: further observation and clinical correlations, Invest. Ophthalmol. **12**:721, 1973.
22. Helveston, E. M.: Cataract aspiration utilizing a constant infusion and shifting needle technique, Ophthalmic Surg. **5**:26, 1974.
23. McKinna, A. J.: Results of treatment of traumatic cataract in children, Am. J. Ophthalmol. **52**: 43, 1961.
24. Binkhorst, C. D., and Gobin, M. H.: Pseudophakoi after lens injury in children, Ophthalmologica **154**:81, 1967.
25. Alpar, J. J.: Guidelines for indications of intraocular lens implantation and selection of the proper lens, Ophthalmic Surg. **6**:31, 1975.
26. Binkhorst, C. D.: The iridocapsular (two-loop) lens and the iris-clip (four loop) lens in pseudophakia, Trans. Am. Acad. Ophthalmol. Otolaryngol. **77**:589, 1973.
27. Binkhorst, C. D.: Iris-clip and iridocapsular lens implants (pseudophakoi), Br. J. Ophthalmol. **51**:767, 1967.
28. Binkhorst, C. D.: Power of the prepupillary pseudophakos, Br. J. Ophthalmol. **56**:332, 1972.
29. Hofer, K. J.: Mathematics and computers in intraocular lens calculation, American Intra-Ocular Implant Society Newsletter **1**:1, 1975.
30. Hiles, D. A., and Wallar, P. H.: Phacoemulsification versus aspiration in infantile cataract surgery, Ophthalmic. Surg. **5**:13, 1974.
31. Kulvin, S. M., Magoon, R. C., and Miller, G. R.: The surgical treatment of postpseudophakos membranes, Ophthalmic Surg. **6**:47, 1975.
32. Binkhorst, C. D., Kats, A., Tjan, T. T., and Loones, L. H.: Retinal accidents in pseudophakia-intracapsular vs. extracapsular surgery, Trans. Am. Acad. Ophthalmol. Otolaryngol. **81**:120, 1975.

CHAPTER 12

Complications and management of intraocular lens implantation

Complications of intraocular lens implantation are conveniently divided into operative, early, early or late, and late complications.

OPERATIVE COMPLICATIONS

Inadequate incision. An incision of 165° to 180° is ideal for intraocular lens implantation in conjunction with an intracapsular cataract extraction. A smaller incision increases the likelihood of damaging the corneal endothelium during the process of inserting the pseudophakos. It also increases the risk of rupture of the lens capsule and operative loss of vitreous. It is far better to err on the side of a larger than a smaller incision, since wound closure complications are probably not more frequent with a 180° incision than a 160° incision. Some surgeons use a smaller incision while implanting the lens under air. An alternative is to partially close the larger incision to permit implantation under air. This is discussed on p. 167.

Excessive bleeding. Excessive bleeding must be controlled, since it not only reduces visibility, but clotted blood in the angle and on the surface of the iris may prevent the pupil from constricting around the optical portion of the implant. Bleeding is usually controlled by irrigation, but if this should fail, a bubble of air in the anterior chamber will tamponade the bleeding vessels and prevent access of blood into the anterior chamber. It is usually unnecessary to tie the safety suture to keep air in the anterior chamber. In addition, in making the incision it is better to approach the anterior limbal zones of cornea at the horizontal extremities of the incision so as to avoid the larger vessels.

The popularization of wet-field cautery (Codman Mentor) has significantly reduced bleeding during surgery. Hemostasis should be complete before the incision is made. Special attention is directed to larger vessels at the extremities of the incision. Epinephrine-soaked cellulose sponges are pressed against the entire upper limbus before making the incision. This area should be completely blanched. After the incision is completed, there may be some troublesome bleeding from the deeper scleral vessels. These vessels should be lightly touched with the tips of the wet-field cautery. There may be some bleeding from the iridectomy sites. If this cannot be controlled by irrigation or air in the anterior chamber, the wet-field cautery may again be used.

The surgeon should not proceed beyond the incision stage until all visible bleeding has ceased.

Iridodialysis. A large, inadvertent iridodialysis occurring during enlargement of the incision or during the performance of the iridotomies or iridectomies is usually not serious. It may also be caused by the posterior loop of an implant inadvertently entering the peripheral iridectomy as the implant is placed in the anterior chamber. It may be repaired at the initial surgery

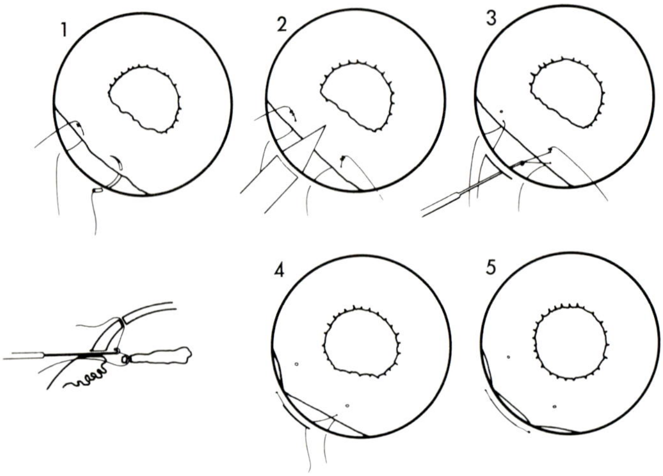

Fig. 12-1. Iridodialysis repair. *1,* A 10-0 monofilament nylon suture on its needle is passed into iris angle under small conjunctival flap opposite dialysis tear. Needle is continued into angle root and, under microscopic view, into posterior chamber up under edge of torn iris, to emerge and proceed vertically across anterior chamber and out through cornea. *2,* Small razor blade incision is made beside suture just placed at corneoscleral junction. *3,* Small, blunt iris hook is slipped through this incision and moved across anterior chamber to engage previously placed vertical suture, which is drawn out in a loop. *4,* Corneal suture is cut flush at its exit, and its loop is pulled out in a single strand. *5,* Two ends are then tied, and as knot is drawn down firmly, it pulls torn edge of iris securely into iris root cleft. A second suture can be placed in a similar manner, and even a third and fourth if iridodialysis is large. (From McCannel, M. A.: Ophthalmic Surg. **7**:98-103, 1976.)

by suturing the iris to the posterior scleral lip of the incision with a 10-0 nylon or polypropylene suture.

On a rare occasion the iridodialysis opening appears much larger postoperatively than it does at surgery. This may result in a markedly displaced pupil, which brings the optical portion of the pseudophakos and its haptic supports dangerously close to the cornea. A simplified method of postoperative repair has been suggested by McCannel (Fig. 12-1). This is done by passing a 10-0 monofilament nylon suture on its needle into the iris angle under a small conjunctival flap opposite the dialysis tear. The needle enters the anterior chamber through the limbus and engages the edge of the dialyzed iris through its posterior surface. The needle continues anteriorly and emerges through the cornea. A small, narrow, limbal stab wound is made with a piece of a razor blade or a No. 57 Beaver blade at the limbus just adjacent to the suture. A small, blunt iris hook is slipped through this incision and moved across the anterior chamber to engage the previously placed vertical suture, which is drawn out in a loop. The corneal suture is then cut flush at its exit, and its loop is pulled out in a single strand by the iris hook. The two ends are then tied, and as the knot is drawn down firmly, it pulls the torn edge of the iris securely into the iris root cleft. Additional sutures may be added as needed if the iridodialysis is large.

Excessive pupillary dilatation. Excessive pupillary dilatation may prevent suitable implantation and favor dislocation. It may be avoided by refraining from preoperative use of cycloplegic-mydriat-

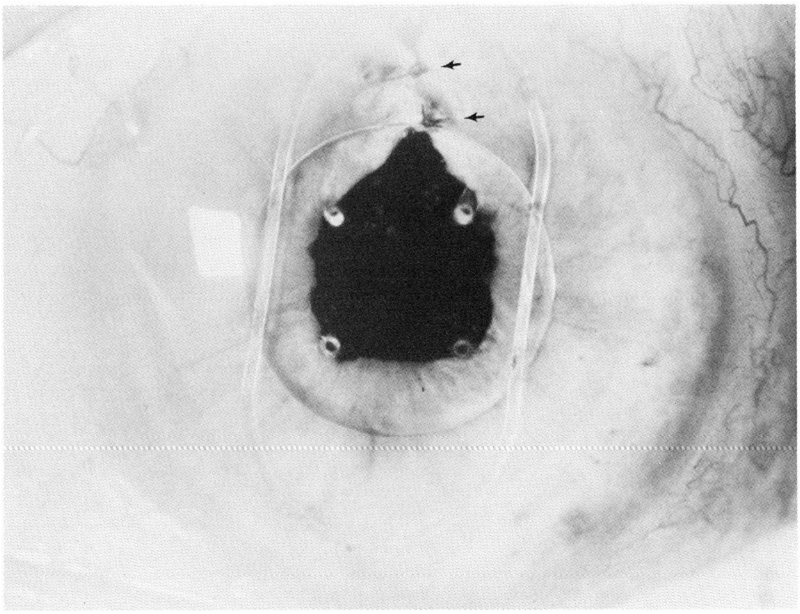

Fig. 12-2. Binkhorst iris-clip implant placed in eye with miotic pupil due to long-term miotic therapy. Iris incision is closed with two 10-0 nylon sutures *(arrows)*.

ics. It is advantageous to depend solely on the retrobulbar injection of the anesthetic solution for pupillary dilatation. If the pupil does not constrict after acetylcholine solution is placed in the eye, gentle stroking of the anterior surface of the iris may irritate the iris sufficiently to produce miosis. If the pupil still fails to constrict, there may have been some iris sphincter damage. In such a case it is probably wise to abandon the implantation. If the surgeon finds difficulty in performing the cataract extraction without preoperative mydriatics, it is better to use them rather than to risk inadvertent freezing of the iris sphincter of an inadequately dilated pupil. The pupil may fail to constrict due to the pressure of a bulging vitreous against the back of the iris. In such a case, filling the anterior chamber with air for a few minutes followed by additional instillation of acetylcholine solution may be helpful.

Inadequate pupillary dilatation. Inadequate pupillary dilatation occurs in eyes with small pupils due to long-term miotic therapy. If cataract extraction is attempted through too small a pupil, one or more ruptures of the iris sphincter usually result. The resulting atonic pupil may preclude lens implantation. To prevent this, a peripheral iridectomy is performed at 12 o'clock. A radial iridotomy through the remaining portion of the iris is performed (p. 139). A 10-0 monofilament nylon or polypropylene suture is passed through the margins of the incised iris just above the sphincter. The suture is looped out of the eye. After lens extraction the suture is tied without crushing the incised iris margins. If necessary, a second iris suture may be placed above the first one (Fig. 12-2). The implant is then inserted. Epinephrine bisulfite solution should not be used to promote mydriasis because of the possible deleterious effect of the bisulfite portion on the corneal endothelium.

Iris sphincter damage. Iris sphincter damage may occur as a result of inadvertent freezing of the iris sphincter with the cryoprobe. It may also occur accidentally while one is performing a partial anterior vitrectomy. If inadequate pupillary constriction results, it may be useful to perform a small radial iridotomy through the damaged sphincter and place a suture, as just described.

Dislocation. Occasionally the implant will dislocate after its insertion. This is managed according to the implant being used. In the case of a Binkhorst iris-clip (4-loop) implant, both inferior loops may be on the same side of the iris at 6 o'clock either in front of or behind the iris. This is corrected by grasping the edge of the optical portion of the implant with suture-tying forceps at either 3, 9, or 12 o'clock (whichever is easier for the surgeon) and withdrawing the implant toward the incision until the distal edges of the inferior loops are visible beyond the iris sphincter at 6 o'clock. The implant is then clipped onto the iris in the usual manner. If the inferior pair of loops had previously dislocated behind the iris, this maneuver might be difficult to perform because of the presence of formed vitreous on the anterior surface of the iris. If the superior pair of haptics have dislocated, it is usually before the placement of the fixation suture. If both loops are anterior to the iris, the situation is easily remedied by passing a spatula between the loops and moving the implant inferiorly. The superior iris is then placed over the posterior loop as described in the section on technique. If both loops are behind the iris, part of the optical portion may also be behind the iris. The iris can be retracted toward the wound until the loops become visible. A spatula is then inserted between the anterior and posterior loop, and the implant is moved inferiorly. The iris is then placed between the loops. If the dislocation is observed after the wound is sutured, one or two sutures should be removed to permit the maneuvers just described.

The Binkhorst iridocapsular (2-loop) implant may dislocate anteriorly. This is easily corrected by using either a spatula, a tying forceps, or a combination of both. If the optical portion should dislocate into the posterior chamber, the iris can be retracted in any convenient location until the edge of the optical portion is visible. If it can be grasped with tying forceps, the implant is easily maneuvered back into position. If this is difficult, a spatula is used to lift one side of the optical portion over the iris. The edge of the optical portion is then grasped with tying forceps, and the implant is maneuvered back into position.

The Worst 2-loop Medallion implant is easily repositioned, since one or both loops can only dislocate anteriorly. The optical portion is usually too large to dislocate posteriorly. However, this may occur. The inferior half of the optical portion may be behind the iris. This is usually corrected by dilating the pupil or by grasping the superior edge of the implant and pulling toward 12 o'clock until the inferior edge of the implant can be brought anterior to the iris. This may occur at the time of surgery by placing an excess amount of air in the anterior chamber. The first situation is corrected by using a spatula to move the implant to one side until the distal end of the dislocated loop can be tucked under the iris. The Worst platinum-clip or titanium-clip implant may dislocate so that the inferior loop is anterior to the iris. A spatula may be introduced from one side of the incision and placed under the inferior part of the optical portion. The implant is moved toward 12 o'clock until the distal end of the inferior loop passes the iris sphincter. It is then tucked under the iris inferiorly. The same result may be accomplished by grasping the extended optical portion of the implant at 12 o'clock as discussed above.

The Copeland implant has no loops or offset haptics. Therefore if three of the four haptics are in front or behind the iris, one haptic is grasped and the implant correctly positioned. This may require a relatively large incision.

Detachment of Descemet's membrane. Detachment of Descemet's membrane is most frequently caused by attempting to implant a pseudophakos through a small opening in the incision. It can often be detected through the surgical microscope. It may unfurl to the level of the corneal center. The detached portion should be rolled back into position using a flat spatula inserted into the anterior chamber from either side of the incision. The eye should temporarily be closed by tying the 12 o'clock retraction suture with a slipknot. A large air bubble is placed in the anterior chamber to tamponade the detached portion of Descemet's membrane. A 10-0 monofilament nylon suture is passed through the full thickness of cornea 2 to 3 mm inside the limbus. The needle engages the detached Descemet's membrane and emerges from the incision without going through the posterior lip of the wound. Two such sutures are placed at 10:30 and 1:30 o'clock. The slipknot of the retraction suture is opened, and the cornea is slightly retracted in order to insert the implant. Great care must be exercised to avoid catching the edge of the detached Descemet's membrane as the implant enters the anterior chamber. The incision is again closed with the retraction suture, and air is placed in the anterior chamber. The needles of the two previously placed 10-0 nylon sutures are passed through the scleral lips of the wound, and the sutures are tied. Additional full-thickness 10-0 nylon sutures are placed so as to engage other areas of the detached Descemet's membrane. The remainder of the wound is closed. The anterior chamber is left completely inflated with air.

Rupture of anterior lens capsule during an intended intracapsular cataract extraction. Unless the rent in the anterior capsule is small, enabling cryoextraction of the entire lens, it is wise to revert to an extracapsular technique. The anterior capsule should be removed with capsulectomy forceps (Schweiger). The nucleus is expressed, and the remaining cortical material should be removed by the surgeon's preferred method. It is far better to leave some residual lens material in the eye rather than risk a rupture of the posterior capsule with its usually associated loss of vitreous. A discission at a later date is a less serious alternative than loss of vitreous. One should be very careful in grasping a large piece of residual anterior capsule, since it will result in removal of posterior cortex, ruptured zonules, and loss of vitreous.

Rupture of posterior capsule. Posterior capsule rupture may occur during the performance of an extracapsular cataract extraction. If the rent in the posterior capsule is small and vitreous loss has not occurred, the procedure need not be altered. If the rupture is large and vitreous has not escaped, it is best to use an implant designed for an intracapsular cataract extraction. If vitreous loss has occurred, a partial anterior vitrectomy should be performed, as well as removal of all retained lens material. The implantation may be abandoned, or an intracapsular type implant may be used.

Vitreous bulge. In spite of all measures to reduce vitreous volume, the vitreous may bulge forward after the cataract is extracted. The surgeon performing his first lens implantations might consider avoiding the risk of vitreous loss or corneal endothelial damage and close the incision. The patient should have been informed preoperatively of this possibility.

The following approaches are suggested for the more experienced lens implant surgeon.

1. Close the eye with a slipknot in the 12 o'clock retraction suture. Add two sutures at 10 and 2 o'clock. Large-gauge sutures should be used such as 7-0 or 8-0 silk. These are also tied with a slipknot. Air is placed so as to completely fill the anterior chamber. It is left in place for 5 minutes. During this time the surgeon might consider using a rapidly administered intravenous solution of 25% man-

nitol (50 ml in 3 minutes) if a hyperosmotic agent was not given preoperatively. This is occasionally useful in reducing the vitreous bulge. A 20 mm Flieringa ring might also be placed at this time. This is useful if the bulge is caused by scleral collapse. The slipknots are released, and the ease with which air escapes enables the surgeon to assess the status of the vitreous bulge and the residual vitreous pressure.

2. Aspiration of retrovitreal fluid may be performed if the vitreous bulge has not lessened significantly (Fig. 12-3). This is performed using a 1.5-inch 22-gauge needle attached to a 2 ml glass syringe with a Luer lock. The needle is passed into the vitreous through the peripheral iridectomy and aimed superiorly and posteriorly. Aspiration pressure is maintained at all times. When the tip of the needle encounters the pocket of retrovit-

A

B

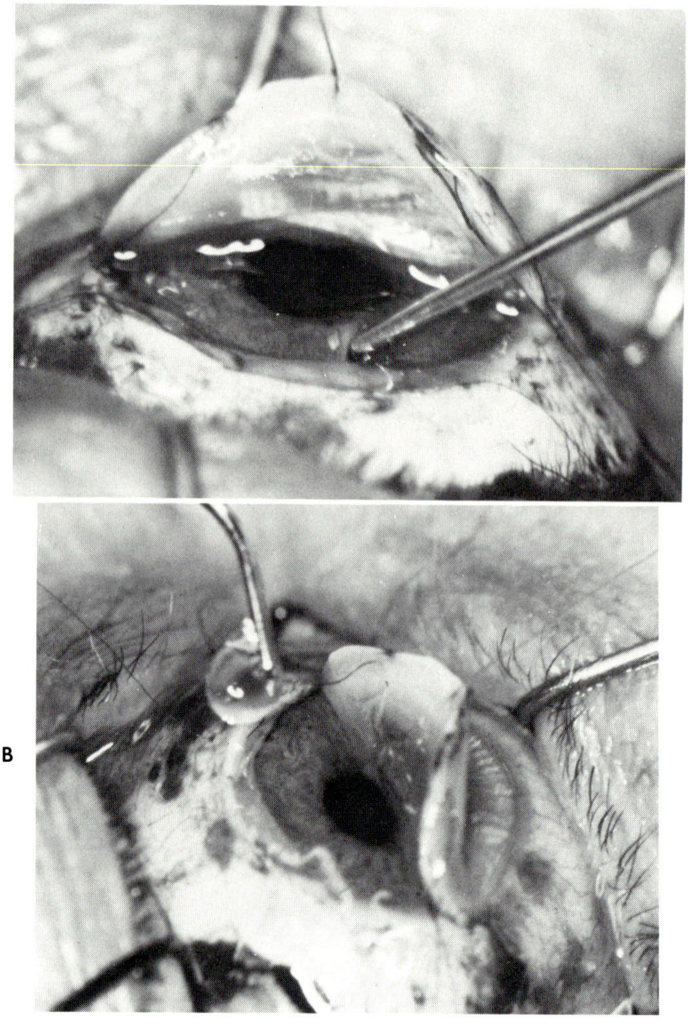

Fig. 12-3. Retrovitreal aspiration of fluid via peripheral iridectomy. **A,** Needle inserted into retrovitreal space through peripheral iridectomy. **B,** Posterior displacement of iris as fluid is aspirated. **C,** Collapsed globe resulting from aspiration of retrovitreal fluid. (From Jaffe, N. S.: Cataract surgery and its complications, ed. 2, St. Louis, 1976, The C. V. Mosby Co.)

real fluid or a liquid cavity, the fluid will rapidly enter the syringe and the iris and vitreous will move posteriorly. Approximately 0.25 to 0.5 ml is aspirated. The needle is then removed, and the implantation may proceed. This entire procedure must be performed with great care not to strike the retina. Although experienced surgeons have found this a useful procedure, it should not be considered innocuous.

3. The implant may be inserted under air. If a Binkhorst iris-clip (4-loop) implant is intended and a large peripheral iridectomy has been placed at 12 o'clock, the following technique is recommended. The 12 o'clock and either the 10 or 2 o'clock sutures are again tied with a slipknot. The anterior chamber is filled with air. The site of entry for the implant into the anterior chamber is oblique so as to avoid the iridectomy, since the posterior loop can easily be caught in it as the implant enters the anterior chamber. As the implant makes its initial entry, there is a tendency for air to escape from the anterior chamber. An experienced assistant is invaluable here, since he can inject air into the anterior chamber through a 27- or 30-gauge cannula between the two tied sutures as air is lost from the implant entry site. It is not too difficult to keep the anterior chamber filled with air as the implant is clipped onto the iris inferiorly at either side of 6 o'clock. The forceps are released, leaving the two superior loops anterior to the iris but under the air bubble. The implant is rotated to the vertical axis using a fine spatula, a Hirschman notched spatula, or a blunt iris hook. A fine spatula enters the anterior chamber from either side and passes between the anterior and posterior loops. The implant is pushed inferiorly until the superior posterior loop clears the upper iris sphincter. The loop is then pushed posteriorly by the spatula so that the superior loops engage the iris. The spatula is then removed. If the implant cannot be pushed sufficiently inferiorly, the iris can be lifted over the posterior loop with a blunt iris hook introduced near the 12 o'clock position. If the peripheral iridectomy is performed according to the surgeon's preference after the implant is in position, the implant can be introduced at the 12 o'clock position by releasing the slipknot of the 12 o'clock suture and leaving the 10 and 2 o'clock sutures tied.

In the case of the Worst platinum-clip

C

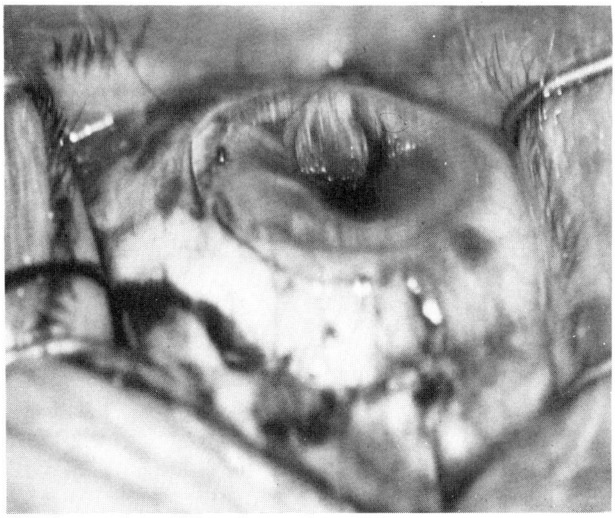

Fig. 12-3, cont'd. For legend see opposite page.

implant, this procedure works well, since the implant is designed to be placed in the vertical position. It is more difficult with the Worst 2-loop Medallion implant. Because the iris suture has already been placed, because it must be passed through the two holes of the implant before the implant is inserted, and because the loops must be in the horizontal position, it is easiest to insert the implant on one side of the 12 o'clock position by releasing the 10 or 2 o'clock sutures. One loop is passed behind the iris in an oblique position. The lens-holding instrument is removed. The implant can be rotated horizontally with one of the instruments described above. The remaining loop is passed behind the iris by pushing the implant toward the correctly positioned side using a spatula. The suture can be tied and cut under air. The biggest problem is to avoid snarling the suture around one of the loops. (See p. 104.)

4. The Sheets glide is a plastic or Silastic instrument that can be used in cases of vitreous bulge (Fig. 12-4). It can be made from the discarded portion of the Steri-Drape (3M Co., Inc.) used at surgery. There should be a 6 mm opening at 12 o'clock between the sutures. The lens glide is slipped into the anterior chamber after the chamber is filled with air. The lens glide passes over the superior iris, across the pupil, and under the inferior iris. This blocks the pupil and keeps the vitreous back. As the implant is grasped in the right hand, the anterior lip of the wound is picked up with forceps to allow passage of the lens into the anterior chamber. The optical portion of the upper edge of the implant is held with fine for-

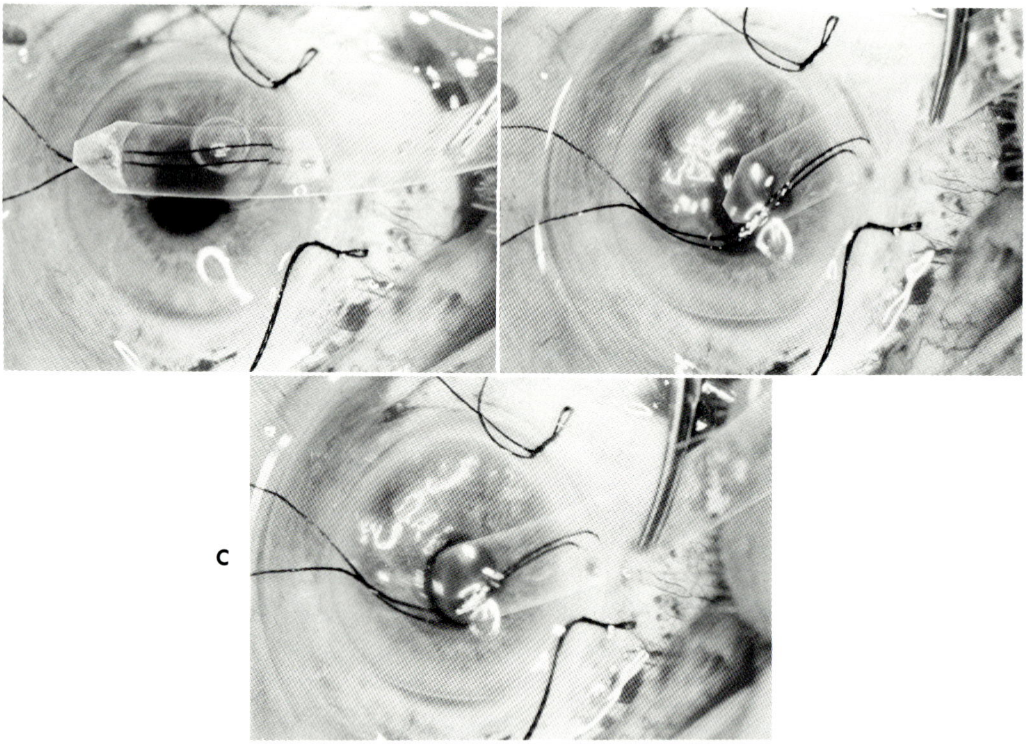

A B C

Fig. 12-4. Use of Sheets glide to permit insertion of pseudophakos under air. **A,** Appearance of glide prior to insertion. **B,** Glide being advanced into anterior chamber. **C,** Glide in situ, with tip under pupillary margin.

ceps or a Shepard forceps. The Binkhorst forceps are too large for this purpose. With moderate pressure against the lens glide and against the posterior lip of the wound, the lens is slid down the glide into the anterior chamber, thus displacing iris and vitreous somewhat posteriorly and allowing further air to pass into the anterior chamber as the lens reaches its position. As the inferior loops reach the lower iris edge, the glide is slowly withdrawn. As it withdraws, the glide pulls slightly on the upper iris to allow clearance of the upper posterior loop and permit it to fall into position behind the iris. If not, the two superior loops will remain anterior to the iris under the air bubble. The implant is maneuvered into position by passing a fine spatula between the two loops and pushing toward 6 o'clock until the posterior loop falls behind the iris.

If the wound is allowed to remain large instead of closed down to approximately 6 mm, the cornea has a tendency to collapse over the lens as it enters the anterior chamber and not retain an air bubble. When it is closed as described, the cornea remains domed and does not have this tendency.

If an iris suture has been previously inserted for a Worst 2-loop Medallion lens, the lens glide is passed so that the sutures through the iris are now beneath the glide and brought to the side of the glide and through the lens, which is lying to the side. The implant is introduced vertically down the glide. As the lower loop passes to the edge of the iris, the lens glide is gradually withdrawn and the loop passed beneath the iris inferiorly. As the glide is withdrawn further, the upper iris is retracted slightly by the glide so that the upper loop is allowed to go beneath the iris. The lens is rotated as described above or by tugging on the suture through the suture holes so that the loops become horizontal. The suture is then tied and cut in the usual manner.

Vitreous loss. In spite of all the prophylactic measures described earlier, vitreous loss is inevitable in a small percentage of cases. If the vitreous loss occurs before implantation, a partial anterior vitrectomy is performed. Although this may be performed with cellulose sponges, there are now available many automated vitrectomy devices that can be made available to the surgeon in a few minutes. These have the advantage of rapidity and less irritation of the iris. The tip of the device can be placed through the pupil and easily remove the anterior vitreous. It is also effective in removing vitreous from the anterior chamber without damaging the iris. If the vitreous escapes during the lens implantation, these devices have the advantage that they can remove the vitreous from around the implant after the implant is in position. If there is vitreous loss through the peripheral iridectomy during the placement of the transiridectomy suture, the tip of the device can be placed through the iridectomy and the vitreous can be removed from this location. Loss of vitreous through the peripheral iridectomy does not require a radical procedure.

Steroids should be used in all cases where the vitreous has been disturbed. One of the numerous available repository steroids is injected into the inferior cul de-sac. This may be accompanied by orally administered steroids if there are no systemic contraindications.

EARLY COMPLICATIONS

Pupillary block. Pupillary block is an uncommon complication. It may occur if the openings in the iris are made too peripherally and the cataract incision too anteriorly. It may also occur if the iris opening is not patent. Air pupillary block is also a possibility. If miotics are being used, they should be discontinued, and careful mydriasis should be attempted along with the systemic administration of a hyperosmotic agent. If this fails, one or more of the following should be tried: peripheral iridectomy, reopening of a closed iridectomy, transfixtion of the iris, or vitreous aspiration through a peripheral iridectomy. If the pupillary block is due to air, repositioning the patient's head may correct the situation. If not, the air should be aspirated.

Flat or shallow anterior chamber due to wound fistula. With a pseudophakos in situ, a flat or shallow anterior chamber due to wound fistula is a surgical emergency, since irreversible corneal damage may result from the implant touching the cornea. The wound should be resutured and a partial bubble of air left in the anterior chamber.

Shallow anterior chamber associated with a ciliochoroidal detachment. A shallow anterior chamber associated with a ciliochoroidal detachment should be managed in the same manner as after a routine cataract extraction with the following exception: if the chamber is sufficiently shallow so that there is danger of the optical portion of the implant touching the cornea, the condition should be remedied without delay.

Striate keratopathy and corneal edema. Striate keratopathy and corneal edema usually are more marked after lens implantation than after a routine cataract extraction due to the greater manipulation of the tissues that occurs in lens implantation (p. 183). It is usually transient, but in some cases it may persist for a long time (Fig. 12-5). There is no effective treatment.

Vitreous in the anterior chamber. Vitreous in the anterior chamber may be due to unrecognized rupture of the anterior face of the vitreous during the surgery or due to residual formed vitreous after a partial anterior vitrectomy. It usually is of no consequence, but occasionally results in a decentered lens (p. 177).

Lens precipitates. There are three types of lens precipitates. One consists of pigment deposits on both surfaces of the implant (Fig. 12-6). They arise from the pigment epithelium of the iris due to dispersion by the loop supports behind the iris. Another consists of grayish white precipitates that are the residue of lens material after an extracapsular cataract extraction. Similar deposits may be seen after recurrent bouts of uveitis. They resemble keratitic precipitates on the back of the cornea (Fig. 12-7). Lens precipitates tend to lessen with time. If the deposits on the implant are heavy, they occasionally lessen with steroid therapy given topically, by sub-Tenon's route, or both.

Endophthalmitis. Endophthalmitis, a rare postoperative complication, does not appear to be more frequent than after routine cataract extraction. At the outset of an intraocular infection one may have a dif-

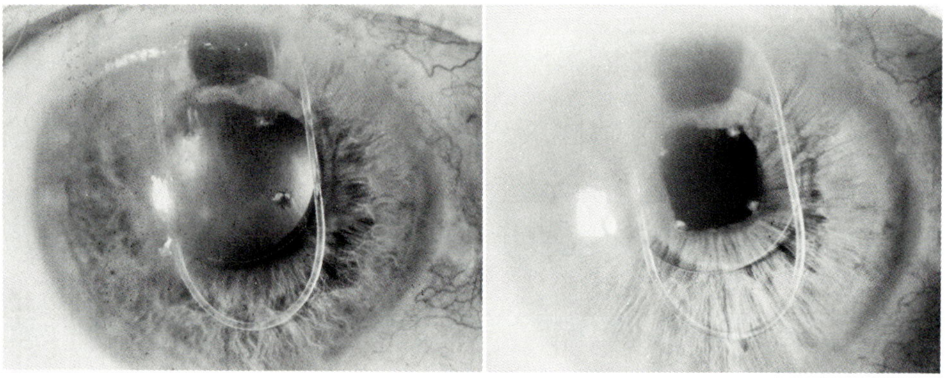

Fig. 12-5. A, Corneal edema resulting from surgical trauma seen 8 weeks postoperatively. (Visual acuity = 20/800.) **B,** Same eye 6 months later. (Visual acuity = 20/20.)

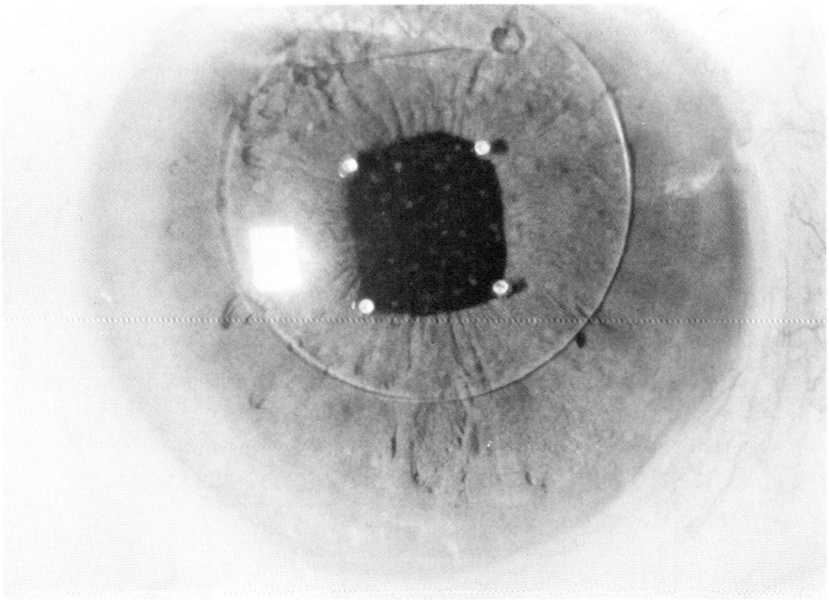

Fig. 12-6. Pigment deposits on posterior surface of Worst Medallion implant.

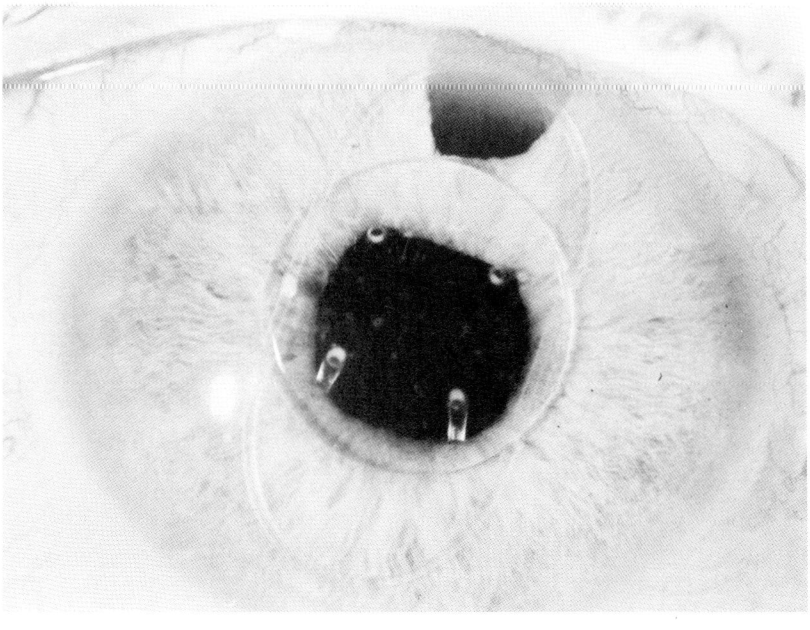

Fig. 12-7. Deposits on posterior surface of Binkhorst iris-clip implant resulting from inflammation.

ficult time differentiating a true infection from an aseptic uveitis even in the presence of a hypopyon. In addition, delaying treatment until the etiologic microorganism is isolated may result in unnecessary damage. Cultures are often negative. Therefore immediate treatment on an empiric basis is mandatory after anterior chamber and vitreous taps, while the results of cultures are being awaited.

There is a growing trend toward pars plana vitrectomy for the treatment of endophthalmitis. It merits careful consideration. The rationale is to treat endophthalmitis as if it were an intraocular abscess. The advantages are that a biopsy is obtained for culture and cytology. Organisms are removed, the matrix for infection is removed, and instillation of intravitreal antibiotics is facilitated.

An anterior chamber tap is performed and the aspirate sent for smear and culture. The vitrectomy should be as total as possible. Material is collected for culture

A

B

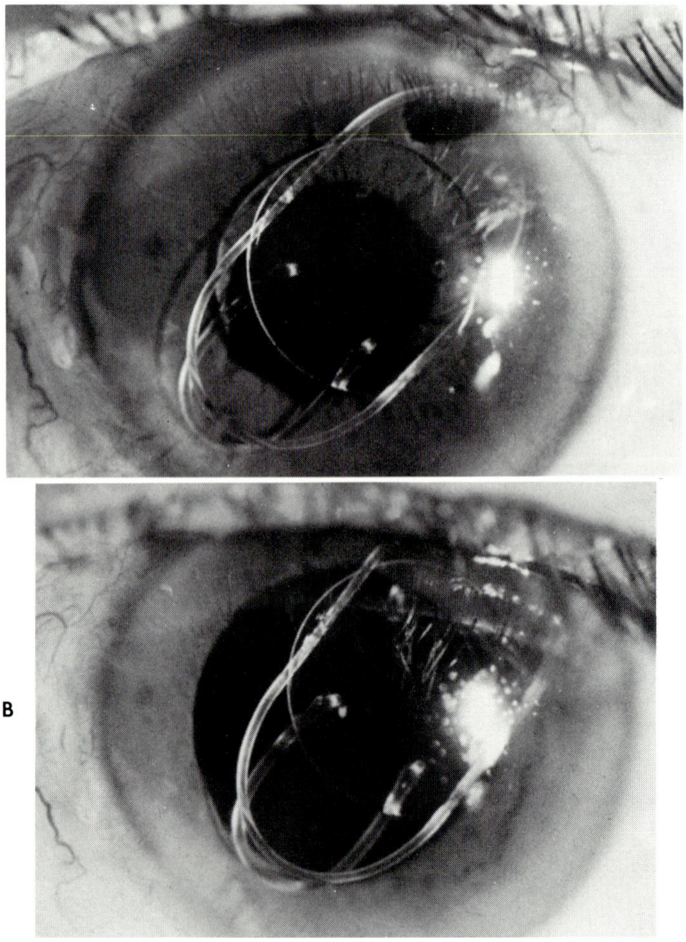

Fig. 12-8. A, Spontaneous dislocation of Binkhorst 4-loop iris-clip implant. Both loops are anterior to iris at 6 o'clock. Condition of eye at diagnosis of dislocation. **B,** Pupil dilated with 10% phenylephrine solution. **C,** Pupil now sufficiently dilated for reposition with echothiophate iodide 0.12% solution. **D,** Implant is now properly positioned. (**A** to **C** from Jaffe, N. S.: Cataract surgery and its complications, ed. 2, St. Louis, 1976, The C. V. Mosby Co.)

and cytology. The implant may be left in situ unless one suspects a fungus contaminant. Fungus organisms tend to cling to surfaces and may remain on the intraocular lens. Intravitreal antibiotics are instilled through the vitrectomy apparatus at the conclusion of surgery. Since the invading organism is unknown at the time of surgery, the following regimen is suggested:

1. Intravitreal: gentamicin, 100 μg, and cephaloridine, 250 μg.
2. Topical: gentamicin, 20 to 40 mg, via sub-Tenon's route daily; cephaloridine, 100 mg, subconjunctivally daily; bacitracin eye drops every 1 to 2 hours; atropine solution four times daily. Kenalog (triamcinolone) is administered via the sub-Tenon's route daily in a dose of 1 ml (40 mg).
3. Systemic: gentamicin, 0.8 mg/kg, initially by intramuscular injection and then 0.4 mg/kg every 6 hours and cephaloridine, 1 g, intravenously or intra-

C

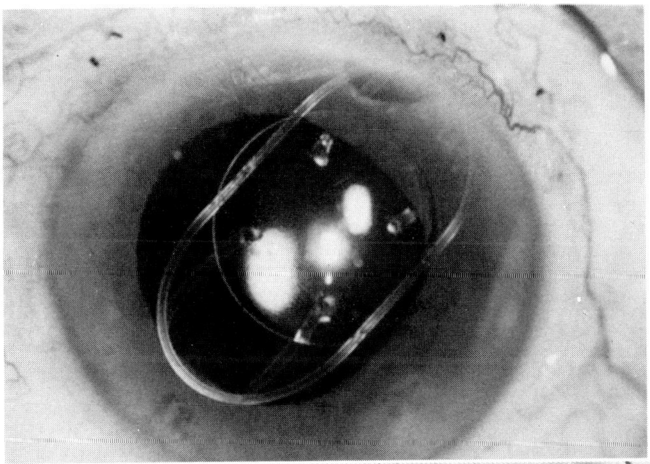

D

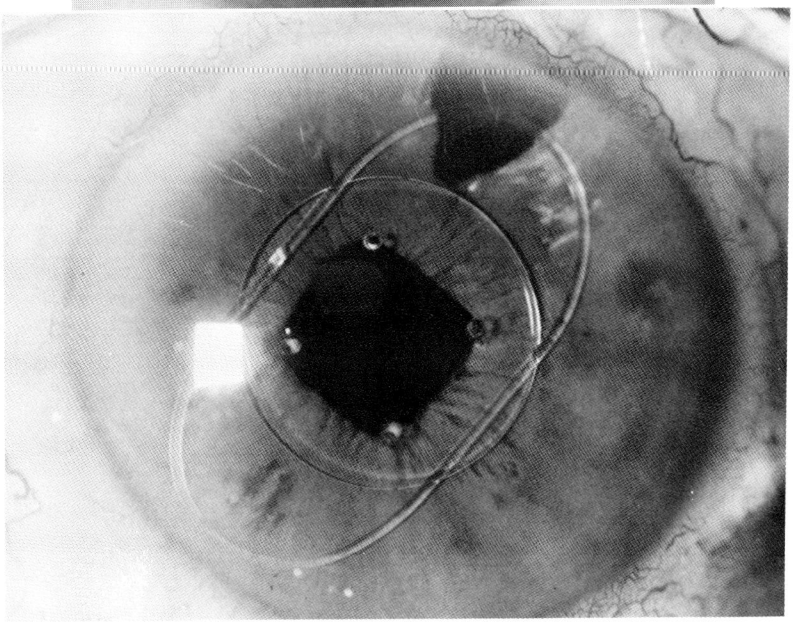

Fig. 12-8, cont'd. For legend see opposite page.

muscularly every 6 hours. Since gentamicin can be nephrotoxic and ototoxic, a baseline blood urea nitrogen determination should be obtained first. If renal status is poor, carbenicillin may be substituted in doses of 2 to 6 g intravenously every 4 hours. Carbenicillin is effective against *Pseudomonas* organisms, but is ineffective against penicillinase-producing staphylococci.

It is difficult to suggest a single regimen, since new antibiotics appear with such regularity that one must expect any discussion of specific antibiotics for the treatment of postoperative intraocular infections to become obsolete within a relatively short period of time. For a complete listing and discussion of all available antibiotics for use in ophthalmology, the reader is referred to one of several books available on ocular pharmacology.

Once the invading organisms have been identified and sensitivity studies made available, specific therapy is administered.

It is repeated that pars plana vitrectomy for the treatment of postoperative endophthalmitis is a new procedure and its effects are still being evaluated. Some will argue that this is a heroic procedure that may not be warranted where the offending organism is only mildly virulent (for example, *Staphylococcus epidermidis*) and may be successfully treated by nonsurgical methods. However, the risk of waiting for identification of the etiologic organism may be even greater than the risk of the surgery. Only too often the retina and choroid are destroyed within a day or two of onset of endophthalmitis. With most invading organisms it appears better to attack the problem surgically if useful vision is to be retained. The performance of a vitreous tap is a surgical procedure in itself and may not secure the responsible organism. Relying on an anterior chamber tap alone is probably no longer valid.

If the initial favorable results of pars plana vitrectomy are continued, this method may prove to be one of the greatest advances in therapeutic ophthalmology.

EARLY OR LATE COMPLICATIONS

Dislocation. Dislocation may be due to the following:

1. Too much air in the anterior chamber
2. Too wide a pupil as a result of rupture of the sphincter of a miotic pupil during cataract extraction or due to sphincter damage by the cryoprobe
3. Premature discontinuation of pilocarpine in those implants that are not secured by a fixation suture or device
4. Accidental use of mydriatrics
5. Pupillary dilatation at night
6. Pupillary dilatation due to excitement
7. Loop length of implant too short
8. Ocular trauma

Reposition is initially attempted pharmacologically. A short-acting mydriatic that is easily reversible, such as 10% phenylephrine solution or 1% Mydriacyl (tropicamide), is instilled. The patient's head is placed in an optimum position determined by the portion that has dislocated. As soon as the pupil dilates sufficiently so that the distal portion of the dislocated haptic clears the iris margin, the patient's head is placed securely in the proper position and a miotic (for example, echothiophate iodide 0.12% solution) is placed in the eye (Fig. 12-8). If this fails (Fig. 12-9), instrumental repositioning must be used. There are a number of fine instruments available. One such instrument is a 25- or 27-gauge Rizzuti-Spizziri cannula needle attached to a 2 ml syringe filled with balanced salt solution or acetylcholine solution. The needle enters the anterior chamber through the limbus and maneuvers the implant into proper position. Disposable needles are very sharp and may also be

A

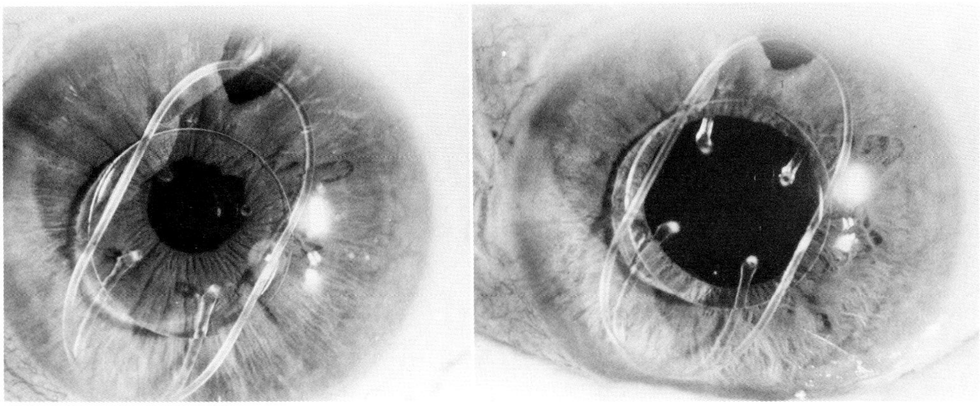

B

Fig. 12-9. A, Dislocation of Binkhorst iris clip implant. **B,** Maximal mydriasis obtained in this eye is insufficient to achieve repositioning by pharmacologic means.

A

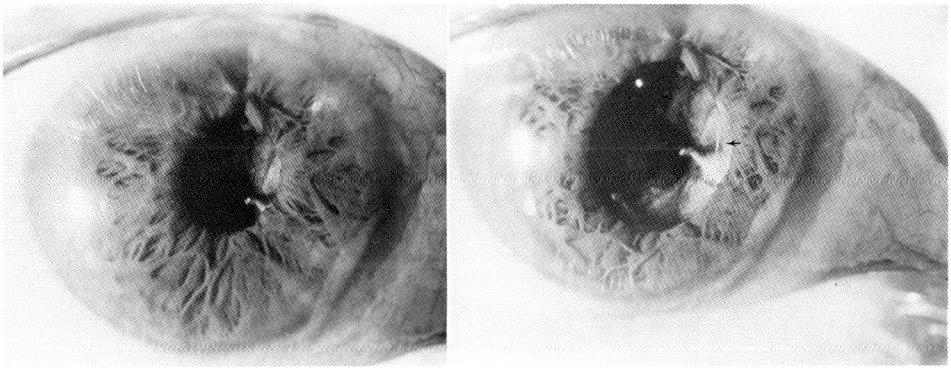

B

Fig. 12-10. A, Extracapsular cataract extraction has been performed in eye with miotic pupil. Superior iris was incised and sutured. Optical portion of Binkhorst iridocapsular implant has dislocated into posterior chamber. **B,** After mydriasis, edge of optical portion *(arrow)* is seen. Capsular fixation is adequate. (Visual acuity 2 years postoperatively = 20/20.)

used for this purpose. If aqueous escapes, it should be replaced with the solution. If dislocation of a capsule-supported lens occurs, it may be possible to reposition it with eye drops, as just described. Pilocarpine solution should be used indefinitely. It may be possible to suture one of the loop supports to the iris. In some instances it may be wise to remove the implant and replace it with an iris-supported lens, for example, a Binkhorst iris-clip (4-loop) pseudophakos. If the optical portion of a capsule-supported implant dislocates behind the iris, it can usually be left in this position as a posterior chamber lens (Fig. 12-10).

If repeated dislocations of an implant with loops occur, in spite of daily miotic medication, a more permanent method of securing fixation must be undertaken. McCannel has suggested a method that has become popular (Fig. 12-11). A stab wound is made just within the limbus through a clear cornea closest to the position where the suture will end up being tied to the iris below. A double-arm 9-0 nylon or polypropylene (Prolene, Ethicon, Inc., Somerville, N.J.) (a half-curve

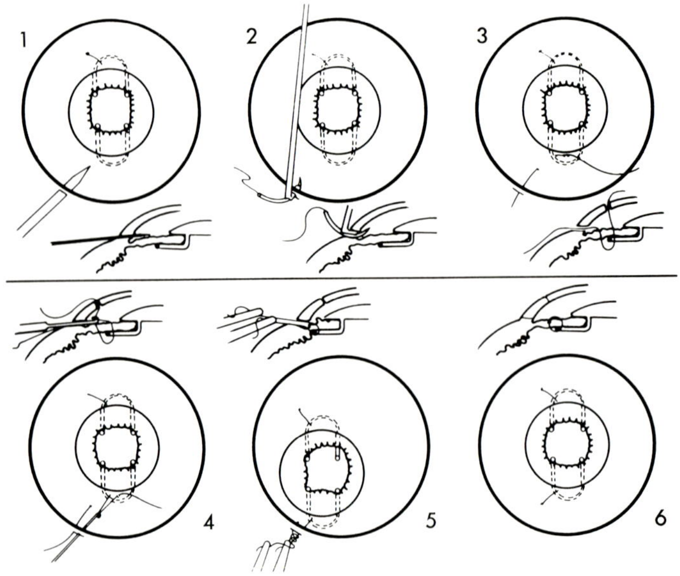

Fig. 12-11. McCannel suture for dislocated intraocular lens fixation. *1,* Following small limbal incision at 8 o'clock position, a long narrow spatula can be used to reposition loop of intraocular lens into its proper place behind iris. *2,* Through this incision, a small, short, grooved 2.5 mm spatula is introduced into incision and acts as guide to 10-0 monofilament nylon suture on half-circle needle, which is directed into anterior chamber under spatula. This prevents needle point from catching on corneoscleral tissues as it enters anterior chamber. *3,* Needle point is then directed down posteriorly through iris and under now properly positioned loop of intraocular lens. Without releasing needle holder grip, needle point is then brought up again through iris and continues vertically across anterior chamber to exit through cornea. *4,* Anterior chamber suture segment is then pulled out in a loop through same stab corneoscleral wound using delicate, blunt iris hook or 26-gauge needle with its point bent into small hook. *5,* Corneal suture is then cut flush on epithelial surface, allowing end to be brought out in single strand at limbus. Triple throw suture tie is placed, using two ends of suture. As knot is drawn down firmly, shift is seen in anterior chamber, intraocular lens, and pupil toward corneal incision. *6,* When knot is fully tied, ends are cut flush at knot, releasing suture tension so iris can then resume its normal shape with intraocular lens and pupil centering again. This results in a tied fixation suture around iris and intraocular lens loop within anterior chamber. A miotic solution may be injected into anterior chamber. (From McCannel, M. A.: Ophthalmic Surg. 7:98-103, 1976.)

needle is best for this purpose) suture is passed through this incision, through the iris, around the loop that may be anterior or posterior to the iris (according to the implant type), back out through the iris, and finally out through the cornea at any point where the needle ends up. At this point we have a suture that is passing through the stab wound, through the iris, around a loop, through the iris again, and out through another area of the cornea. The needle is cut off from the leading end of the suture that has emerged from the cornea. Five to 7.5 cm of suture are left outside the cornea after the needle is cut off. A small iris hook is introduced through the stab wound, and the free end of the suture is grasped and withdrawn from the eye through the stab wound. Both ends of the suture are now emerging from the stab wound. These two ends are then tied together with four knots. This brings the loop and iris up to the stab wound. The suture is cut close to the knot. The iris and the sutured loop will then retract into the anterior chamber.

Decentration. When decentration occurs, it nearly always does so within the first 6 postoperative months. This may be caused by an asymmetric adhesion of the loop supports to residual capsulolenticular material after an extracapsular cataract extraction. It may also be caused by iris incarceration, peripheral anterior synechiae, an atonic pupil, too tight a suture used for fixation to the iris, and vitreous strands in the anterior chamber. The implant may not only decenter but tilt. This usually does not require treatment, since vision is not at all or only minimally altered. This may be due to the fact that the optical portion of the lens rests close to the first principal plane of the eye. The most frequent cause of decentration is fibroplasia of vitreous left in the anterior chamber when operative loss of vitreous has occurred. If there is extensive incarceration of vitreous in the wound, the implant may become decentered so that the optical portion or an anterior loop (iris-clip lens) may touch the cornea or be dangerously close to it. This must be surgically corrected by removing the offending vitreous and repositioning the implant.

Uveitis. Uveitis may be a reaction to surgical trauma. It may be sufficiently exaggerated to be considered a sterile endophthalmitis. It may be a response to retained lens material (phacoanaphylaxis). The first two causes respond well to steroid therapy. The last is much more difficult. It may require evacuation of all lenticular remains. It is somewhat surprising that the repopularization of the extracapsular cataract extraction has not yet brought forth a reappearance of phacoanaphylactic uveitis as a serious postoperative problem. Recurrent uveitis might also cause opacification of the anterior vitreous (p. 181).

Cystoid macular edema. The cause of this complication is still speculative. It occurs between 1 and 4 months after surgery but in some instances does not appear until years later. Studies are currently under way to compare the incidence of angiographically proven cystoid macular edema in age-matched groups of patients undergoing intracapsular cataract extraction without lens implantation, intracapsular cataract extraction with implantation of a Binkhorst iris-clip (4-loop) lens, and extracapsular cataract extraction (not by phacoemulsification) with implantation of Binkhorst iridocapsular (2-loop) lens (see p. 83). The treatment of cystoid macular edema is difficult to assess because of the tendency to spontaneous resolution. A trial of steroids or other antiinflammatory drugs might be tried. One regimen consists of three injections of 40 units (1 ml) of triamcinolone by sub-Tenon's route at weekly intervals. Indomethacin, 25 mg three times daily after meals, might be tried for 2 weeks. The efficacy of these agents is still questionable.

Secondary membranes. After a planned extracapsular cataract extraction, an excess of unevacuated lens material may migrate into the pupillary space. With the implant in situ, the passage of this material into the anterior chamber, where absorption is more likely, is retarded. This encourages dense secondary cataracts that occasionally vascularize due to migration of iris vessels. In most of these cases one need not be concerned about dislocation due to attempted dilatation of the pupil. The pupil should be kept dilated as much as possible with hyoscine or atropine solution. This helps prevent pupillary block and aids in absorption of the retained lens material. If the secondary cataract membrane shows no tendency to absorb or becomes severely involved in adherence to the iris, surgical intervention is indicated.

Surgery designed to create an adequate pupillary aperture in a secondary membrane must be carefully planned. It is easy to underestimate the difficulties one might encounter with a very thick capsulolenticular membrane. Although capsulotomy at the time of surgery is frequently employed with phacoemulsification, it is safer to perform this at a later date when implanting an intraocular lens. It is nearly impossible to open the posterior capsule at the time of implantation without rupturing the anterior hyaloid membrane, since they are in apposition. However, at a later date there is usually an easily demonstrable space between these two structures. A relatively thin secondary membrane lends itself easily to surgery. If the membrane has disturbed the patient's vision and appears to be getting progressively more dense, surgery should not be delayed. Early surgery is more effective and less complex. The surgeon should assure himself that the decline in vision is in accord with the view of the fundus (direct ophthalmoscope or Hruby lens). For most thin secondary membranes the following procedure has been found useful (Fig. 12-12). A stab wound is made just inside the limbus with a Beaver No. 75 disposable razor blade fragment or some other similar instrument. This location for the initial entry into the anterior chamber is selected to avoid bleeding from a more

A B

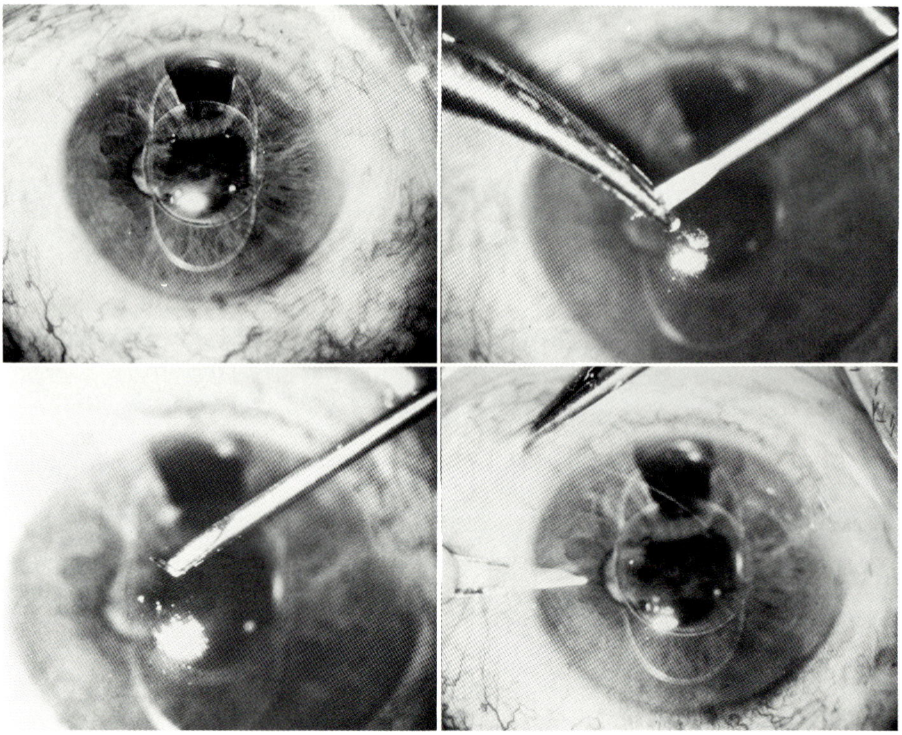

C D

Fig. 12-12. A, Secondary membrane after extracapsular cataract extraction (12 weeks) with implantation of a Binkhorst iris-clip lens. Maximum mydriasis shown. (Visual acuity = 20/400.) **B,** Hook created at tip of 25-gauge disposable needle using needle holder. **C,** Bent tip shown. **D,** Limbal stab wound made with No. 75 Beaver blade. **E,** Needle is attached to irrigating solution and enters anterior chamber, passing behind implant. **F,** Tip of needle engages membrane as irrigating flow is stopped. **G,** Hole in membrane is created as irrigating flow resumes. **H,** Membrane is drawn toward limbal wound. **I,** Opening in membrane is enlarged still further. **J,** Final result. Visual acuity improved to 20/25 3 months later.

peripheral location. It is mandatory to maintain clear visibility for this procedure. A tiny hook is made at the tip of a disposable 25-gauge needle by bending it with a needle holder so that the opening is at the inside of the bent tip. The angle of the bend may be from 45° to 90°. The needle is attached to an irrigating handle such as the Cavitron irrigation-aspiration handle. The handle is attached to the plastic tubing of a container of irrigating solution. The irrigating container is elevated sufficiently for free flow through the needle. All air should be evacuated from the tubing. The needle is passed through the stab wound, under the optical portion of the implant, until the opposite edge of the pupil is reached. The continuous flow of fluid pushes the posterior capsule posteriorly. When the hook of the needle is in the correct position, the plastic tubing is pinched closed by the surgeon or an assistant. This permits the posterior capsule to float forward against the tip of the needle. A tiny tear is made in the posterior capsule, and the irrigation

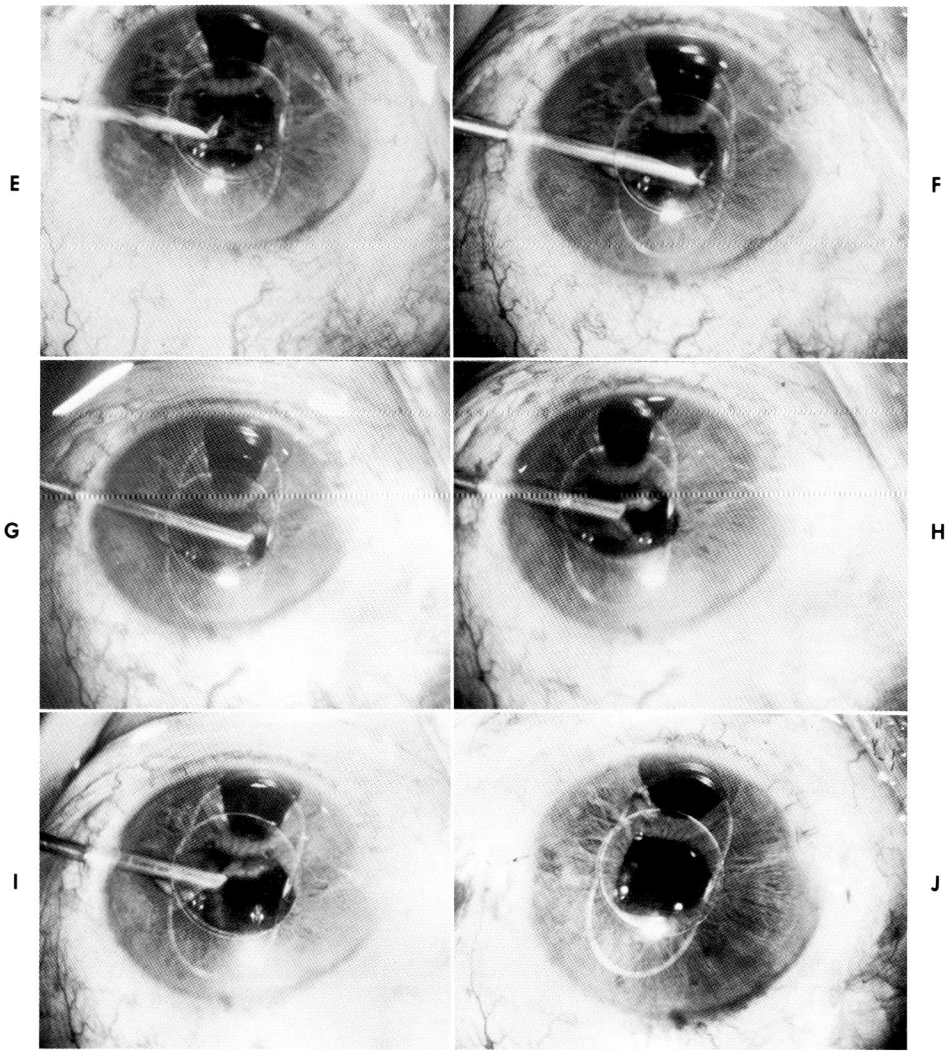

Fig. 12-12, cont'd. For legend see opposite page.

flow is permitted to resume. The fluid passes through the hole and pushes the vitreous posteriorly. The tear in the posterior capsule is then completed across the entire pupil. The needle is withdrawn from the eye. The stab wound may be left unsutured, or a single 10-0 nylon suture may be used to close the small opening.

This procedure works very well for thin secondary membranes and for thin membranes that develop on the surface of the vitreous after an intracapsular cataract extraction. Thick membranes are much more difficult and often impossible to manage by this technique. These membranes may be so extensive as to adhere to the ciliary processes. It would be dangerous to pull on such a membrane. Another approach is recommended in this situation. One of the various types of vitrectomy instruments may be used, for example, Douvas Roto-Extractor, Machemer Vitreous Infusion Suction Cutter, Girard ultrasonic fragmentor, or Berkeley Ocutome. In these cases the iris on all sides of the pupil is often pulled centrally except at the origin posts of the posterior loops or at the apices of the Copeland implant. The pupil may have the shape of a vertical and horizontal hourglass. The cutting instrument is usually passed through a pars plana incision until it appears in the pupillary space. If the membrane is confined to the posterior capsule or the anterior vitreous, fiber optics illumination is not required. The dense membrane is removed. The pulled-in portions of iris may also be resected. This will usually not result in undue mydriasis. The iris is resected until a square-shaped pupil is fashioned (Fig. 12-13). The surgeon may elect to create a V-shaped notch in the inferior border of the pupil. The surgery is concluded when a clear fundus reflex is visible through the surgical microscope. Some surgeons prefer to perform the surgery through the anterior chamber via a limbal incision. The advantage of avoiding an incision through the pars plana is somewhat offset by the increased possibility of dislocating the implant and the lessened freedom of maneuvers behind the implant. When properly performed, this technique rarely damages or dislocates the implant.

In summary, a discission is recommended for thin, postlental membranes and a membranectomy using a vitrectomy instrument for thick membranes.

Retinal detachment. Fortunately, with

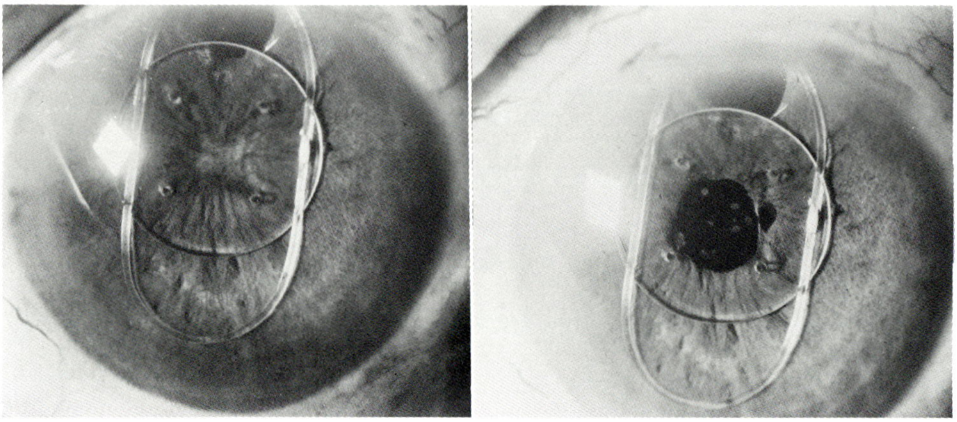

A B

Fig. 12-13. A, Dense retrolental membrane in patient who suffered hypopyon uveitis 3 days after intracapsular cataract extraction and implantation of Binkhorst iris-clip lens. (Visual acuity = hand motion at 1 foot.) **B,** Membrane and anterior vitreous removed with Douvas Roto-Extractor. Pupil reshaped. Visual acuity 4 months later was 20/40.

improved methods of examining the fundus, a satisfactory examination for retinal detachment is usually possible. However, reattachment of the retina may be more difficult with than without an implant due to an undilatable pupil, optical distortion from metal loops, and optical discontinuity between the implant and the aphakic portion of the dilated pupil. Moreover, a dense intraocular lens membrane or a dense secondary membrane would be serious obstacles to satisfactory localization of retinal breaks. These obstacles may be eliminated at the time of retinal surgery by the methods just discussed.

LATE COMPLICATIONS

Secondary membranes. Secondary membranes have been discussed on p. 177.

Intraocular lens membrane. The intraocular lens membrane appears to be more common with the iris-plane (Copeland) implant, since it lies closer to the vitreous face (Figs. 12-14 and 12-15). Vitreous may contact the posterior surface of the optical portion of the implant and proliferate on this surface. The iris may migrate over the back or front of the implant. Recurrent iritis may also cause such a membrane. Retained lens remnants may do likewise, but this tends to lessen with time.

Opacification of the anterior face of the vitreous. Opacification of the anterior face of the vitreous usually results from a severe hyphema or recurrent iritis. If it interferes with vision, it can be incised as in performing a discission of a secondary membrane.

Cystoid macular edema. Cystoid macular edema may appear some years after implantation for no apparent reason.

Retinal detachment. Retinal detachment may occur as a late complication and is managed in the same manner as after routine cataract extraction.

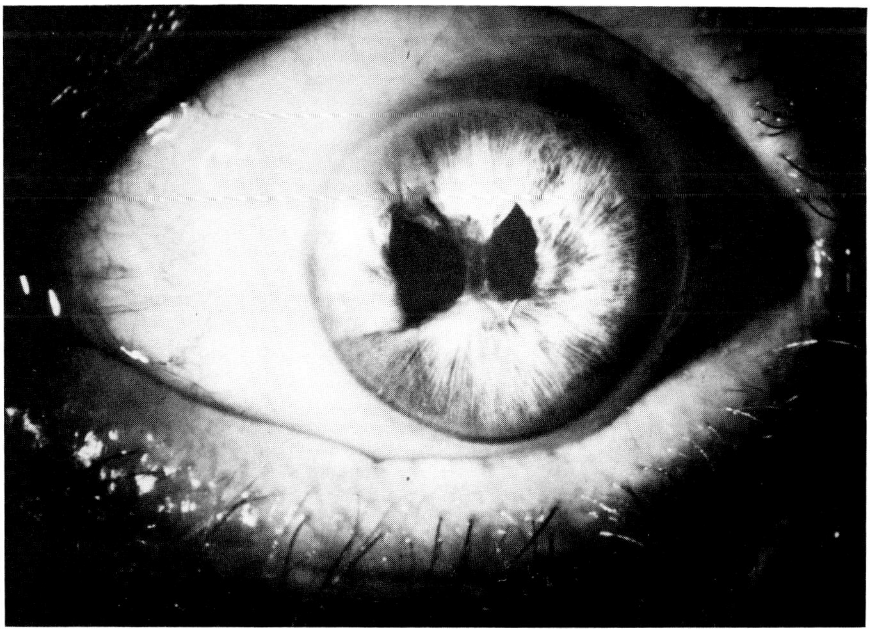

Fig 12-14. Membrane behind Copeland iris-plane implant. (Visual acuity = 20/25.) (From Jaffe, N. S.: Cataract surgery and its complications, ed. 2, St. Louis, 1976, The C. V. Mosby Co.)

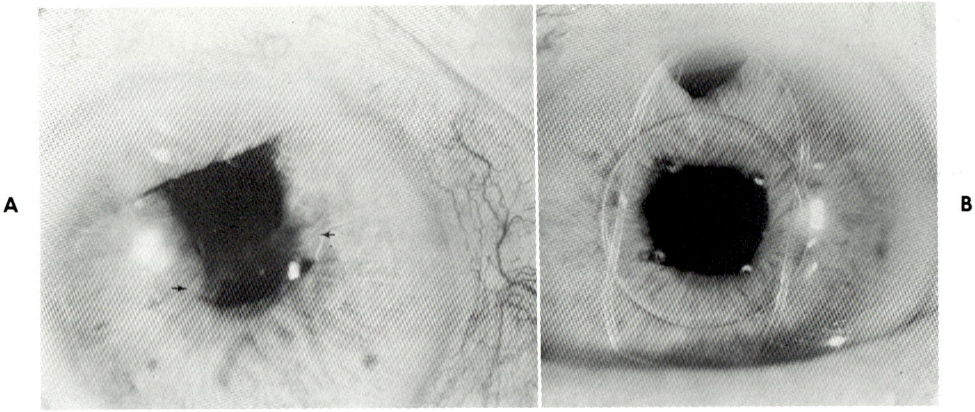

Fig. 12-15. A, Right eye of patient 6.5 years after implantation of Copeland lens. Note membrane *(arrows)*. (Visual acuity = 20/25.) **B,** Left eye of same patient 6 months after implantation of Binkhorst iris-clip lens. Pupil is dilatable. (Visual acuity = 20/25.)

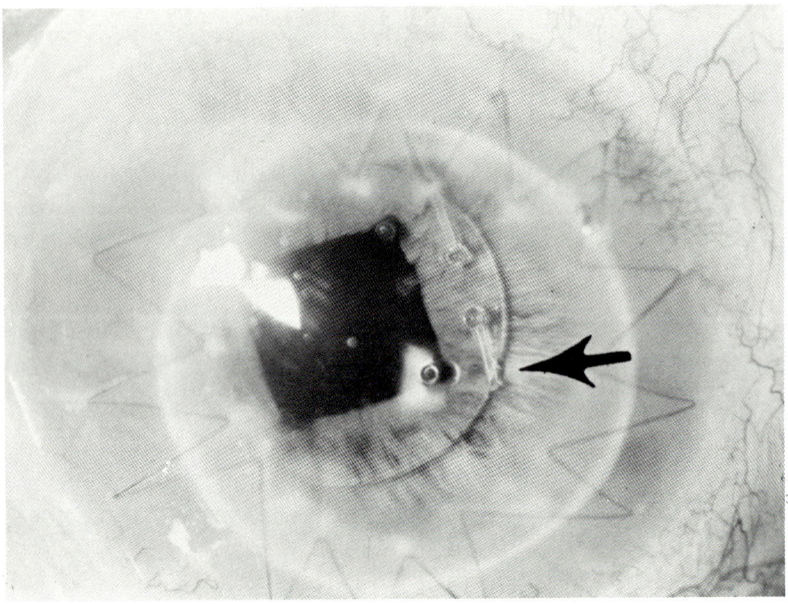

Fig. 12-16. Corneal edema resulted from contact of lower loop of Fyodorov-Binkhorst implant with cornea. Penetrating keratoplasty and amputation of loop *(arrow)* performed.

Corneal edema. Corneal edema has become far less frequent than in the days of anterior chamber angle implants. It may occur due to intermittent contact between the anterior loops of the implant or the optical portion of the implant and the cornea. It is theoretically possible for this to result from degradation of the plastic implant, although this has never been documented. It is more likely to result from senescent corneal degeneration, especially in eyes with endothelial abnormalities. It may follow repeated attacks of iritis, especially with secondary glaucoma. If mild, localized corneal edema results from a defective or malformed loop support touching the cornea, the situation should be corrected immediately. Procrastination in this situation usually leads to total corneal edema. The defective loop may be excised (Fig. 12-16). In irreversible corneal edema the only treatment for visual restoration is a penetrating keratoplasty. This usually has a favorable prognosis, since the implant prevents the vitreous from contacting the cornea.

Nevertheless, from the inception of lens implant surgery, corneal edema has been the most dreaded complication related to the surgery. It has also been the one most responsible for the seemingly endless number of changes in implant design and techniques of surgery. Postoperative corneal edema is not restricted to implant surgery, since it has also been a significant complication of both intracapsular and extracapsular cataract extraction without lens implantation.

It would be illogical to assume that corneal edema is merely a sign of senescence and the surgery is just a minimal cause. If one were to compare a large population of patients with clinically normal corneas who have never had cataract surgery with an equal number with normal corneas who have had cataract surgery, one would expect to find a higher incidence of corneal edema in the latter group at a particular age level. One relates this directly to the trauma of surgery and the alteration in the intraocular morphology. For example, some patients have unusually traumatic surgery and some have problems related to a particular postoperative occurrence, such as vitreocorneal adherence. The eye that has never had surgery has not been exposed to these events. Carrying this logic further, it would appear justified to anticipate a higher incidence of corneal edema after lens implant surgery than after routine cataract extraction. The reason for this is simple. Implant surgery begins where routine cataract surgery ends. Even the most skillful insertion of an intraocular lens involves an additional number of surgical manipulations not required in a routine cataract extraction. In addition, there are a number of postoperative complications related specifically to the implant, and these probably outweigh those that are not seen after implant surgery, for example, corneal edema due to vitreocorneal adherence.

In general, one might expect lens implant surgery rather than conventional cataract surgery more likely to be followed by corneal edema for the following reasons:

1. Improper selection of cases (for example, preexisting corneal disease, severe diabetes)
2. Greater risk of operative and postoperative endothelial damage
3. Use of a badly designed implant that can make contact with the cornea (Fig. 12-16)
4. Toxic influence of degenerative products of the implant, although this has never been demonstrated

Probably the single most important factor in causing corneal edema after lens implant surgery (or after any intraocular surgery) is a lowered endothelial vitality. This term appears nebulous only because we do not yet possess reliable clinical means of grading corneal endothelial health. The slit lamp is of some help in pointing out certain degenerative changes such as cornea guttata, but is of little help when the cornea appears normal. It has been shown that there is a decreasing endothelial cell population with age, but until recently there have been no reliable clinical indicators of this. Pachymetry is occasionally useful but is probably not yet a significant tool. Specular microscopy of the endothelial cells holds far greater promise (see below), but its widespread use will certainly require some time.

Endothelial vitality varies greatly among individuals, which leads one to suspect that it might be inborn. Note how susceptible some eyes are to corneal edema after minor trauma such as a simple needling or during an attack of iritis. Some eyes show a strong tendency to striate keratopathy or edema of the wound margins. In this there is a strong tendency to bilaterality. This is a warning that endothelial vitality has exceeded its critical level of decompensation. On the other hand, some corneas fare remarkably well after the most difficult surgical procedures. That there are individual differences in endothelial vitality is certain on the basis of clinical experience. This probably explains why some eyes develop persistent corneal edema immediately after surgery, while others do not develop it for many years with the origin being the surgery itself. There is no such thing as atraumatic surgery; it is merely a matter of degree. Every eye subjected to a cataract extraction suffers some damage from instruments, retraction of the cornea, inflammation, toxic and mechanical effects of intraocular solutions and medications, alterations of intraocular pressure (high and low), and so on. Conditions occur immediately following the surgery that favor decreased endothelial vitality. A certain amount of iritis is inevitable. The intraocular pressure may be elevated for several days. This may be due to the use of alpha-chymotrypsin or to the current tendency to tight wound closure. Epithelial corneal edema is frequent and may be due to these factors as well as others. A wound leak or pupillary block associated with a flat or shallow anterior chamber may cause vitreocorneal or iridocorneal contact, which damages corneal endothelium. As stated previously, the response of the eyes of different individuals to these surgical and postoperative traumas vary. Even among those eyes that appear to make a complete clinical recovery, there will be marked differences in the residual endothelial cell population. It would be naive to consider these corneas to have resumed their preoperative health. Support of this concept is to be seen in eyes that develop an unexplained

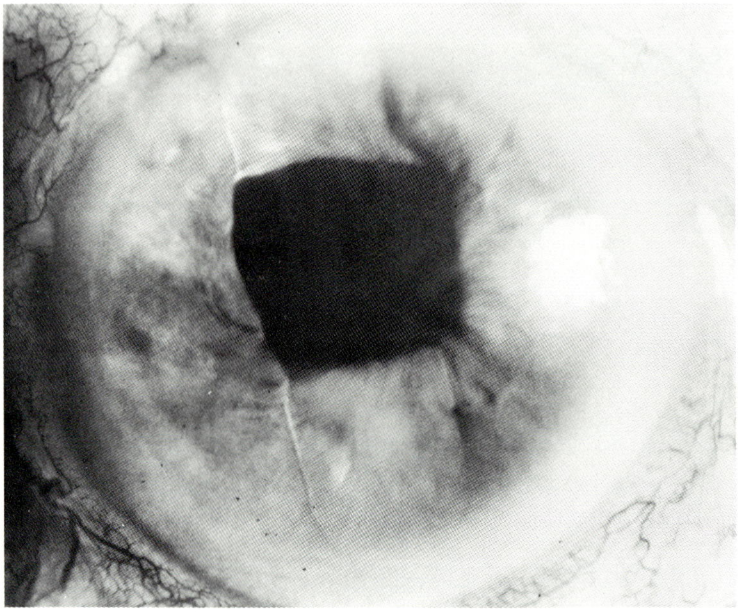

Fig. 12-17. Corneal edema occurring 6.5 years after implantation of Copeland iris-plane lens.

iritis months or years after surgery. In some there is an associated corneal edema, indicating endothelial decompensation, while in others there is no clinical evidence of corneal edema.

Binkhorst listed the following three causes as the most frequent etiologic factors (in nearly equal frequency) in a survey of intracapsular cataract extractions with a 4-loop implant: (1) low endothelial vitality before surgery, (2) surgical and postoperative complications, and (3) late contact of implant with cornea.

It is not difficult to accept that corneal edema may result from surgical trauma or postoperative problems. However, late corneal edema remains a problem in etiology, especially when there are no postoperative problems such as recurrent iritis, secondary glaucoma, or corneal contact. Such an example is illustrated in Fig. 12-17. Corneal edema occurred in this eye 6½ years after an uneventful intracapsular cataract extraction with implantation of an iris-plane (Copeland) lens. The postoperative course was entirely normal. Of interest is that pachymetry performed on this eye revealed a corneal thickness of 0.74 mm and 0.54 mm in the fellow eye. The latter showed no slit-lamp evidence of corneal abnormality, although pachymetry suggested the possibility of lowered corneal vitality. Occurrences such as this have been observed after routine cataract extraction without implantation. However, when it occurs after lens implant surgery, the cause is usually related to poor behavior of the implant, in spite of no evidence to support this.

A recent attempt was made to explain the apparent higher incidence of late corneal edema after lens implant surgery as compared to routine cataract surgery. This was done with the aid of the specular microscope, which was described in

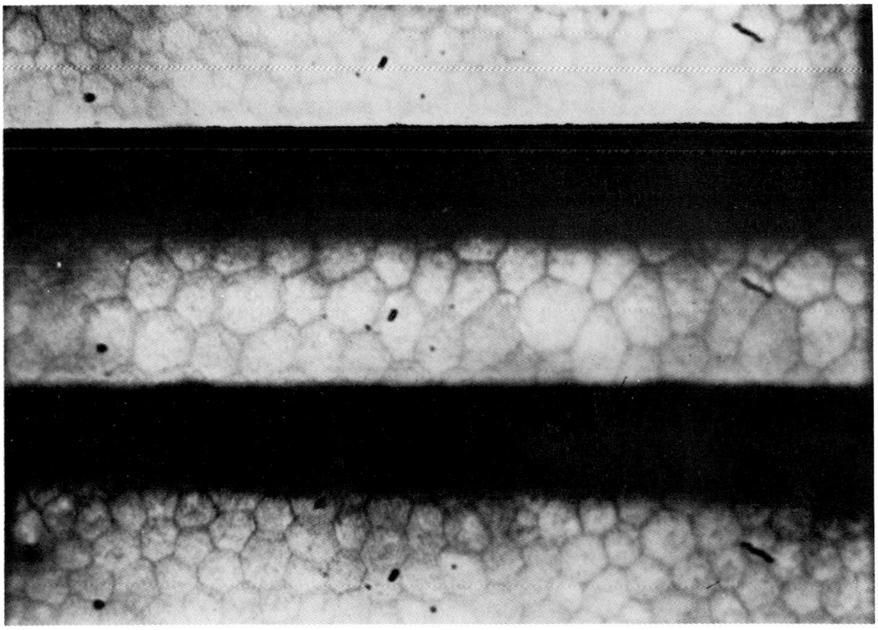

Fig. 12-18. Specular microphotograph. *Upper*, Endothelial cells in 21-year-old woman. *Middle*, Endothelial cells in 79-year-old woman 4 years after uneventful intracapsular cataract extraction. *Lower*, Opposite, unoperated eye of same patient in middle section of this figure.

1968 for observing corneal endothelium in vitro and modified later for clinical examination of the human corneal endothelium in vivo. Using this technique, an extensive evaluation of the effect of cataract extraction and lens implantation on the central endothelial cell density is possible.

Forstot and co-workers studied a series of patients operated on by one surgeon, Norman Jaffe (Fig. 12-18). All patients examined had clear corneas without edema or scarring. The 76 patients included in the study were divided into four groups.

Group I included 12 consecutive patients, studied prospectively, who had lens implantation after intracapsular cataract extractions. Preoperative and postoperative cell counts (measured 7 to 15 days postoperatively) were compared. Ten of these were uncomplicated. The average decrease in cell density preoperatively to postoperatively was 28.6%. One patient had a sterile hypopyon postoperatively that cleared; the cell density was 57.6% less postoperatively (Fig. 12-19). The second patient had vitreous loss at surgery requiring an extensive sponge vitrectomy; the cell density was 84.1% less postoperatively. Overall the decrease in cell density in this prospective group was 35.7%. Group IA was a similar prospective study of five additional consecutive patients undergoing intracapsular cataract extraction without lens implantation; the average decrease in cell density was only 8%.

Group II consisted of 38 monocular pseudophakic patients studied retrospectively. All cell counts of pseudophakic eyes were compared to the unoperated phakic fellow eye. These patients were subdivided into groups by lens type. There were five patients with an iris-plane (Copeland) lens inserted following intracapsular cataract extraction. The time from surgery varied from 3 to 7

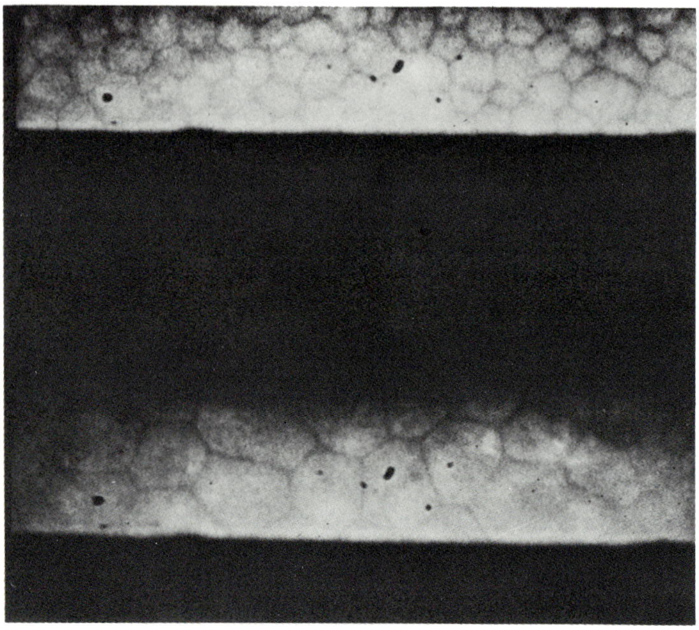

Fig. 12-19. *Upper,* Endothelial cells in 81-year-old man preoperatively. *Lower,* Same eye 11 days after implantation of Binkhorst iris-clip implant. Hypopyon uveitis occurred on second postoperative day. This cleared with aid of steroid therapy.

years. The average cell density was 47.9% less in the implant eye. Nine patients had a Binkhorst 2-loop implant inserted following planned, conventional extracapsular cataract extraction. The time from surgery varied from 7 months to 4 years. The average cell density was 47.5% less in the implant eye. Twenty-one patients with Binkhorst 4-loop implants inserted after an intracapsular cataract extraction, the time from surgery varying from 1 week to 15 months, had a cell density in the implant eye averaging 43.5% less than the fellow eye. One patient had a Fyodorov-Binkhorst lens implanted after an intracapsular cataract extraction 2.5 years previously; the difference in cell count was 84.1%. Two monocular pseudophakic patients with Binkhorst 4-loop lenses had postoperative dislocations. One patient's lens was repositioned pharmacologically. The difference in cell count between his unoperated and implant eye was 54.5%. The second patient required surgical repositioning and had 72.2% less cells in the implant eye compared to the unoperated eye. An analysis was performed to determine any correlation between the percent differences in cell density (unoperated eye and implant eye) and the time from surgery (1 week to 7 years) in the 36 uneventful implant procedures. There was no correlation to indicate progressive endothelial damage.

Group III was a study of eight patients comparing a standard uneventful cataract extraction in one eye with an uneventful intracapsular cataract extraction with an implant in the fellow eye. There were six patients with iris-plane (Copeland) lenses and two with Binkhorst 4-loop lenses. All implant eyes had less cells (six of eight significantly less cells). The average difference in cell density was 41.4%.

Group IV retrospectively compared the eyes of seven bilateral aphakic patients to those of eight bilateral pseudophakic patients. Of the bilaterally pseudophakic patients, two had an iris-plane lens in one eye and a Binkhorst 4-loop lens in the fellow eye, and one had an iris-plane lens in one eye and a Binkhorst 2-loop lens in the fellow eye. The average cell count for aphakic eyes was 1882 cells per square millimeter. The average cell count in the pseudophakic eyes was 1078 cells per square millimeter. The difference between these average cell counts was 42.7%.

This study is not represented as a statistical analysis, but the trend of the results is overwhelming. The most obvious conclusion is that an intraocular lens implantation procedure is more traumatic to the corneal endothelium than an uneventful cataract extraction. A striking similarity was observed in the monocular pseudophake series. Comparing three lenses (iris-plane, Binkhorst 2-loop, and Binkhorst 4-loop), the average difference between phakic unoperated and pseudophakic eyes was 47.9%, 47.5%, and 43.5%.

The cell loss associated with lens implantation is probably related to several factors. The first and probably most obvious is contact between the intraocular lens and the cornea, however brief this contact might be. A second factor is the increased manipulation required by this procedure. Folding of the cornea occurs with routine cataract extraction but is greater with lens implantation. In the case of the Binkhorst 4-loop lens the cornea must be retracted for placement of the transiridectomy suture. In addition, there is more drug use. In this series, alpha-chymotrypsin was always used with the intraocular lens implantations (except in extracapsular extraction), and acetylcholine was used to constrict the pupil. There was also more use of irrigating solutions, greater with extracapsular extractions. It is by no means clear at this time which of these factors may be the most significant contributor to cell loss, but the endothelial microscope should make it possible to define the role of these separate maneuvers.

The data also suggests that the lens itself appears to cause no further endothelial damage or cell loss with time, once it is implanted. Analysis of cell loss versus time from surgery (1 week to 7 years) in the monocular pseudophakic patient group showed no greater comparative loss with time. This evidence is not as conclusive as consecutive measurements on the same patient over many years, but it does provide evidence for good tolerance of the lens by the eye following the surgical procedure. Further cell loss probably does occur with intraocular inflammation or mechanical trauma (lens dislocation).

Cell counts in the implant eyes varied from 2900 to 380 cells per square millimeter. In all eyes the corneas were clear and without edema. This clearly indicates that eyes can tolerate the procedure well, and corneas can remain clear with significant reductions in endothelial cell numbers. As yet it cannot be determined what is the minimum number of central endothelial cells per square millimeter required to maintain corneal dehydration. Eyes with less cells, however, may be more susceptible to corneal edema due to inflammation or trauma, and the possible effect of further cell death with age is unknown.

This study should not serve as an incrimination of the intraocular lens implant procedure. At the outset it was stated that it is only logical to anticipate a higher incidence of corneal edema after lens implant surgery than after routine cataract surgery simply because there are greater manipulations required in the former. The study tends to point to endothelial cell damage at the time of surgery, rather than toxic degradation of the implant, as the principal cause of late corneal edema. However, the study serves as a challenge to all implant surgeons. Every step of the operation must be guided by the most fundamental principle of surgery, minimal trauma. Assiduous attention to details, such as avoidance of corneal endothelial contact, minimal folding back of the cornea, less irrigation, better irrigating solutions, less intracameral drugs, and so on will protect the cornea against undue trauma. In the meantime, it appears justified to assume a conservative approach to surgical indications since, as shown, the cornea may not show clinical evidence of degeneration in spite of lowered endothelial vitality. It is possible that as the patients age, any further loss of cells may be enough to result in corneal edema.

Returning to Binkhorst's three most frequent causes of corneal edema (p. 185)—low endothelial vitality, surgical and postoperative complications, and late contact of implant with cornea—only the latter requires further comment. Contact between the optical portion of the implant can only result from some abnormality in anterior chamber depth such as wound leak, pupillary block, and so on. If this is not corrected rapidly, corneal edema will inevitably result. More insidious is intermittent contact between the haptic supports of the implant and the cornea. Since the contact is usually made with the periphery of the cornea and is often intermittent, the edema may not appear until quite late in the postoperative course. A portion of the blame rests directly with improper implant design and a portion with improper methods of implantation.

A good illustration of this is seen if one follows the evolution of the Binkhorst implant. This has been discussed in Chapter 4 so that some of what follows will be repetitive. Early designs of the iris-clip (4-loop) lens included anterior loops that measured only 7.5 to 8.0 mm in length. Suture fixation was unknown at that time. The result was a high incidence of dislocations. Therefore the length of the anterior loops was increased to 8.5 to 9.0 mm. This caused less dislocations but increased the incidence of corneal edema because of loop contact with the periphery of the cornea. Another unfavorable element appeared to be the fact that the loops were placed in a horizontal position. Since horizontal ocular rotations predominate over movements in other directions, the possibility of intermittent corneal contact became more than theoretical. In order to lessen the chance of corneal edema due to loops contact, the length of the anterior loops was shortened again to 7.5 to 8.0 mm, the anterior and posterior loops were angled posteriorly 10° to 15°, and the implant was inserted in a vertical position. In order to prevent dislocation, a method of secure fixation was adopted. The transiridectomy suture is discussed on p. 78. The current implant design and method of insertion are likely to result in a far lessened tendency to corneal contact.

It was further reasoned that an implant without loops in the anterior chamber would lessen the possibility of corneal edema due to corneal contact. This is partly (not wholly) responsible for the genesis of the 2-loop iridocapsular Binkhorst implant and the Worst 2-loop Medallion implant. Support for this concept is usually cited in the research of Nordlohne who ingeniously measured the depth of the anterior chamber with the patient prone and supine. Comparing the 4-loop and 2-loop Binkhorst implants, he observed that the anterior chamber was shallower with the former when the patient lay flat on his face. The difference was only 0.12 mm. The validity of these findings in incriminating loop contact remains speculative with currently designed implants. No one would argue with this thesis if the loops are too long or if they are defective in manufacture so that they bend anteriorly.

One might safely conclude from this discussion that the most important causes of corneal edema resulting from implant surgery are lowered endothelial vitality and surgical trauma to the endothelial cells of the cornea.

SUMMARY

The implant surgeon of today owes a debt of gratitude to those pioneers who carefully analyzed their data and made changes in implant design and methods of implantation to the end that the safety of the procedure has increased enormously. However, this again outlines the challenge that faces all implant surgeons. Vigilance must not lessen. The surgeon must assume the posture of watchdog over industry. It is likely that new implant designs will be introduced. These should not be endorsed and used by surgeons without painstaking scrutiny.

CHAPTER 13

Results of pseudophakos surgery

BINKHORST IMPLANTS

A relatively short-term follow-up series of 800 eyes with Binkhorst implants is available from Jaffe. The series commenced on May 14, 1974. The patient most recently operated on had a 6-month follow-up. The follow-up ranged from 6 to 42 months.

Patient population (Table 13-1)

The series includes 800 Binkhorst implants in 765 patients (35 bilateral cases). The patients ranged in age from 54 to 94 years. The mean age was 73.86 years; 5% were less than 65 years of age, 5% were 85 years of age or older, and 90% were between 65 and 84 years of age.

Table 13-1. Binkhorst implants: patient population

Age (years)	No. eyes	Percent
50-54	1	0.1
55-59	6	0.8
60-64	36	4.5
65-69	162	20.3
70-74	229	28.6
75-79	219	27.4
80-84	108	13.5
85-89	33	4.1
90-94	6	0.8
TOTAL	800	

Type of cataract surgery (Table 13-2)

The series was heavily weighted toward the intracapsular cataract extraction (ICCE) (87%) rather than the extracapsular cataract extraction (ECCE) (14%).

Table 13-2. Binkhorst implants: type of cataract surgery

Surgical technique	No. eyes	Percent
Intracapsular	698	87
Extracapsular	102	13
TOTAL	800	100

Visual acuity (Tables 13-3 and 13-4)

A total of 722 (90.3%) eyes achieved 20/40 corrected visual acuity or better. Only 1.5% had less than 20/400. It is not surprising that patients under 75 years of age achieved slightly better than the overall average visual acuity, and those 75 years of age or more, slightly poorer.

Table 13-3. Binkhorst implants: visual acuity

Visual acuity	No. eyes	Percent
20/15 to 20/40	722	90.3
20/50 to 20/80	34	4.3
20/100 to 20/400	32	4.0
<20/400	12	1.5
TOTAL	800	100.0

Table 13-4. Binkhorst implants: visual acuity of 20/40 or better by age groups in 722 of 800 eyes

Age (years)	No. eyes	Percent
50-54	1	100.0
55-59	5	83.3
60-64	34	94.4
65-69	154	95.1
70-74	214	93.4
75-79	191	87.2
80-84	92	88.0
85-89	25	75.8
90-94	6	100.0
TOTAL	722	MEAN 90.3

Causes of visual acuity of less than 20/40 (Table 13-5)

Seventy-eight of the 800 eyes (9.8%) achieved less than 20/40 visual acuity. Senile macular choroidal degeneration was the most frequent cause, with 33 eyes (4.1%) having this disorder. Cystoid macular edema was the cause much less frequently (1.5%). Corneal edema caused less than 20/40 visual acuity in 0.6% of eyes. The remaining causes are listed in Table 13-5.

Table 13-5. Binkhorst implants: causes of visual acuity of <20/40 in 78 of 800 eyes

Causes	No. eyes	Percent of 800	Percent of 78
Senile macular choroidal degeneration	33	4.1	42.3
Cystoid macular edema	12	1.5	15.4
Corneal edema	5	0.6	6.4
Retinal detachment	4	0.5	5.1
Venous thrombosis	3	0.4	3.8
Diabetic maculopathy	2	0.3	2.6
Secondary membrane	1	0.1	1.3
Macular hole	1	0.1	1.3
Macular hemorrhage	1	0.1	1.3
Ischemic optic neuropathy	2	0.3	2.6
Glaucomatous atrophy	1	0.1	1.3
Optic atrophy	1	0.1	1.3
Retinitis pigmentosa	1	0.1	1.3
Amblyopia	6	0.8	7.7
Unknown	5	0.6	6.4

Bilateral implants (Table 13-6)

Sixty-three patients in this series had bilateral implants. Their ages ranged from 66 to 91 years, and their mean age was higher (78.7 years) than the overall mean age of the series (73.86 years). Thirty-five patients had some type of Binkhorst implant in both eyes, while 28 patients had a Binkhorst implant in one eye and another type of implant in the opposite eye.

Table 13-6. Binkhorst implants: bilateral implants

Type of implants	No. patients
Copeland—Binkhorst ICCE	18
Copeland—Binkhorst ECCE	2
Worst—Binkhorst ICCE	7
Fyodorov I—Binkhorst ICCE	1
Binkhorst ICCE—Binkhorst ICCE	23
Binkhorst ICCE—Binkhorst ECCE	8
Binkhorst ECCE—Binkhorst ECCE	4
TOTAL	63

Iris suture (Table 13-7)

It was necessary to suture the iris in 34 eyes (4.3%). This was usually due to a miotic pupil that had undergone chronic miotic therapy for glaucoma control (16 eyes) or a miotic pupil associated with a previously performed peripheral iridectomy (13 eyes). In two eyes it was necessary to close a previously performed sector iridectomy. This technique was also used in one eye each because of a previously performed iridencleisis, a trabeculectomy, and senile iris sphincter rigidity. Only two of the 34 eyes had less than 20/40 visual acuity, both due to senile macular choroidal degeneration.

Table 13-7. Binkhorst implants: iris suture in 34 of 800 eyes (4.3%)*

Cause	No. eyes
Miotic therapy	16
Previous peripheral iridectomy	13
Previous sector iridectomy	2
Previous iridencleisis	1
Previous trabeculectomy	1
Senile miosis	1
TOTAL	34

*Visual acuity of two eyes was <20/40 due to senile macular choroidal degeneration.

Vitreous problems (Table 13-8)

There was some type of operative vitreous problem in 57 eyes (7.1%). There was vitreous loss in 10 eyes (1.4%) during an intracapsular cataract extraction and in 10 eyes (9.8%) during a planned extracapsular cataract extraction. The latter incidence is high and is probably due to early experience with automated devices for extracapsular cataract extraction. The vitreous face was ruptured during the implant insertion in 19 eyes. There was vitreous loss through the peripheral iridectomy during the placement of the transiridectomy suture in 10 eyes. Aspiration of retrovitreal fluid was performed in seven eyes due to a vitreous bulge after lens extraction. In no instance was the implant insertion aborted because of a vitreous disturbance. This was because of satisfactory management of the vitreous problem in all cases.

The visual acuity in these eyes (82.5% achieved 20/40 visual acuity or better) was poorer than that in the overall series (90.3%). The causes of visual acuity of less than 20/40 in the 10 eyes are shown in Table 13-8. The comparative incidence of clinically significant cystoid macular edema (less than 20/40 visual acuity) with an operative vitreous disturbance was 2/57 (3.5%) and without a vitreous disturbance 10/743 (1.3%). One eye with an operative vitreous disturbance achieved less than 20/40 visual acuity due to a retinal detachment.

Table 13-8. Binkhorst implants: vitreous problems in 57 of 800 eyes (7.1%)*

Occurrence	No. eyes	Percent
During ICCE	10	1.4
During ECCE	10	9.8
Before ICCE	1	
During implantation	19	
Through peripheral iridectomy	10	
Aspiration for bulge	7	

*Causes of visual acuity <20/40: senile macular choroidal degeneration, 5; cystoid macular edema, 2; retinal detachment, 1; diabetic maculopathy, 1; amblyopia, 1.

Additional surgery (Table 13-9)

Forty-eight eyes (6.0%) required additional surgery. Of these, 28 eyes had surgery to correct a secondary membrane. A penetrating keratoplasty was performed in five eyes. Five eyes required surgery for a retinal detachment. Wound dehiscence occurred in three eyes, necessitating repair. Two implants were removed, both in eyes that had undergone extracapsular cataract extraction. This was done because of presumed severe inflammatory response to retained lenticular remnants. Both eyes recovered completely following removal of the implant. Other types of additional surgery are listed in Table 13-9.

Table 13-9. Binkhorst implants: additional surgery in 48 of 800 eyes (6.0%)

Type of surgery	No. eyes
Discission of secondary membrane	22
Trans pars plana membranectomy and partial anterior vitrectomy	6
Trans pars plana vitrectomy for endophthalmitis	1
Penetrating keratoplasty	5
Retinal detachment	5
Wound repair	3
Implant removal	2
Reposition of implant dislocated into vitreous	1
Repair Descemet's membrane	1
Implant replaced	1
Malinsertion corrected	1

Table 13-10. Binkhorst implants: surgery for secondary membranes

Technique	No. eyes	Discission	Trans pars plana membranectomy and partial anterior vitrectomy	Total
ECCE	102	14	1	15 (14.7%)
ICCE	698	8	5	13 (1.9%)
ECCE and ICCE	800	22	6	28 (3.5%)

Secondary membranes (Tables 13-10 and 13-11)

Secondary membranes appeared in 28 eyes (3.5%) that required surgery to improve vision. These occurred in 15 of 102 eyes (14.7%) after an extracapsular cataract extraction and in 13 of 698 eyes (1.9%) after an intracapsular cataract extraction. These were treated by simple discission of the secondary membrane in 22 eyes (14 extracapsular, eight intracapsular). None of these eyes failed to achieve 20/40 visual acuity. Because of a dense secondary membrane that also involved the iris, a membranectomy and partial anterior vitrectomy were performed in six eyes (one extracapsular, five intracapsular) via a trans pars plana route.

Table 13-11. Binkhorst implants: visual acuity of <20/40 after surgery for secondary membrane*

Technique	Discission	Trans pars piana membranectomy and partial anterior vitrectomy
ECCE	0/14	0/1
ICCE	1/8	3/5

*Causes of visual acuity of <20/40: cystoid macular edema, 2; ischemic optic neuropathy, 1.

Three of the five eyes that had an intracapsular cataract extraction failed to achieve 20/40 visual acuity. Two of these had cystoid macular edema, and one had ischemic optic neuropathy.

Dislocations (Tables 13-12 to 13-14)

In considering dislocations, the series of 800 Binkhorst implants was expanded to 939 cases. This made it possible to study the incidence of dislocations in a variety of situations. The overall series was divided into a series of 108 extracapsular cataract extractions and 831 intracapsular cataract extractions.

From the results shown in Table 13-12, it is seen that there were three dislocations among the 33 iridocapsular (2-loop) implants (9.1%). Fifty-eight extracapsular cataract extractions were performed using a Binkhorst iris-clip (4-loop) implant with a transiridectomy suture, and there were no dislocations. Seventeen extracapsular cataract extractions were performed using a Binkhorst iris-clip (4-loop) implant without a suture, and there was one dislocation (5.9%).

From the results shown in Table 13-13, it is seen that there were 10 dislocations among the 429 intracapsular cataract extractions using a Binkhorst iris-clip implant with a transiridectomy suture (2.3%). There were 13 dislocations among the 402 intracapsular cataract extractions using a Binkhorst iris-clip (4-loop) without a suture (3.2%). Four implants rotated to the horizontal or oblique position in those eyes in which no suture was used. Most disturbing, however, was the fact that three implants among the 13 dislocations in the series without a suture dislocated completely into the vitreous. In one instance the implant became lodged at the vitreous base at the 6 o'clock position. It was left in this position. Visual acuity with a contact lens has been 20/20 for the 8 months following this occurrence. It was possible to correctly reposition the implant in the other two cases using a trans pars plana approach. One of these patients has 20/20 and the other has 20/25 visual acuity.

The methods of treating the 27 dislocations are presented in Table 13-14. In 19 instances the dislocation was corrected by maneuvering the dislocated loop into normal position using a sharp disposable needle in the anterior chamber. In two instances the implant was repositioned using a mydriatic agent followed by a miotic, both applied topically. In three instances the dislocation was not treated: in one case the implant became lodged in the vitreous base; in another case the optical portion of an iridocapsular (2-loop) implant slipped behind the iris so that the entire implant was in the posterior chamber, but because visual acuity was excellent and good capsular fixation existed, it was decided not to treat the eye; in the third case both inferior loops were behind the iris, but the implant repositioned itself spontaneously. Two instances of dislocation into the vitreous with subsequent repositioning using a trans pars plana approach are discussed above. In a final case a dislocation of an iridocapsular implant into the anterior chamber occurred. The implant was removed and an iris-clip implant was substituted using a transiridectomy suture.

Before drawing absolute conclusions from these results, we are reminded that this is a short-term series. The follow-up periods for the implants with no suture are shorter than those with a transiridectomy suture. In Jaffe's experience, however, dislocations usually occur early in the postoperative period. There was only one dislocation in the suture series, which occurred more than 6 months after surgery. There was not a single case of permanent corneal edema as a result of dislocation. There were only two patients whose implant dislocated two times. No other patient had more than one dislocation, and it was not necessary to use a McCannel suture in any case. The alarming occurrence of three dislocations into the vitreous among the intracapsular cataract extraction cases without a suture must be seriously considered in spite of the fortunate results attained in these patients.

Table 13-12. Binkhorst implants: extracapsular cataract extraction dislocations

Technique	No. cases	Dislocations	Percent
ECCE (iridocapsular implant)	33	3	9.1
ECCE (iris-clip implant with suture)	58	0	0.0
ECCE (iris-clip implant without suture)	17	1	5.9
TOTAL	108	4	MEAN 3.7

Table 13-13. Binkhorst implants: intracapsular cataract extraction dislocations

Technique	No. cases	Dislocations	Percent
ICCE (iris-clip implant with suture)	429	10	2.3
ICCE (iris-clip implant without suture)	402	13	3.2
TOTAL	831	23	MEAN 2.8

Table 13-14. Binkhorst implants: treatment of dislocations in 27 of 939 eyes (2.9%)

Treatment	No. eyes
Needle	19
Pharmacologic	2
Repositioned from vitreous	2
2-loop removed and 4-loop inserted	1
None	3

Retinal detachment (Table 13-15)

A comparison between the incidence of postoperative retinal detachment in the first 650 Binkhorst implants and in two combined series of routine intracapsular cataract extractions was available. In the latter group there was a total of 2304 consecutive cataract extractions. There were 40 (1.74%) postoperative retinal detachments compared to three (0.46%) in the implant series. The mean age of patients with retinal detachments was significantly lower than that in both overall series. Another significant factor in the routine cataract extraction group was the presence of myopia (characterized by an aphakic correction of +9 D or less) in 18 of 40 patients (45%). It would be expected that the incidence of postoperative retinal detachment would be lower in the implant series, since young patients and those with significant myopia were not subjected to lens implant surgery.

Table 13-15. Binkhorst implants: retinal detachment

	ICCE	Percent	IOL	Percent
Cases	2304		650	
Retinal detachment	40	1.74	3	0.46
Mean age RD	62.23		67.00	
Myopia (aphakic correction +9 D or less)	18/40	45.0		
Time				
0-6 mo	27/40	67.5	1/3	33.3
6-12 mo	4/40	10.0	1/3	33.3
>1 yr	9/40	22.5	1/3	33.3

MATCHED RETROSPECTIVE SERIES OF 500 ROUTINE INTRACAPSULAR CATARACT EXTRACTIONS (ICCE) AND 500 BINKHORST IMPLANTS (IOL)

The series of Binkhorst implants includes the first 512 cases of the 650 discussed above. Twelve were omitted for reasons outlined below. An attempt was made to match as closely as possible a series of routine intracapsular cataract extractions and Binkhorst implants. The surgery in both series was predominantly performed by Jaffe and some by his associates with Jaffe assisting.

Patient population (Table 13-16)

Both series had a minimum age requirement of 60 years. The age ranges were nearly identical for both groups. The average ages were very close, 72.72 years in the ICCE series and 73.95 years in the Binkhorst implant series. The surgery in both series occurred during a similar time span and comprised 30 months for the ICCE group and 31 months for the Binkhorst implant group. Therefore the surgery occurred at a time when the principal surgeon was performing implants in close to 50% of his cataract operations.

Table 13-16. Routine ICCE versus IOL: patient population

Patient population	ICCE	IOL
No. patients	500	500
Age range	60-90	60-91
Mean age	72.72	73.95
Time span	30 mo	31 mo

Visual acuity (Table 13-17)

The percentage of patients in each series who achieved 20/15 to 20/40 visual acuity was similar: 85.4% in the ICCE group and 89.0% in the Binkhorst implant group. The percentage of those who attained less than 20/400 in each group was also similar: 1.6% in the ICCE group and 1.8% in the Binkhorst implant group.

Table 13-17. Routine ICCE versus IOL: visual acuity

Visual acuity	ICCE		IOL	
	No. patients	Percent	No. patients	Percent
20/15 to 20/40	427	85.4	445	89.0
20/50 to 20/80	42	8.4	22	4.4
20/100 to 20/400	23	4.6	24	4.8
<20/400	8	1.6	9	1.8
TOTAL	500	100.0	500	100.0

Visual acuity according to age groups (Table 13-18)

The patients in both series were subdivided into five-year age categories starting with the youngest (60 to 64 years) and ending with the oldest (over 90 years). The number and percent of those achieving 20/15 to 20/40 visual acuity were compared in each age category. The number of patients was greatest in the four subgroups between 65 and 84 years. As would be expected there was a decline in visual acuity results with increasing age.

Table 13-18. Routine ICCE versus IOL: visual acuity of 20/15 to 20/40

Age (years)	ICCE			IOL		
	No. patients	20/15 to 20/40	Percent	No. patients	20/15 to 20/40	Percent
60-64	47	40	85.1	25	24	96.0
65-69	106	99	93.4	95	87	91.6
70-74	132	117	88.6	151	139	92.1
75-79	132	117	88.6	134	117	87.3
80-84	70	47	67.1	65	56	86.2
85-89	12	7	58.3	27	19	70.4
>90	1	0	00.0	3	3	100.0

Causes of visual acuity of less than 20/40 (Table 13-19)

Special attention is directed toward four of the more frequently discussed complications associated with intraocular implant lens surgery: senile macular choroidal degeneration, cystoid macular edema, corneal edema, and retinal detachment. It is noted that senile macular choroidal degeneration was easily the most frequent cause of failure to achieve 20/40 visual acuity: 7.6% in the ICCE group and 4.2% in the Binkhorst implant group. Cystoid macular edema was the cause in 2.2% in the ICCE group and 1.4% in the Binkhorst implant group. Corneal edema was the cause in 0.4% in the ICCE group and 1.2% in the Binkhorst implant group. Retinal detachment was the cause in 0.8% in the ICCE group and 0.6% in the Binkhorst implant group. It is also of interest to examine what percentage of those eyes that did not achieve 20/40 visual acuity is attributed to each of these causes. Of the 73 eyes in the ICCE group and the 55 eyes in the Binkhorst implant group, senile macular choroidal degeneration was the cause in 52% in the ICCE group and 38% in the Binkhorst implant group. Cystoid macular edema was the cause in 15% in the ICCE group and 13% in the Binkhorst implant group. Corneal edema was the cause in 3% in the ICCE group and 11% in the Binkhorst implant group. Retinal detachment was the cause in 5% in both groups. The most important difference was corneal edema, which occurred three times as frequently in the Binkhorst implant group although the incidence was low in both groups. The remaining causes are listed in Table 13-19.

Table 13-19. Routine ICCE versus IOL and causes of visual acuity of <20/40

	ICCE			IOL		
Causes	No. cases	Percent of 73	Percent of 500	No. cases	Percent of 55	Percent of 500
Senile macular choroidal degeneration	38	52.0	7.6	21	38.0	4.2
Cystoid macular edema	11	15.0	2.2	7	13.0	1.4
Corneal edema	2	3.0	0.4	6	11.0	1.2
Retinal detachment	4	5.0	0.8	3	5.0	0.6
Venous thrombosis	0	0.0	0.0	4	7.3	0.8
Diabetic maculopathy	3	4.1	0.6	1	1.8	0.2
Vitreous hemorrhage	2	2.7	0.4	0	0.0	0.0
Macular pucker	1	1.4	0.2	1	1.8	0.2
Macular hole	0	0.0	0.0	1	1.8	0.2
Retinitis pigmentosa	1	1.4	0.2	1	1.8	0.2
Optic atrophy	0	0.0	0.0	1	1.8	0.2
Glaucomatous atrophy	1	1.4	0.2	1	1.8	0.2
Ischemic optic neuropathy	1	1.4	0.2	2	3.6	0.4
Amblyopia	2	2.7	0.4	3	5.0	0.6
Congenital nystagmus	1	1.4	0.2	0	0.0	0.0
Secondary membrane	1	1.4	0.2	2	3.6	0.4
Expulsive hemorrhage	1	1.4	0.2	0	0.0	0.0
Unknown	4	5.0	0.8	1	1.8	0.2
TOTAL	73			55		

Causes of visual acuity of less than 20/40 according to age groups (Table 13-20)

Once again, senile macular choroidal degeneration (SMCD), cystoid macular edema (CME), corneal edema (CE), and retinal detachment (RD) are given emphasis. Table 13-20 compares the number of eyes in each age group that did not achieve 20/40 visual acuity due to these conditions. It also gives the percentage of those that did not achieve 20/40 visual acuity (not the percentage of the total patients) due to these conditions in each age group. As expected, the incidence of senile macular choroidal degeneration increases with age. There is no consistent age relationship with cystoid macular edema and corneal edema. It is of interest that all retinal detachments occurred in patients less than 70 years of age.

Table 13-20. Routine ICCE versus IOL in achieving visual acuity of <20/40

Age (years)	ICCE				IOL			
	SMCD	CME	CE	RD	SMCD	CME	CE	RD
60-64	0 (0.0%)	4 (8.5%)	0 (0.0%)	3 (6.4%)	0 (0.0%)	1 (4.0%)	0 (0.0%)	0 (0.0%)
65-69	2 (1.9%)	1 (0.9%)	0 (0.0%)	1 (0.9%)	3 (3.2%)	0 (0.0%)	1 (1.1%)	3 (3.2%)
70-74	6 (4.5%)	2 (1.5%)	2 (1.5%)	0 (0.0%)	2 (1.3%)	1 (0.7%)	2 (1.3%)	0 (0.0%)
75-79	8 (6.1%)	2 (1.5%)	0 (0.0%)	0 (0.0%)	5 (3.7%)	4 (3.0%)	3 (2.2%)	0 (0.0%)
80-84	19 (27%)	0 (0.0%)	0 (0.0%)	0 (0.0%)	6 (9.2%)	1 (1.5%)	0 (0.0%)	0 (0.0%)
85-89	2 (17%)	2 (17%)	0 (0.0%)	0 (0.0%)	5 (19%)	0 (0.0%)	0 (0.0%)	0 (0.0%)
>90	1 (100%)	0 (0.0%)	0 (0.0%)	0 (0.0%)	0 (0.0%)	0 (0.0%)	0 (0.0%)	0 (0.0%)

COPELAND IMPLANTS

A relatively long-term follow-up of two series of Copeland implants performed by Jaffe is available. The first series consists of the first 81 Copeland implants inserted between May 13, 1968, and October 1, 1969. On the latter date a lens implant moratorium was agreed upon in the Miami, Florida, community in order to ascertain the short- and medium-range safety of the first group of implants (Chapter 14). The moratorium was lifted on October 1, 1971. The second series consisted of the next 81 consecutive Copeland implants. Thus the two series are identical as to the number of eyes in each. All cataract extractions were intracapsular.

Patient population (Table 13-21)

The follow-up periods in series 1 and 2 for those patients who were not dead (18 in series 1 and four in series 2) or lost to follow-up (two in series 1 and four in series 2) were 75 months in the former and 32 months in the latter. The mean age of patients in series 1 was 70.3 years, and 76.3 years in series 2.

Table 13-21. Copeland iris-plane implant study: patient population

Patient population	Series 1		Series 2	
	No. patients	Follow-up months	No. patients	Follow-up months
Dead	18	32	4	13
Lost to follow up	2	48	4	12
Patients available	61	75	73	32
Follow-up range		7-86		1-45
Total patients	81		81	
Mean age	70.3		76.3	

Visual acuity (Table 13-22)

Seventy-five percent of patients in series 1 who had not had the implant removed attained 20/40 visual acuity. The corresponding figure for series 2 was 79%.

Table 13-22. Copeland iris-plane implant study: visual acuity

Visual acuity	Series 1		Series 2	
	Lens inserted	Lens removed	Lens inserted	Lens removed
20/20 to 20/40	55 (75.3%)	5	63 (79.7%)	1
20/50 to 20/400	15 (20.5%)	2	13 (16.5%)	1
<20/400	3 (4.1%)	1	3 (3.8%)	0

Causes of visual acuity of less than 20/40 (Table 13-23)

The most common cause of failure to achieve 20/40 visual acuity was senile macular choroidal degeneration, which was present in 13.6% in series 1, 4.9% in series 2, and 9.3% in both series combined. The next most common cause was cystoid macular edema or macular pucker. Macular pucker was present in some cases following resolution of cystoid macular edema. There was no instance in which this was present without cystoid macular edema where the patient had less than 20/40 visual acuity. Therefore they were grouped together. This complication was present in 9.9% in series 1, 4.9% in series 2, and 7.4% in both series combined. Note the marked difference in incidence of senile macular choroidal degeneration and cystoid macular edema and their frequency in relation to each other in this series compared to the series of 650 Binkhorst implants described earlier (see Table 13-5). In the latter series, senile macular choroidal degeneration was the cause of failure to achieve 20/40 visual acuity in 4.5%, and cystoid macular edema in 1.4%. Corneal edema was present in 1.2% in series 1, 2.5% in series 2, and 1.9% in both series combined. This is a greater incidence than that (0.9%) which occurred in the Binkhorst 650 implant series.

Implants removed

A total of 10 implants were removed from the 162 eyes in the combined series (6.2%) (see Table 13-22). This may be partly due to insecurity on the part of the surgeons, since this occurred early in their lens implant experience and there

Table 13-23. Copeland iris-plane implant study: causes of visual acuity of <20/40

Causes	Series 1		Series 2	
	Lens inserted	Lens removed	Lens inserted	Lens removed
Senile macular choroidal degeneration	11 (13.6%)	0 (0.0%)	4 (4.9%)	0 (0.0%)
Cystoid macular edema or pucker	6 (7.4%)	2 (2.5%)	4 (4.9%)	0 (0.0%)
Diabetic maculopathy	0 (0.0%)	0 (0.0%)	1 (1.2%)	0 (0.0%)
Ischemic optic neuropathy	0 (0.0%)	1 (1.2%)	2 (2.5%)	1 (1.2%)
Corneal edema	1 (1.2%)	0 (0.0%)	2 (2.5%)	0 (0.0%)
Intraocúlar lens membrane	0 (0.0%)	0 (0.0%)	2 (2.5%)	0 (0.0%)
Glaucoma	0 (0.0%)	0 (0.0%)	0 (0.0%)	0 (0.0%)
Unknown	0 (0.0%)	0 (0.0%)	1 (1.2%)	0 (0.0%)

were few other surgeons performing the procedure in the United States. In support of this is the fact that eight implants were removed in series 1 but only two in series 2. However, the percentage is extraordinarily high when compared to the Binkhorst series experience described earlier where only two implants were removed from 650 eyes (0.3%). Thus implant removal occurred 21 times more frequently in the Copeland series.

Causes of implant removal and final visual acuity

1. Uveitis in six eyes. The corrected visual acuities after implant removal were 20/20 (2), 20/25 (2), 20/40 (1), and 20/400 (1). The latter was associated with cystoid macular edema.
2. Recurrent hyphema in one eye. Final visual acuity was 20/30.
3. Cystoid macular edema with partial corneal edema in one eye. Final visual acuity was 20/70.
4. Flat anterior chamber in one eye. The eye could not be treated adequately, since the patient suffered a cardiac arrest at the time of onset of the flat anterior chamber (two weeks postoperatively). The final visual acuity was no light perception due to glaucomatous optic atrophy.
5. Dislocation of the implant in one eye. Final visual acuity was 20/60 due to ischemic optic neuropathy.

Results in young patients

Copeland implants were placed in 13 eyes of 12 patients in series 1 who were less than 60 years of age. By the time series 2 commenced, more rigid criteria for case selection were in force in Miami. Therefore no patients in series 2 were less than 60 years of age. The results in these patients are as follows:

1. Five implants (38%) were removed.
2. The cause of implant removal was uveitis in all eyes.
3. The times of implant removal were 4 weeks, 13 months, 18 months, 36 months, and 48 months.
4. Four of the five patients who had an implant removed had a routine intracapsular cataract extraction in the opposite eye. All eyes had 20/25 or better visual acuity.
5. Of the eight eyes of patients under 60 years of age with the implant in situ, six (75%) had cystoid macular edema. All six of these eyes had less than 20/40 visual acuity. Three of the six eyes with cystoid macular edema had a routine intracapsular cataract extraction in the opposite eye. None developed cystoid macular edema.

The reason for the unsatisfactory results in patients under 60 years of age is uncertain. It may be that this is peculiar to the Copeland implant, since this has not been reported with other types of iris-supported implants.

CYSTOID MACULAR EDEMA STUDY

A cystoid macular edema study has been in progress at the Bascom Palmer Eye Institute since May 14, 1974. The study has not yet reached its conclusion. The participants include N. S. Jaffe, A. Allen, J. C. Johnson, N. Zakov, J. McBeath, D. S. Light, H. M. Clayman, D. M. Eichenbaum, J. D. M. Gass, and E. W. D. Norton.

Material

All cataract extractions were performed by Jaffe and his associates on patients 67 years of age or older between May 14, 1974, and December 16, 1975. Both intracapsular and extracapsular procedures were performed utilizing the Binkhorst implant as well as some intracapsular extractions without implants.

Technique

Fundus angiograms were taken at 4, 8, and 16 to 24 months postoperatively. At each visit the pupils were dilated with 0.5% or 1% tropicamide (Mydriacyl). Two stereo color pair photographs were taken, and angiograms were taken at 5 and 30 minutes post injection.

Analysis of data

The angiograms were read primarily by retinal subspecialists. All angiograms were read without knowledge of the type of surgery performed. The surgeons did not see the angiograms.

Cases were excluded for the following reasons: (1) poor quality angiogram, (2) age less than 67 years, (3) presence of other macular disease, and (4) lack of reviewer agreement in questionable cases. Some patients did not complete the study because of (1) nonparticipation, (2) death or severe illness, (3) reaction to intravenous fluorescein injection, (4) onset of other fundus disease, and (5) poor quality angiogram.

Table 13-24. Incidence of cystoid macular edema—pseudophakia versus aphakia (746 angiograms)

Procedure	4 months	8 months	16 to 24 months
Pseudophakia	22/186 (14.0%)	16/165 (9.7%)	19/166 (12.9%)
Aphakia	16/106 (15.1%)	13/88 (14.8%)	8/96 (8.3%)

Table 13-25. Incidence of cystoid macular edema in pseudophakia according to type of cataract extraction

Procedure	4 months	8 months	16 to 24 months
Intracapsular	22/141 (15.6%)	13/115 (11.3%)	17/119 (14.3%)
Extracapsular	4/45 (8.9%)	3/50 (6.0%)	2/47 (4.3%)

Conclusions (Tables 13-24 to 13-26)

The following conclusions hold true for this particular age group of patients, with this surgical team, and with these types of implants.

1. Standard intracapsular cataract extractions and all implants have comparable incidence of cystoid macular edema at 4, 8, and 16 to 24 months postoperatively.

2. Extracapsular cataract extractions with Binkhorst implants appear to have a significantly lower incidence of cystoid macular edema than either intracapsular cataract extractions without an implant or intracapsular cataract extractions with a Binkhorst implant. A larger number of extracapsular cataract extractions will be added to establish statistical significance.

3. Visual function as measured by visual acuity is good in all groups with cystoid macular edema, although the acuity did not take into account the problem of distortion.

Table 13-26. Final visual acuity of eyes with cystoid macular edema at any time during the study

Procedure	No. with positive study	Visual acuity <20/40
Pseudophakia	34	6 (17.7%)
Aphakia	26	5 (19.2%)

WORST MEDALLION IMPLANTS
(Table 13-27)

Clayman began a Worst lens implant series on September 3, 1975. The series has available 140 cases for study with a follow-up ranging from 3 to 21 months. This is an ongoing retrospective study with a short follow-up. The data presented is current but may be revised later as the series enlarges and the follow-up lengthens.

In 138 cases the implant inserted was the Worst Medallion 2-loop model, requiring an iris suture (Fig. 8-51). Of these, in the first 55 cases a 9-0 or 10-0 nylon suture was used intracamerally, and a 9-0 or 10-0 polypropylene suture was utilized in the remaining 83 cases. To date, no cases of suture failure have been observed in either group, and neither has loop failure occurred. In one case each a Worst circular loop and a Worst platinum-clip lens implant were used. Intracapsular cataract extraction was the preferred technique in 95.7% of cases.

Table 13-27. Worst Medallion implants: type of surgery

Procedure	No. cases	Percent
Intracapsular	134/140	95.7
Extracapsular	6/140	4.3

Patient population (Table 13-28)

The patients ranged from 61 to 90 years of age, with a mean age of 75.4 years. There were 140 implants in 135 patients, five cases being bilateral with an appropriate interval between operations. Five percent of patients were less than 64 years of age, 10% were 84 years or older, and the majority (85%) between 65 and 84 years. In this elderly patient population no serious medical problems were encountered during surgery or in the immediate postoperative course. All surgery was performed under local anesthesia.

Table 13-28. Worst Medallion implants: age distribution

Age (years)	No. patients	Percent
60-64	7	5.0
65-69	13	9.3
70-74	46	32.9
75-79	38	27.1
80-84	22	15.7
85-89	13	9.3
90-94	1	0.7
TOTAL	140	100.0

Visual acuity (Tables 13-29 and 13-30)

In 84.4% of patients the visual acuity was 20/40 or better (Table 13-29). Two patients (1.4%) had less than 20/400. The predominant cause of visual acuity of less than 20/40 was senile macular choroidal degeneration. This and other causes are listed in Table 13-30. The one case of corneal edema occurred with the platinum-clip implant.

Table 13-29. Worst Medallion implants: visual acuity

Visual acuity	No. patients	Percent
20/15 to 20/40	118	84.4
20/50 to 20/80	10	7.1
20/100 to 20/400	10	7.1
<20/400	2	1.4

Table 13-30. Worst Medallion implants: causes of visual acuity of <20/40 in 22 of 140 cases (15.7%)

Cause	No. cases	Percent
Senile macular choroidal degeneration	8	5.7
Cystoid macular edema	3	2.2
Corneal edema	1	0.7
Retinal vein occlusion	3	2.2
Vitreous hemorrhage	1	0.7
Retinal detachment	1	0.7
Macular cyst (preexisting)	1	0.7
Amblyopia	2	1.4
Unknown	2	1.4
TOTAL	22	15.7

Bilateral implants (Table 13-31)

Bilateral implant surgery was performed in 18 patients (12.9% of series), and of these, five patients (3.6%) had bilateral Worst Medallion lens implants. Four patients had routine cataract surgery several years earlier in the first eye and Worst Medallion 2-loop lens implant surgery in the second eye. The interval between operations was at least one year in all cases.

Table 13-31. Worst Medallion implants: bilateral intracapsular cases in 22 of 140 patients (15.7%)*

First eye	Second eye	No. patients
Binkhorst	Worst Medallion	9
Worst Medallion	Worst Medallion	5
Copeland	Worst Medallion	3
Worst Medallion	Choyce Mark VIII	1
Aphakia/contact lens	Worst Medallion	4
TOTAL		22

*Mean age bilateral implants: 74.1 yrs.

Iris suture

Iris surgery concomitant with implant insertion was required in seven (5%) cases. In all cases the cause was a miotic pupil. The technique was to perform a radial iridotomy, which was repaired after cataract extraction but before implant insertion, in an attempt to avoid multiple sphincter ruptures. The postoperative visual acuity was 20/40 or better in all cases.

Vitreous loss

Vitreous loss during surgery occurred in five patients (3.6%). In the intracapsular group all three cases occurred during implant insertion. Obviously, if routine cataract surgery was performed or implant surgery had been aborted, vitreous would not have been lost. Nevertheless, two of the patients are currently 20/40 or better, and the other was 20/30 but sustained a retinal vein occlusion 6 months after surgery, and the visual acuity dropped to 20/100. The role of vitreous loss in the latter is questionable. In two extracapsular cases vitreous was lost during aspiration of cortical remnants. Considering there were only six extracapsular cases in the series, the incidence is high and a reflection of initial attempts to perform extracapsular cataract surgery using automated irrigation-aspiration systems.

Additional surgery (Table 13-32)

Further surgery was performed for several reasons (Table 13-32). Both cases of pupillary membranes occurred after intracapsular surgery. One case of lens implant dislocation followed successful repair of a retinal detachment.

A dislocated loop of a Worst Medallion 2-loop lens implant may not be readily reposited by pharmacologic means. All five dislocations had one loop anterior to the iris and required surgery. Each of the five cases were noted within one week of initial surgery (four followed cataract surgery and one followed a scleral buckling procedure). Three of these cases occurred in the same week, demonstrating how suddenly incidence percentages and statistics can fluctuate with a small series.

Table 13-32. Worst Medallion implants: additional surgery

Surgery	No. cases
Keratoplasty/Implant removal	1
Implant removal	1
Discission pupillary membrane	2
Wound dehiscence	1
Retinal detachment	2
Implant dislocation	5

FYODOROV SPUTNIK LENS IMPLANT

Galin's series of 300 cases with implantation of a Fyodorov sputnik lens implant has been followed for a minimum of 5 years, the follow-up ranging from 5 to 10 years. In this series Galin excluded any patient with preexisting macular disease, or a history of such, when the fundus could not be visualized. All patients with any preexisting corneal disease were also excluded. Lens implantation was aborted in all cases where the anterior hyaloid face, vitreous loss, or other technical factors precluded easy implant insertion. All cases were intracapsular extractions.

Patient population

There were 300 patients, ranging in age from 62 to 86 years, with a mean age of 72 years. No bilateral cases were included in this series.

Table 13-33. Fyodorov implants: visual acuity

Visual acuity	No. patients	Percent
20/20 to 20/40	264	88.0
20/50 to 20/60	18	6.0
20/70 to 20/200	12	4.0
20/200 or less	6	2.0
TOTAL	300	

Visual acuity (Tables 13-33 and 13-34)

Eighty-eight percent of patients achieved a visual acuity of 20/40 or better, and 2% were 20/200 or worse (Table 13-33). All identifiable cases of visual acuity of less than 20/40 were on the basis of disease of the posterior segment (Table 13-34). It is not surprising in this series that cystoid macular edema has a higher incidence of failure to achieve 20/40 or better visual acuity than senile macular degeneration, since patients with preexisting macular disease were excluded.

Table 13-34. Fyodorov implants: causes of visual acuity of <20/40

Cause	No. cases	Percent
Senile macular choroidal degeneration	5	1.7
Cystoid macular edema	9	3.0
Corneal edema	0	0.0
Ischemic optic neuropathy	3	1.0
Retinal detachment	4	1.3
Vein occlusion	3	1.0
Diabetic maculopathy	2	0.7
Macular hole or pucker	3	1.0
Amblyopia	3	1.0
Unknown	4	1.3
TOTAL	36	12.0

Postoperative complications (Tables 13-35 to 13-39)

From 1969 to 1971 Galin routinely used topical miotics during the postoperative course. In 1972 he discontinued this practice and noted a decrease in the incidence of pupillary membrane formation. When *mild* mydriatics were prescribed in the postoperative period, the incidence of pupillary membrane formation decreased further (Table 13-35).

Table 13-35. Fyodorov implants: percent membrane formation

Year	Postoperative treatment	Percent cases
1969	Miotics	8
1970	Miotics	11
1971	Miotics	10
1972	No miotics	4
1973	No miotics	2
1974-1976	Mydriasis	1

Table 13-36. Fyodorov implants: percent dislocations

Year	Postoperative treatment	Strut or loop	Optic	Medically treated	Surgically treated	Un-treated
1969	Miotics	10	1	3	6	2
1970	Miotics	11	0	4	4	3
1971	Miotics	10	0	5	2	3
1972	No miotics	6	0	3	1	2
1973	No miotics	6	0	3	0	3
1974-1976	Mydriasis	5	0	2	1	2

Table 13-37. Fyodorov implants: increase in intraocular pressure in first postoperative week (over preoperative level)

Intraocular pressure	Implant	Nonimplant
> 6 mm Hg	20%	15%
> 10 mm Hg	8%	5%

Table 13-38. Fyodorov implants: striate keratopathy in first postoperative week

Striate keratopathy	Implant	Nonimplant
Severe	20%	3%
Moderate	30%	5%
Mild to none	50%	92%

Table 13-39. Fyodorov implants: other first-week postoperative complications

Postoperative complications	Implant	Nonimplant
Shallow anterior chamber (nonsurgically treated)	3%	4%
Shallow or absent anterior chamber (surgically treated)	0%	0%
Iris prolapse	0%	0%
Pupillary block	0%	0%
Endophthalmitis	0%	0%
Sterile hypopyon	2%	0%
Retinal detachment	2%	2%

Paradoxically the incidence of implant dislocation also decreased when postoperative miotics were discontinued (Table 13-36), and decreased further with postoperative mydriasis. For this type of lens, eccentric synechia formation often leads to a strut going behind or getting into the iris. Consequently, mydriasis significantly prevents this event from occurring, since the lens will move symmetrically on dilatation from any cause.

Galin and his associates compiled a series of 600 routine intracapsular cataract extractions, age matched to the implant series, but not directly comparable inasmuch as preexisting corneal disease and maculopathy were not excluded, as in the implant series. Nevertheless, some of the postoperative observations are of interest. The preoperative intraocular pressures ranged from 16 to 22 mm Hg in both groups. Table 13-37 shows the elevation of pressure over preoperative levels during the first postoperative week. It is higher in the implant group, a finding unrelated to alpha-chymotrypsin, since this enzyme was not used in any case, regardless of whether an implant was inserted. Striate keratopathy was more common in the lens implant series during the first postoperative week (Table 13-38), even though preexisting corneal disease precluded implant insertion. Table 13-39 summarizes other postoperative complications, and the 2% incidence of sterile hypopyon in the lens implant series is thought provoking.

VARIOUS LENS TYPES (Tables 13-40 to 13-43)

Hirschman has tabulated data on 1784 lens implantations he performed between 1967 and 1977 (Table 13-40). Patients under 20 years of age accounted for 0.3% of the series, and 73.3% of patients were over 60 years (Table 13-41). There were 751 cases of extracapsular cataract surgery, comprising 349 phacoemulsifications and 402 standard planned extracapsular extractions. Intracapsular cataract extraction was performed in 882 cases (Table 13-42). Five percent of the series were secondary lens implantations (Table 13-43), and this with other surgical situations made up the balance of the series.

Table 13-40. Various lens types (Hirschman): distribution of cases

Year	No. operations
1967	1
1968	42
1969	59
1970	59
1971	62
1972	87
1973	152
1974	420
1975	404
1976	396
1977 (first 3 months)	92
TOTAL	1784

Table 13-41. Various lens types (Hirschman): age distribution

Age (years)	No. patients
20	6 (0.3%)
20-40	42 (1.4%)
40-60	446 (25.0%)
60	1290 (73.3%)
TOTAL	1784 (100.0%)

Table 13-42. Various lens types (Hirschman): surgical distribution

Type of operation	No. patients	Percent
ICCE	882	49.4
ECCE	402	22.6
Phacoemulsification	349	19.6
Secondary implantation	95	5.3
Unplanned ECCE	52	2.9
Lens removal/replacement	4	0.2
TOTAL	1784	100.0

Table 13-43. Various lens types (Hirschman): secondary implantation*

Initial surgery	No. cases
ICCE	58
ECCE	16
Phacoemulsification	21
TOTAL	95

*Secondary implantations = 5.3% of series.

Lens types (Table 13-44)

Hirschman has used several types of implants. The bulk of his cases were Worst Medallion, Worst platinum-clip, and Binkhorst iridocapsular lens implants. Of the latter, approximately half had metal loops and the remainder plastic loops, either nylon or polypropylene.

Table 13-44. Various lens types (Hirschman): lens distribution

Lens type	No. cases	Percent
Worst Medallion 2-loop	612	34.4
Binkhorst 2-loop irido-capsular	426	23.9
Worst platinum-clip	356	19.9
Binkhorst 4-loop iris-clip	174	9.7
Fyodorov-Binkhorst	133	7.4
Fyodorov sputnik	30	1.7
Epstein	14	0.8
Choyce Mark VIII	13	0.7
Worst circular loop	9	0.5
Worst 3-loop clover leaf	6	0.3
Leonard 4-loop iris-clip	5	0.3
Copeland	5	0.3
Worst small incision	1	0.1
TOTAL	1784	100.0

Postoperative visual acuity (Tables 13-45 to 13-49)

Follow-up in this series ranged from 3 months to 10 years (Table 13-45). The data is incomplete or irretrievable in 124 patients (7% of series). Table 13-46 shows the visual acuities obtained in 1660 cases after implant surgery, and 83.4% of patients achieved 20/40 or better. The comparison of visual acuity versus implant type and patient age is shown in Tables 13-47 and 13-48, respectively. The relationship of the final visual acuity to the type of surgery was obtainable in 1714 patients (Table 13-49).

Table 13-45. Various lens types (Hirschman): length of follow-up

Years	No. cases	Percent
1 or less	832	46.6
1-2	445	24.9
2-3	257	14.5
3-5	144	8.1
5-10	106	5.9
TOTAL	1784	100.0

Table 13-46. Various lens types (Hirschman): most recent visual acuity recorded

Visual acuity	No. patients	Percent
20/40 or better	1385	83.4
20/50 to 20/200	144	8.7
<20/200	121	7.3
No light perception	10	0.6
TOTAL	1660	100.0

Table 13-47. Visual acuity compared to lens types (1669 patients)

Visual acuity	Binkhorst lenses								Worst lenses				Fyodorov lenses			
	2-loop (metal)		2-loop (plastic)		2-loop (unspecified)		4-loop		Medallion 2-loop		Platinum-clip		Fyodorov-Binkhorst		Sputnik	
	No.	Percent	No.	Percent	No.	Percent	No.	Percent	No.	Percent	No.	Percent	No.	Percent	No.	Percent
20/25 or better	84	48.3	89	54.9	36	50.8	47	27.0	210	35.7	160	47.2	39	29.5	11	27.9
20/30 to 20/40	75	43.1	62	38.3	29	40.8	71	40.8	275	46.8	138	40.7	59	44.7	9	31.1
20/50 to 20/200	12	6.9	7	4.3	4	5.6	22	12.6	54	9.2	27	8.0	18	13.6	7	24.1
<20/200	3	1.7	4	2.5	2	2.8	32	18.5	44	7.5	13	3.8	15	11.4	2	6.9
No light perception	0	0.0	0	0.0	0	0.0	2	1.1	5	0.8	1	0.3	1	0.8	0	0.0
TOTAL	174	100.0	162	100.0	71	100.0	174	100.0	588	100.0	339	100.0	132	100.0	29	100.0

Table 13-48. Visual acuity according to age (1714 patients)

Visual acuity	<20 years		20 to 40 years		41 to 60 years		>60 years	
	No.	Percent	No.	Percent	No.	Percent	No.	Percent
20/25 or better	1	16.7	15	60.0	263	61.9	410	32.6
20/30 to 20/40	1	16.7	7	28.0	130	30.6	596	47.4
20/50 to 20/200	2	33.2	1	4.0	18	4.2	137	11.0
<20/200	1	16.7	2	8.0	13	3.1	106	8.4
No light perception	1	16.7	0	0.0	1	0.2	8	0.6
TOTAL	7	100.0	25	100.0	425	100.0	1257	100.0

Table 13-49. Various lens types (Hirschman): visual acuity according to type of surgery

Visual acuity	ICCE	ECCE	KPE*	Secondary	Unplanned ECCE	Vitreous loss
No light perception	6	1	2	0	1	2
≤20/200	86	16	6	9	5	20
>20/50 to 20/200	93	30	15	11	9	23
20/25 to 20/40	388	164	118	39	25	73
≤20/20	278	168	199	32	12	48

*Kelman phacoemulsification.

Causes of decreased visual acuity
(Table 13-50)

In the 1660 cases with adequate follow-up, various lens types were represented. The major causes of visual acuity of less than 20/40 are listed in Table 13-50. In common with Jaffe's and Clayman's series, the predominant cause of decreased visual acuity was senile macular choroidal degeneration. Galin excluded preexisting macular disease in selecting patients for implant surgery.

Table 13-50. Various lens types (Hirschman): main causes of visual acuity of <20/40

Cause	No. cases	Percent series
Senile macular choroidal degeneration	87	5.2
Cystoid macular edema	43	2.5
Corneal edema or dys-trophy	53	3.2
Retinal detachment	32	1.9
Secondary pupillary membrane	15	0.9
Uveitis	13	0.8
Amblyopia	17	1.0
Unknown	45	2.7

Intraoperative complications
(Table 13-51)

The high incidence of vitreous loss is attributable to prophylactic aspiration of vitreous in cases of vitreous bulge early in Hirschman's series. He now uses a Sheets glide (p. 168) to manage this contingency.

Table 13-51. Various lens types (Hirschman): intraoperative complications

Complication	No. cases	Percent
Descemet's detachment	33	1.9
Inadvertent rupture of posterior capsule	34	1.9
Vitreous loss	172	9.6

Postoperative complications
(Tables 13-52 to 13-58)

Hirschman has data on iris sphincter erosion and has shown the frequency of this in various lens types (Table 13-52). It is of interest that the majority of cases occurred with a *metal* 2-loop Binkhorst iridocapsular lens implant.

In the 612 Worst Medallion lens implants inserted, there was failure of the iris suture remote from surgery in 29 patients, 4.7% of this group. This was presumably due to chemical degradation or chafing of the nylon, a problem that may be lessened now that polypropylene suture material is available for intracameral use.

Table 13-52. Various lens types (Hirschman): erosion of iris sphincter*

Lens type	No. cases	Percent
Binkhorst iridocapsular (metal loops)	16/213	7.5
Binkhorst iris-clip	3/174	1.7
Fyodorov-Binkhorst	3/133	2.3
Fyodorov sputnik	2/30	6.7
Worst 2-loop Medallion	2/612	0.3
Worst platinum-clip	1/356	0.3
Epstein	1/14	7.1
Binkhorst iridocapsular (plastic loops)	1/213	0.5

*Incidence 1.7% (29/1660 cases)

Table 13-53. Dislocation of various lens types (Hirschman): relationship of lens type and type of surgery

Surgery	Binkhorst 2-loop metal	Binkhorst 2-loop Supramid	Binkhorst 2-loop unspecified	Binkhorst 4-loop	2-loop with sutures
ICCE				14 (4 had 2 to 3 dislocations)	13 (8 had 2 to 5 dislocations)
ECCE	11 (1 dislocated 2×, 1 dislocated 7×)	2	1	1	2 (1 dislocated 3×)
KPE*	5 (1 dislocated 2×, 1 dislocated 5×)	1	5 (2 dislocated 2×)		4 (1 dislocated 3×)
Secondary	2			2 (1 dislocated 3×, 1 dislocated 4×)	
Unplanned ECCE				2	
TOTAL	18	3	6	19	19

*Kelman phacoemulsification.

Table 13-54. Various lens types (Hirschman): removal of lens implant

Implant type	Reason for removal: Corneal touch	Inflammation	Dislocation
Binkhorst iris-clip	4	3	2
Fyodorov-Binkhorst	4	6	1
Binkhorst iridocapsular (metal loop)	0	1	4
Worst platinum-clip	1	0	0
Epstein	0	1	0
Choyce Mark VIII	0	0	1
Worst Medallion 2-loop (plastic loop)	2	0	0
Worst Medallion 2-loop (metal loop)	0	2	1
TOTAL	11	13	9

Table 13-55. Various lens types (Hirschman): retinal detachment*

Initial surgery	No. cases
ICCE	16
ICCE (vitreous loss)	4
ECCE	2
ECCE (vitreous loss)	2
Phacoemulsification	7
Phacoemulsification (vitreous loss)	2
Secondary inplantation	2
TOTAL	35

*Incidence: 2.1% (35/1660 cases)

Lens dislocation was noted in 98 of 1660 patients (5.9%), 50% of which were repositioned pharmacologically, while the other 50% required further surgery. The relationship of the lens type and type of surgery to subsequent lens dislocation is shown in Table 13-53. Several of these patients had multiple dislocations, which were ultimately repaired with a McCannel suture (p. 176).

The implant was removed in 33 eyes, and the reasons for this are shown in Table 13-54, together with the lens types. Of the cases in which the implant was removed due to corneal touch, six eyes had vitreous loss at the initial surgery with resultant lens displacement due to synechiae formation, and three eyes had shallow anterior chambers preoperatively.

Fyodorov-Binkhorst	Fyodorov II	Epstein	Worst platinum-clip	Worst circular loop	Total
3 had 2 to 4 dislocations)	2 (1 dislocated 4×)	1	6 (3 had 2 to 5 dislocations)	2	45/882 (5.1%)
			3		20/402 (5.0%)
			6 (3 dislocated 2×)		21/349 (6.0%)
			3 (1 dislocated 2×; 1 dislocated 3×)		7/95 (7.4%)
dislocated 2×)			2 (1 dislocated 2×)		5/52 (9.6%)
8	2	1	20	2	98

Table 13-56. Various lens types (Hirschman): retinal detachment—time of occurrence after implant surgery

Months	No. cases
1	1
2	3
3	2
4	6
5	2
6	6
7	1
8	0
9	3
10	2
11	0
12	1
12-18	3
19-24	1
25-48	2
Over 48	2
TOTAL	35

Table 13-57. Various lens types (Hirschman): retinal detachment—age at occurrence*

Age (years)	No. patients
46-50	2
51-55	3
56-60	6
61-65	6
66-70	7
71 75	4
76-80	5
81-85	2
TOTAL	35

*Mean age: 65.5 years.

Pupillary block developed in 1.1% of patients, (18/1660 cases), and of these, 55.6% occurred with the Worst platinum-clip lens implant. The importance of the peripheral iridectomy with this type of implant was discussed in Chapter 8. Thirteen of the patients required surgical intervention for relief of the pupillary block.

The incidence of retinal detachment was 2.1% (35/1660 cases), as shown in Table 13-55, which well demonstrates the relationship of vitreous loss to retinal detachment. Of the patients with retinal detachment, 43.7% had an antecedent history of vitreous loss or other surgery. Table 13-56 shows when the detachment occurred after implant surgery; 27/35 cases (77%) were noted within the first postoperative year. The mean age of pa-

Table 13-58. Various lens types (Hirschman): secondary membranes

Lens type	Planned extracapsular		Unplanned extracapsular		Phacoemulsification		Intracapsular		Total	Incidence of lens type (%)
	Discission	Repeat discission	Discission	Repeat discission	Discission	Repeat discission	Discission	Repeat discission		
Binkhorst iridocapsular metal loop	35	2	—	—	20	3	—	—	55/176	31.2
Binkhorst iridocapsular plastic loop	19	4	—	—	17	0	—	—	36/179	20.1
Binkhorst iridocapsular loop (unspecified)	4	0	—	—	20	4	—	—	24/71	33.8
Binkhorst 4-loop	1	0	—	—	—	—	1	—	2/174	1.1
Worst Medallion 2-loop	9	2	2	1	11	0	6	—	28/612	4.6
Worst platinum-clip	18	1	1	—	12	4	—	—	31/356	8.7
Worst circular loop	1	—	—	—	—	—	—	—	1/9	11.1
Worst clover leaf	—	—	—	—	1	—	—	—	1/4	25.0
Fyodorov-Binkhorst	—	—	—	—	—	—	2	—	2/133	1.5
Fyodorov sputnik	3	1	1	—	1	—	2	—	7/30	23.3
Epstein	1	—	1	—	1	—	—	—	3/14	21.4
TOTAL	91/402		5/52		83/349		11/882		190/1758	
Incidence of type of extraction	22.6%		9.6%		23.8%		1.2%		10.8%	

tients with retinal detachments was 65.5 years (Table 13-57).

A secondary pupillary membrane was noted in 226 eyes and followed extracapsular cataract extraction or phacoemulsification in the majority of cases. Discissions were ultimately required in 10.8% of the series (190/1758 cases), and in some of these patients the membrane reoccurred. Table 13-58 relates the incidence of secondary membrane formation to lens type and type of surgery. It would be erroneous to assume that the 2-loop Binkhorst lens implant "causes" secondary membranes even though it accounts for 115/426 cases (27.0%). This figure is an indication of the type of surgery, since the 2-loop lens is only inserted after an extracapsular extraction. Of the 190 secondary membranes requiring discission, 94% occurred after extracapsular surgery or phacoemulsification. The incidence of discissions following planned extracapsular surgery was 22.6% (91/402 cases) and 23.8% (83/349 cases) after phacoemulsification. This compares unfavorably with the low incidence of 1.2% (11/882 cases) following intracapsular surgery.

CONCLUSION

The results we have presented show that 80% to 90% of patients with pseudophakoi will attain a visual acuity of 20/40 or better and maintain this over a reasonable follow-up period, predicated on suitable case selection. Complications do occur, and some of these may be compounded by the presence of an implant. Obviously the cases presented need to be followed over a prolonged period with scrupulous accumulation of data.

The results do not entirely show whether a given patient would have benefited in the long run from a routine cataract extraction instead of an implant or perhaps no surgery. A prospective study is required to answer this question, and this is currently being devised under the auspices of the National Eye Institute of the National Institutes of Health.

CHAPTER 14

Surgical education

By surgical education we mean the process by which a surgeon can acquire the knowledge to select suitable patients for lens implantation, choose the implant, and perform the surgery. If a complication should arise at or after surgery, there should be sufficient depth of knowledge to manage and prevent progression of the problems to serious proportions.

Indications are discussed in Chapter 5. There is no consensus on these among implant surgeons, but the beginning implant surgeon should be conservative both in age criteria and the need for cataract surgery. It would be prudent initially to exclude any patient with degenerative or dystrophic corneal disease. The pupil should both dilate and constrict easily. There should be no history of retinal detachment or retinal holes, even in the contralateral eye. Controlled glaucoma is not a contraindication to lens implantation (Chapter 10), but the beginner would be well advised to start with ocular normotensive patients. Additionally the patient should have the desire for lens implant surgery and be expected to follow the surgeon's postoperative instructions.

Prior to the selection of the implant, an essential part of the surgeon's education is a knowledge of the history of lens implantation. It tells us how and why we arrived at the present state of the art and is discussed in Chapter 4. Certain aspects of the history bear reemphasis. The family tree of lens implants (Fig. 4-18) is not a tribute to illustrious ancestors, as is the case with most family trees, but rather a testimony to past failures. Intrinsic in the evolution of currently used lenses were complications in their predecessors. Modifications of design, dimensions, and weight have resulted in the present generation of lens implants. Most of the pioneers of lens implant surgery were extremely capable surgeons, and their disastrous complications were usually attributable to the lens implant design rather than the surgery. The beginning implant surgeon should remember the sensitivity of the intraocular tissues and the problems that could be caused by a relatively large, mobile foreign body placed within the eye. After studying the history of lens implantation and design, the beginning surgeon will have some concept of what constitutes an acceptable implant. It is recommended that the beginner use implants with a proven record in regard to quality and reliability of power and that he be aware of methods of sterilization and their limitations. Calculation of lens power is discussed elsewhere (Chapter 6), and for the first few cases the beginning surgeon should select eyes in which the required power may be easily determined so that the predicted result produces minimal anisometropia.

A surgeon who is insecure with his surgical expertise should not contemplate lens implantation. The lens implant phase of the operation begins where normally the surgeon would be closing the incision. As such it can engender its own set of intraoperative complications that would compound preexisting inadequacies. The beginning implant surgeon should not stray too far from his accustomed technique when he starts implant surgery. An extreme example of impending disaster would be the intracapsular loupe surgeon who begins microsurgery, phacoemulsification, and lens implantation, all in the same week.

For the intracapsular lens implant surgeon the difference between a gratifying or difficult lens implant insertion rests largely with the behavior of the anterior hyaloid face. The old dictum "as the incision goes, so goes the cataract operation" can be updated to "as the anterior hyaloid face goes, so goes the implant insertion." Steps can be taken prior to entering the anterior chamber to facilitate reduction in vitreous volume and a resultant concave anterior hyaloid face following cataract extraction. These are described in Chapter 8 and can be summarized as the concept of "surgery on the soft eye."

In spite of all precautions a substantial vitreous bulge can occur. The beginning implant surgeon should be prepared for this contingency, and the patient should be aware that implant surgery may be aborted. There are techniques for dealing with this situation described in Chapter 12, but the beginner should be cautious in his initial cases lest they turn into unforgettable experiences.

In extracapsular surgery a soft eye is not as critical, but it is helpful in avoiding endothelial damage as the implant is inserted. An extracapsular surgeon should perform competent surgery before embarking on implant insertion. Next to the anterior hyaloid face and the corneal endothelium, the most important structure for the implant surgeon is the pupillary sphincter. Extracapsular surgeons should be wary of causing sphincter damage with cystotomes or irrigating-aspirating tips.

The vast majority of cataract surgeons perform cataract surgery well. Should they now start inserting implants, or go through some sort of educational process? History and indications are amenable to

Table 14-1. Criteria for an overview course

Surgery	Complications	Miscellaneous
Copeland technique	Corneal	Indications
Binkhorst intracapsular and extracapsular techniques	Macula Retinal	Contraindications Extracapsular versus intracapsular
Worst implant techniques	Glaucoma	
Fyodorov techniques	Dislocations	Lens power selection
Choyce techniques	Pupillary membranes Infections	

self-study, but additional surgical training is required. Suggested changes in surgical technique may be tried on routine cataract extractions, so that the surgeon may be satisfied with their feasibility and efficacy. Smooth and consistent implant surgery comes only with experience, and the beginner can only acquire this by the teaching of more experienced colleagues.

It is recommended that an overview course be the initial step. The contents of the course should deal with the principal types of currently used implants, indications, contraindications, and most impor tantly, complications. A suggested course outline is described in Table 14-1. The caliber and integrity of the faculty are of crucial importance in selecting an overview course. It is unconscionable for a teacher to minimize pitfalls and complications to enhance his own image.

A practical laboratory course is then advisable in which an animal laboratory is available. The need for supportive veterinarian care and humane considerations speak against unnecessary live animal surgery. Though human eye bank eyes are excellent for training purposes, they are not always readily available. Consequently, animal eyes, such as postmortem pig eyes, are quite satisfactory. A useful technique for all iris-supported implants is to completely remove the

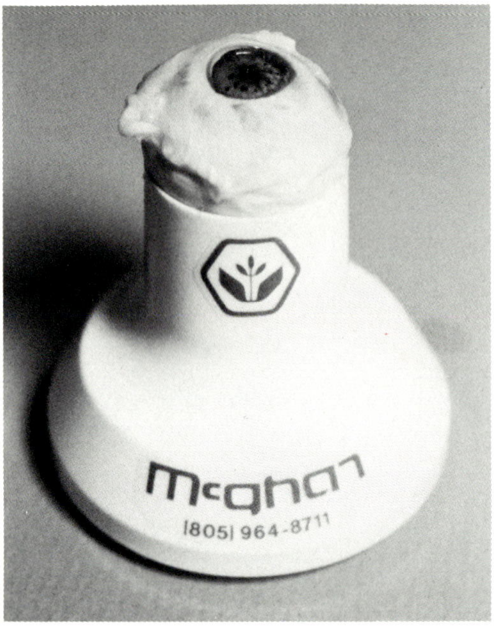

Fig. 14-1. Postmortem eye with cornea removed at limbus, in practice holder. (Courtesy McGhan Medical.)

cornea of the postmortem practice eye at the limbus. A practice holder (McGhan Medical) is used to mount the eye (Fig. 14-1). The crystalline lens does not have to be removed, and various types of lens implants can be inserted into the pupillary aperture with and without iris sutures (Fig. 14-2). If the pupil becomes vacuous from manipulation, it can be tightened with a 7-0 black silk suture placed in the sphincter.

The course should also have the opportunity to observe live surgery, either on videotape or in the operating room. Ideally, one-on-one surgical assistance is the ultimate, but is difficult to accomplish due to legal restrictions. The practical laboratory should be supplemented by didactic lectures germane to teaching the techniques of lens implantation; that is, how the surgeon inserts the lens and how complications are avoided and managed. It is understandable that the courses reflect the personal bias of their sponsors, and the aspiring implant surgeon should be sure that the contemplated course is adequate. Earlier in this chapter the beginner was advised not to change technique drastically when implant surgery is first begun, and any practical course should fulfill this criterion.

Implant surgery may now be started, preferably with an experienced assistant. In spite of assiduous education and preparation, questions and problems usually arise in the first few cases. The beginner should have available an experienced colleague with whom to consult, if only by phone. After the initial cases, a visit to observe a more experienced implant surgeon with a sizeable surgical load and compatible technique will be an enriching experience and will permit refinement of technique. The American Intra-Ocular Implant Society has been an invaluable source of information to the implant surgeon, and the beginner is urged to join this organization.

The role of implant surgery in a residency training program is a problem dependent on several factors. First, the departmental chairman should decide if the surgical load is adequate to permit this specialized type of cataract surgery and whether implant surgery is compatible with departmental philosophy. Then there are the perennial problems of any teaching program, which include frequent turnover of residents, surgical inexperience, and poor patient compliance. On the other hand, most residents are familiar with the surgical microscope, their colleagues provide an instantaneous and ongoing peer review, and attending surgeons are available for guidance and advice.

If implant surgery is instituted as part of a residency program, common sense dictates that not all implants and techniques be taught in the fleeting span of time. The residents should be taught a technique and implant type compatible with their technical capabilities and which will form a basis for later progression and innovation.

The combination of lectures, animal

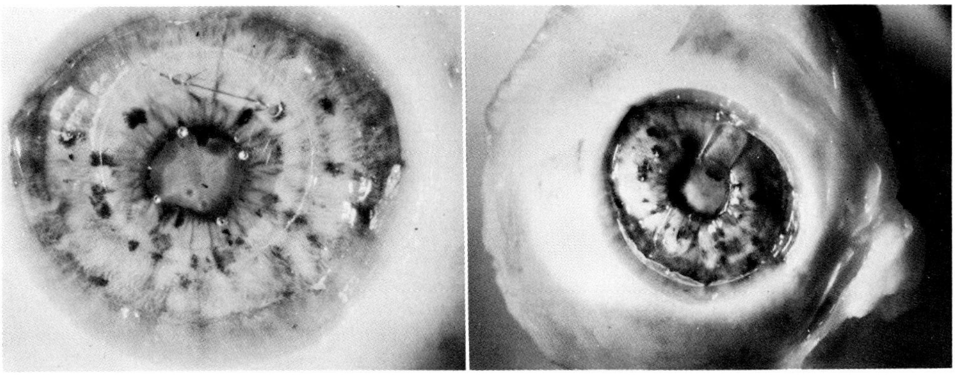

Fig. 14-2. Practice lens implants inserted *over* crystalline lens in postmortem eye with cornea removed at limbus. (Courtesy McGhan Medical.)

laboratory, and observation or assisting for the beginning postgraduate implant surgeon has value for the resident in training. If sufficient talent is available in the community and department, an ongoing course of instruction may be incorporated into the official teaching program. Where local resources are not adequate, guest lecturers could be invited to augment the educational experience on a regular basis.

It is recommended that an experienced implant surgeon supervise the residents' lens implantation program. If a resident does not do creditable cataract surgery, then he should not be permitted to perform lens implantation. The concept of using indigent patients as clinical material is to be deprecated. The program supervisor should arrange for lectures and courses and be responsible for case selection. No patient should be scheduled for lens implantation without the supervisor's prior approval. Ultraconservatism should be emphasized in case selection, which hopefully will develop good habits in the neophyte surgeon. The program supervisor should assist on all resident cases and correct deficiencies in technique. Videotapes are also helpful, and replay will often show errors amenable to easy correction.

A record documenting pertinent data of resident implant surgery should be kept on all cases. The data should be periodically updated, and review will show how much was gained or lost by lens implantation. A department that develops a viable implant instruction program would probably benefit the community by making it available to ophthalmologists beyond the residency level.

There are personal attributes of realism and honesty that cannot be taught in medical schools or residencies, nor can they be legislated. The surgeon who is truly interested in the welfare of his patients must face the question of whether he is capable of performing the surgery, and if so, does he have the fortitude to live with the complications that occur even in the most experienced hands. There is obviously a difference in individual abilities and judgment. Circumstances also vary; some surgeons have large surgical practices, in contradistinction to the occasional surgeon. Even the more experienced ophthalmologist must accept the fact that more complications are likely with implant surgery than with routine cataract surgery. Further, there is nothing wrong in requesting consultation, and in specific cases, referring the patient until adequate expertise is reached.

In digesting the increasing literature on lens implantation the beginning surgeon should distinguish between opinions, anecdotes, and facts. The quest should be for the latter, and all implant surgeons should keep scrupulous data on

A

SOUTH FLORIDA
PSEUDOPHAKOS REGISTRATION

Type of Implant Used ____________________

Date of Implant ____________ Surgeon ____________
(Please Print)

Patient's Name ____________________

(Or Initials plus I.D. No.) ____________________

Date of Birth ____________

If Unavailable, Age at Time of Implant ____________

Color of Iris: Brown ____________ Sex ____________

Blue ____________ Race ____________

Type of Extraction: Intracapsular ____________

Planned Extracapsular ____________

Unplanned Extracapsular ____________

Vitreous Loss: Yes ____________

No ____________

Other Surgical Complications ____________________

____

Other Preexisting Eye Disease ____________________

Remarks: ____________________

____

Phone: 324-4340

(FOLD IN HALF, SEAL AND MAIL POSTAGE FREE)

B

FIRST CLASS
PERMIT NO. 10132
MIAMI, FLORIDA

BUSINESS REPLY MAIL
NO POSTAGE STAMP NECESSARY IF MAILED IN THE UNITED STATES

POSTAGE WILL BE PAID BY

FLORIDA LIONS EYE BANK
P.O. Box 520009
Biscayne Annex
Miami, Florida 33152

REGISTRY

Fig. 14-3. Patient registration form for Miami Pseudophakos Community Protocol.

their cases for their own education and that of their colleagues. If the size of the community permits, a collective implant study is an excellent project. The ideal model is the Miami Community Protocol.[1]

The sequence of events leading to the protocol began in December 1967 when Jaffe performed the first intraocular lens implant in the Miami area. The procedure was taken up by other ophthalmic surgeons in the community, but it was soon realized that, in spite of patient acceptance, long-term results and complications were unknown. The ophthalmic community responded with wisdom and foresight by declaring a two-year moratorium, during which time no lens implantations were performed, with a few minor exceptions.

The patients operated on prior to the moratorium were studied on a continuing basis by senior residents of the Bascom Palmer Eye Institute, University of Miami School of Medicine. Predicated on favorable results, lens implantation was resumed in October 1971 with some reservations, primarily as to patients' age. All patients operated on were registered with the Florida Lions Eye Bank, using a preaddressed form (Fig. 14-3). These forms were annually reviewed by a senior resident of the Eye Institute who then *personally* examined the patient at the operating surgeon's office and audited the office record. Due to the tact and professional demeanor of those senior residents involved in the study, patient and professional acceptance were excellent. Reports were made to the ophthalmic community in June at the annual scientific meetings of the Bascom Palmer Alumni Association.[2,3] Satisfactory results led to a partial relaxation in criteria for patient selection. The study continued through 1974, by which time more than 600 patients were studied.

Apart from the valuable data collected, the protocol fostered an enviable spirit of cooperation and goodwill in the community. It also provided a respectable and believable basis from which implant surgery in the United States could grow. It showed lens implantation to be a meaningful contribution to ophthalmology, when correctly applied. In fact, the quantity of information offered by this and similar studies acted as a strong stimulus for critical review of many accepted, but not investigated, techniques.

REFERENCES

1. Duffner, L. R.: The Miami pseudophakos study—a suggested community study protocol, Trans. Am. Acad. Ophthalmol. Otolaryngol. **81**:OP128-131, 1976.
2. Forster, R. K.: Bascom Palmer Eye Institute residents' day, Am. J. Ophthalmol. **71**:765-766, 1971.
3. Bedotto, C.: Bascom Palmer Eye Institute seventh annual residents' day, Am. J. Ophthalmol. **72**:1153-1154, 1971.

CHAPTER 15

Role of regulatory agencies in intraocular lens implant surgery

ALEXANDER B. McDONALD
EDWARD J. PULASKI

Almost unnoticed by those most directly affected, a "regulatory revolution" has taken place in America. Regulatory authority over many aspects of daily life has been delegated to a host of regulatory agencies that can enact laws, enforce those laws, and in many instances adjudicate the dispute. The experience encountered by patients, physicians, and manufacturers of intraocular lenses with two regulatory bodies, the Food and Drug Administration (FDA) of the U.S. Department of Health, Education, and Welfare and the California Department of Health, during the efforts of those bodies to expand their control over this medical device is illustrative.

The Federal Food and Drug Act[1] originated in a burgeoning of public awareness of appalling conditions in the food and drug industries that had evolved in the late nineteenth century. It empowered the secretaries of the treasury, agriculture, and commerce and labor to administer the provisions of the legislation and directed the United States attorney of the particular district where a violation occurred to enforce the law.[2] A driving force leading to this legislation was the series of abuses documented and publicized by Upton Sinclair and other "muckrakers" in the early years of the twentieth century. Immediate and grave threats to the public health were posed by the untrammeled free-enterprise system then operative in most basic industries in the United States. At that time medical devices were few in number and could be divided into two categories: devices used by physicians as an adjunct to their practice and other devices directly touted to the public as cures for a variety of ills. Mail-order catalogs of the era are replete with quack devices such as rings to cure rheumatism and the like. Understandably, then, early efforts at enforcing the provisions of the new food and drug act were directed principally at adulterated food and mislabeled or impure medicine introduced into interstate commerce. The legislation easily survived a number of attacks on its constitutionality.[3]

In 1938 the Food, Drug, and Cosmetic Act[4] was enacted to expand federal regulatory authority over food, drugs, and cosmetics. A critically important change was the addition of the "new drug" provisions of the act,[5] which precluded introduction of a new drug into interstate commerce without approval of the secretary of agriculture.[6] Still the act limited its efforts to regulate medical devices to removal of offending products from the market. Litigated cases involved some

□ McDonald, Pulaski and Harlan, Attorneys at Law, San Diego, California (Counsel, American Intra-Ocular Implant Society).

truly remarkable monuments to man's inventiveness: phonograph records designed to induce sleep;[7] mechanical hearts that would treat ailments from headaches to asthma to sexual weakness (male and female),[8] and a cabinet producing colored lights similar to neon lights, which was alleged to be effective in treating disorders of the "liver, eyes, female trouble, asthma, nervousness and sinus trouble."[9] Significantly the FDA's efforts against these devices were centered on its powers to prohibit introduction into interstate commerce of mislabeled devices.[10] That in turn meant that devices whose advertising was false or misleading in any particular respect could be seized, but only after they were produced and sought to be introduced into interstate commerce.

Thus, under the provisions of the Food, Drug, and Cosmetic Act of 1938 the FDA could require premarket approval of drugs but not of devices. The remedy available to federal authorities was to attack a device as misbranded or adulterated and thus secure its removal from the interstate market by seizure or injunction.

With the major post–World War II technological innovations in medicine came an increasing desire by regulatory agencies to regulate medical devices, as well as drugs. In the absence of legislation granting the FDA express authority to require premarket clearance of the devices, the FDA appeared limited to its traditional approach of litigating, on a case-by-case basis, the issue of whether given medical devices were misbranded or adulterated, and were therefore contraband in interstate commerce.

In 1967 a new approach to the regulation of medical devices occurred. Administratively the FDA declared a locking ligature of new design to be a "new drug."[11] The rationale for this appeared to be based upon two significant factors, first, a rapid expansion in the number of medical devices on the American market, and second, the corresponding inability of the FDA to regulate those devices before market introduction. The legal definition of "drugs" and "devices" was so broad as to allow the argument that virtually anything used in a medical context could be a drug.

> The term "drug" means . . . (B) articles intended for use in the diagnosis, cure, mitigation, treatment or prevention of disease in man or other animals; and (C) articles other than food intended to affect the structure or any function of the body of man or other animals.
>
> The term "device" means . . . instruments, apparatus, and contrivances, including their components, parts and accessories, intended (1) for use in the diagnosis, cure, mitigation, treatment or prevention of disease in man or other animals or (2) to affect the structure of any function of the body of man or other animals.[12]

This vague statutory language allowed the FDA to expand existing legislative authority to meet new challenges calling for a regulatory response. Another landmark case in this approach occurred when the FDA declared an antibiotic sensitivity disk to be a drug.[13] The U.S. Supreme Court upheld the FDA'S action, concluding that Congress had granted broad discretion to the FDA to classify articles as drugs or devices; it therefore declined to interfere. Running counter to the FDA's approach, a federal appeals court held that surgical nails, even though implanted in the body, were devices.[14] Thus by 1975, federal law appeared to be hopelessly confused regarding what was a drug or a device.

Although most public attention over the years had been directed toward the actions of the FDA, the states had maintained an active and comprehensive role in the regulation of food, drugs, and cosmetics. This role was specifically approved by the U.S. Supreme Court in 1912, and again in 1915 and 1919.[15] One of the more comprehensive state regulatory schemes was enacted in California in 1970.[16] It provided, among other things, for premarket control and approval of both new drugs and new devices.[17]

Into this regulatory setting came a rapidly developing industry concerned with manufacture of the intraocular lens. Although the intraocular lens, in various designs, had been manufactured in Europe since 1949, manufacture in the United States was of relatively recent origin; moreover, nearly half the American manufacturers were located in California. Finally, intraocular lens implantation had, by 1975, won increasing acceptance in medical circles as one of the treatments for cataract.

The California Department of Health became actively involved with the intraocular lens in the spring of 1975. A panel of ophthalmologists was called together in Los Angeles on April 25 by officials of the Food and Drug Section of the California Department of Health. In attendance also were two representatives of the California Department of Health and one representative of the FDA. A discussion ensued regarding the intraocular lens. In a letter dated May 21, 1975, and sent to intraocular lens manufacturers, the California Department of Health declared that the intraocular lens was a "new drug" and could be distributed in California only under the terms of an approved new drug application or a notice of claimed investigational exemption.

Why, one may ask, would the California Department of Health classify the intraocular lens as a new drug when it had existing statutory authority to regulate devices pursuant to the California Health and Safety Code? The answer is found in a little-noted section of the code[18] that exempts from state regulation medical devices used by a physician within the scope of his license. Thus if the California Department of Health were to regulate intraocular lenses directly, rather than by inspecting labeling and packaging, they could do so only by declaring the intraocular lens to be a new drug; for drugs, unlike devices, were not exempted from state regulation even when used by physicians acting within the scope of their license.

A particularly alarming aspect of the California Department of Health's declaration was that any physician distributing an intraocular lens, whether he knew of the declaration or not, could be charged with a crime.[19] Belatedly addressing this issue, the California Department of Health on June 20, 1975, dispatched a letter to ophthalmologists in California warning them that the department had determined intraocular lenses were drugs and that such products could not be sold, delivered, or given away in California without an approved new drug application or notice of claimed investigational exemption. The letter urged ophthalmologists to contact manufacturers to determine the status of each manufacturer's lens. It did not warn the doctors that continued implantation of lenses already in possession of the physicians would be a criminal act, possibly with grave consequences to the physician resulting from disciplinary action, which could be initiated by the Board of Medical Examiners following conviction. This situation effectively terminated lens implant surgery in California.

Two experienced implant surgeons, together with a hospital, a lens manufacturer, and an individual patient who had been denied implants by the California Department of Health's declaration of May 21, 1975, retained counsel in late July 1975. Preliminary legal analysis of the actions of the California Department of Health raised fundamental questions of procedure, of statutory interpretation, and of constitutional rights of the plaintiffs. Several intraocular lens manufacturers were contacted, and all who had spoken with California Department of Health personnel related that the department appeared to have made a firm decision to label the intraocular lens a new drug. At least two[20] California manufacturers had applied to the California

Department of Health for approval to manufacture intraocular lenses, but their applications elicited neither approval nor rejection.

There appeared to be only two practical alternatives to the complete cessation of intraocular lens implantation in California: (1) some type of negotiated settlement that would allow resumption of intraocular lens manufacturing and distribution coupled with such reasonable safeguards as the California Department of Health might require to discharge its responsibilities, or (2) litigation seeking judicial relief. To pursue the former, on August 6, 1976, an attorney representing the plaintiffs met in Sacramento with house counsel for the California Department of Health and representatives of the Food and Drug Section. The considered position of the California Department of Health at that meeting was that the intraocular lens was a new drug, that the California Department of Health had the power to make that determination, and that the classification would not be changed.[21] Furthermore, despite what appeared to be an unmistakable legislative instruction requiring regulations to be issued to interpret the statutory scheme of the Sherman Food, Drug, and Cosmetic Act,[22] the California Department of Health argued that it had the "inherent power" to determine what was or was not a drug or device and that the issuance of regulations, with their safeguards of notice to interested parties and the opportunity for a hearing,[23] was therefore not required. Litigation followed.

The most expeditious manner to obtain judicial relief from the actions of the California Department of Health was through the vehicle of a petition for injunctive relief. The vagueness of the California Department of Health's letters of May 21 and June 20 presented a difficult problem of pleading, for specific types of relief were dependent upon the characterization of the letters: Were they regulations? Were they orders restricting licenses of the plaintiff physicians, hospital, and manufacturer? Were they adjudications that sale, delivery, or gift of the intraocular lens in California are criminal acts? Different types of relief are specifically appropriate for each theory. Thus if the letters were viewed as an attempt to revoke or restrict the licenses of the plaintiff physicians, hospital, and manufacturer, administrative mandamus was the proper remedy.[24] If the letters were regulations, declaratory relief was proper.[25] If, on the other hand, the letters amounted to an invalid or overbroad administrative order, injunctive relief was proper.[26] Failure to approach all these theories alternatively as a basis for relief would raise the risk of denial of relief simply because a reviewing court might disagree with the plaintiffs' characterization of the nature of the California Department of Health's actions.

On August 22,1975, the petition for relief was heard in the Superior Court of California for the County of Los Angeles by Judge Harry Hupp. Satisfied by the showing made by the plaintiffs that great or irreparable injury would result unless immediate relief was granted, Judge Hupp issued a temporary restraining order preventing the California Department of Health from enforcing its decisions of May 21 and June 20, 1975, declaring the intraocular lens to be a new drug. This, however, was but the first step in the legal proceedings. Further hearings to determine whether a preliminary injunction should issue were scheduled for October 8, and subsequently continued to December 8, 1975. Extensive preparation was required for this hearing because the burden of proof lay upon the plaintiffs to demonstrate that they were entitled to injunctive relief until a full trial could be held. Depositions of central figures in the controversy were scheduled, many knowledgeable surgeons volunteered their assistance, and manufacturers provided invaluable technical and test data to assist in presenting the most comprehensive possible case at the hearing on December 8. Supplemental pleadings totaling more than 600 pages, with 44 additional affidavits, were filed with the court to assist in its deliberations. In addition, oral argument was presented both by the plaintiffs' attorneys and the California Attorney General's Office regarding the propriety of the relief sought. On the afternoon of December 8, 1975, the court issued a preliminary injunction preventing the California Department of Health from regulating the intraocular lens as a new drug on the grounds that it was a device;[27] since the legislature had precluded the California Department of Health from regulating devices dispensed by a physician acting within the scope of his license, irreparable harm would result to the plaintiffs if the California Department of Health were allowed to proceed with this plan. Although trial on the merits of the issues raised in this litigation is still possible, it is unlikely because of changes in *federal* legislation that occurred soon after the December 8 hearing.

On May 28, 1976, President Ford signed the Medical Devices Amendment Act of 1976.[28] This legislation expanded the power of the FDA to regulate medical devices. Several years in the drafting, the new legislation consists of a complex regulatory scheme to extend premarket and postmarket controls to medical devices in much the same manner as those controls now apply to drugs. An obviously thorny problem was presented by devices such as the intraocular lens, which had been on the market for years but which the FDA wished to regulate. Some of these devices had been declared drugs (as in the locking-ligature case), while other devices (such as pacemakers) had been regulated on a different theory—labeling. The new legislation clarified the distinction between drugs and devices by defining devices as follows:

> The term "device" . . . means an instrument, apparatus, implement, machine, contrivance, implant, in vitro reagent, or other similar or related articles, including any component, part, or accessory, which is—
>
> 1. recognized in the official *National Formulary*, or the *United States Pharmacopoeia*, or any supplement to them,
> 2. intended for use in the diagnosis of disease or other mitigation, treatment, or prevention of disease in man or other animals, or
> 3. intended to affect the structure or any function of the body of man or other animals, and
>
> which does not achieve any of its principal intended purposes through chemical action within or on the body of man or other animals and which is not dependent upon being metabolized for the achievement of any of its principal intended purposes.[29]

Although the FDA had issued a notice declaring the intraocular lens to be a new drug on April 6, 1976,[30] that determination was not to become effective, so far as requiring a new drug application or claimed exemption for investigational use, until October 7, 1976. The purpose of this notice, which was published when the new medical device legislation was in final House/Senate Conference Committee and assured of passage, becomes clear when one examines section 520(1) of the bill, entitled "Transitional Provisions for Devices Considered as New Drugs or Antibiotic Drugs." That section provides, in pertinent part, that any device which had been declared a new drug in a *Federal Register* statement published after March 31, 1976, was required to have in effect an approved premarket approval application 18 months after enactment of the legislation unless the device had been exempted for investigational use.[31] To our knowledge there was only one device that met this criterion: the intraocular lens. All other medical devices on the market on the date of enactment of the medical device amendments of 1976, similarly classified into category III (requiring premarket approval) were allowed 36 months before an approved premarket approval application was required.[32] Thus the motivation to publish the *Federal Register* statement was to bring the intraocular lens within an 18-month "grandfather rights" period, rather than the 36-month period accorded all other similarly classified devices.

The new federal regulatory scheme is complex and poses problems for the medical profession, intraocular lens manufacturers, and the FDA alike. Effective 180 days after enactment of the new legislation, only "experts qualified by scientific training and experience" may use the intraocular lens.[33]

The FDA has consistently taken the position that while the manufacturer of any device is responsible for applying for such exemption, the FDA has final control over the qualifications of the "investigators," raising the question of direct federal control over the determination of which surgeons will be allowed to implant intraocular lenses. In the new act, Congress expressly declared its intent that devices, such as the intraocular lens, which might be placed in an investigational status, should nevertheless be made reasonably available to physicians meeting appropriate qualifications prescribed by the secretary of the U.S. Department of Health, Education, and Welfare.[34] The potential conflict between the congressional intent that intraocular lenses be reasonably available to physicians and the FDA's responsibility to administer a comprehensive and time-consuming regulatory scheme may strain relations between the regulators and the regulated. At the present time, new drug applications require some 5 to 7 years to process to completion, despite long-standing procedures and personnel both within the FDA and the drug industry who are thoroughly familiar with these rules and procedures. Massive increases in staff and budget will be required by the FDA's Bureau of Medical Devices and Diagnostic Products just to handle the volume of paperwork required for a premarket approval application. Although the intraocular lens has the shortest grandfather rights period of any of the class III medical devices now on the market, large numbers of other devices presently on the market must comply with the requirements of the new legislation by May 28, 1979. When one considers the number of new medical devices falling into category III being prepared for marketing by manufacturers, it is apparent that the Bureau of Medical Devices and Diagnostic Products will be faced with an avalanche of premarket approval applications for both new and existing medical devices within a short time after passage of the new act. If these difficulties were not enough, the Bureau of Medical Devices and Diagnostic Products was shorthanded at the time the act was passed; given the best of intentions and effort by the FDA, it is most questionable that staff in adequate numbers and qualifications can be added to the Bureau of Medical Devices and Diagnostic Products in time to process and approve submitted premarket approval applications for intraocular lenses by December 28, 1977, let alone other class III devices 18 months thereafter.

Some administrative flexibility exists in the length of time a device such as the intraocular lens may be subject to an exemption for investigational use.[35] By continuing a device in an investigational status beyond expiration of the grandfather rights period, additional time may be provided to process and approve the premarket approval application. Unfortunately, any widespread use of this tactic will only result in an even more massive jam of unprocessed premarket approval applications as time goes on than otherwise would have occurred. Therefore this expedient appears to be of limited utility.

The objectives of the Medical Devices Amendment Act, to provide safer and more reliable medical devices for the public, are laudable and have attracted wide support from industry, medicine, and the public. It would be wry, indeed, if this legislation resulted instead in a diminution of the quality of medical care available to Americans because of inflexible procedures and deadlines written into law. Some concern has been voiced by alarmed individuals that the Medical Devices Amendment Act will effectively shut down, by mid-1979, at least that portion of the medical device industry responsible for the innovation and manufacture of the most sophisticated new products.

Although the new federal legislation and the role of the FDA has attracted the most attention, the states have not been precluded from regulatory role regarding medical devices. The secretary of Health, Education, and Welfare has the express power to publish regulations allowing states or localities to impose more stringent requirements on medical devices than those required by federal law.[36]

Certain key decisions must be made, principally by FDA officials, in 1977 and 1978. These decisions will have a fundamental bearing upon the availability, sophistication, and cost of all medical devices both to the medical profession and its patients. Because it has the shortest grandfather rights period, the intraocular lens seems likely to be the guinea pig upon which most initial experiments in the workability of the medical legislation will be performed.

What then is the future likely to hold for the intraocular lens manufacturer, the surgeon, and, most important, the patient? Prognosticating is a risky business, particularly at so early a stage in the life of significant new legislation; nevertheless, unresolved questions that will have a major bearing on the impact of the legislation may be discerned. They include:

1. To what extent will the FDA regulate the selection and qualifications of surgeons chosen by manufacturers as "investigators" on or before December 28, 1977? How extensively will the FDA monitor the activities of these investigators, and what standards will it adopt to disapprove or disqualify an investigator?

Only tentative answers to these questions have been forthcoming. The FDA's Ophthalmic Panel has recommended that investigators be licensed ophthalmologists in addition to having served a residency in ophthalmology; the selection, the panel contends, should otherwise be made by the manufacturer. No modification of this position has, at this writing, been proposed by the FDA. Direct intrusion by the FDA into the qualifications of surgeons electing to perform an intraocular lens implant obviously is an exceedingly sensitive matter. In view of the imminence of required premarket approval applications, the FDA simply may elect not to move into this area to any measurably important degree at this time as a result of other administrative burdens and the certainty of virulent opposition from the medical profession.

If the FDA elects to act in this area, it might very well require a review of the qualifications and selection of investigators selected by manufacturers prior to their approval by the FDA. The extent of FDA scrutiny would in all likelihood be limited initially to ascertaining an investigator's biographical data with the assurance that general intraocular lens experience, such as that recommended by the FDA Ophthalmic Panel, would suffice as qualification of an investigator. But inherent in such a scheme is the authority to criticize or reject a surgeon's qualifications or the selection process itself, a development that would place a federal administrative agency directly in position to determine who may perform a specific surgical procedure. The only limitation on the exercise of the FDA's power would then appear to be the restriction that its authority may not be arbitrarily or capriciously excercised.

2. How closely will the FDA pattern premarket approval applications on the new drug application model.

The recent developments in premarket applications for devices indicate that the drug application model will be closely assimilated. To date, the FDA has proposed guidelines for good manufacturing practices (GMP) and good laboratory practices (GLP). A vast reporting system is currently in draft form and is expected to be implemented. The proposed GMP's and GLP's suggest that the FDA considers medical devices on the same level as drugs. Unfortunately, the closer the approximation of premarket approval applications to new drug applications, the greater will be the time required to process and approve such lengthy documents.

3. How willing will Congress be to appropriate funds for the hundreds of new staff positions needed for the FDA's Bureau of Medical Devices and Diagnostic Products if it is to process the anticipated flood of claimed exemptions for investigational use and premarket approval applications by May 1979?

Any effort to predict congressional action can be an invitation to error. However, the absence of a concerted plan to staff and fund the needs posed by the new Medical Devices Amendment Act bodes ill for an orderly approach to lessening the impact of the legislative mandate that premarket approval applications be effectuated not later than May 28, 1979.

4. What methods, if any, will be devised to ease the financial burden on small manufacturers of preparing exhaustive premarket approval applications, which may cost upwards of $1 million to compile? Will the result be to confine new medical device pioneering to an oligopoly of large, heavily capitalized manufacturers?

The costs of complying with the new legislation are sure to condemn a significant percentage of small firms to failure or withdrawal from the market. To another important segment of the industry, increased costs will make business operation significantly less profitable and therefore less desirable. Entry of new firms into the medical device industry will undoubtedly decrease.

This ominous note has been struck by many small manufacturers who have stressed the legislation's impact on their ability to survive. To lessen this impact, the Medical Devices Amendment Act provided for an office to give technical and other nonfinancial assistance to small manufacturers. The FDA is also considering the payment of attorney's fees for participation in its hearings and proceedings. While these aids may alleviate some of the strain, a small manufacturer will still incur major costs in amassing the reports necessary for a premarket application that may be beyond its ability to fund. It is doubtful that present or predictable FDA methods will satisfactorily resolve the problem of financial assistance to small manufacturers.

5. Will the public become aware of the implications (both as to cost and availability of medical devices) of extended processing of premarket approval applications by the FDA? If so, will public awareness of these problems generate remedial legislation?

It is certain that the public will experience one impact of the medical device amendments through increased costs of medical care. It is also certain that the application process will slow or interrupt the delivery of existing and new medical devices. Fortunately, events surrounding the enactment of the Medical Devices Amendment Act have amply demonstrated the responsiveness of government to active participation by the medical profession and the public.

NOTES

1. Food and Drug Act, June 30, 1906, c. 3915, 34 Stat. 768.
2. Food and Drug Act, June 30, 1906, c. 3915, ss. 3-5, 34 Stat. 768.
3. *Weeks* v. *United States* (1917) 245 U. S. 620; *United States* v. *Sweet Valley Wine Co.* (1913) 208 F. 85; *United States* v. *Seventy-Four Cases of Grape Juice* (1910) 181 F. 629.
4. Food, Drug, and Cosmetic Act, June 25, 1938, c. 675, 52 Stat. 1040.
5. 21 U. S. C. ss. 321 (p), 355.
6. The FDA, which was charged with administration of this act, was transferred from the U.S. Department of Agriculture to the Federal Security Agency in 1940, and then to the newly established Department of Health, Education, and Welfare in 1953.
7. *United States* v. *23 Articles, etc.* (1951) 192 F. 2d 308.
8. *United States* v. *6 Devices "Electrical Mechanical Heart"* (1941) 38 F. Supp. 236.

9. *United States* v. *4 Devices, Labelled in Part "Colortherm"* (1949) 176 F. 2d 652.
10. 21 U. S. C. ss. 331, 352.
11. *Amp, Inc.* v. *Gardner* (1968) 389 F. 2d 825.
12. 21 U. S. C. ss. 321 (g) (1), 321 (b).
13. *United States* v. *Bacto-Unidisk* (1969) 394 U. S. 784.
14. *Orthopedic Equipment Co. Inc.* v. *Eustler* (1960) 276, F. 2d 455.
15. *Savage* v. *Jones* (1912) 225 U. S. 501; *Sligh* v. *Kirkwood* (1915) 237 U. S. 52; *Weigle* v. *Curtice Bros. Co.* (1919) 248 U. S. 285.
16. Sherman Food, Drug, and Cosmetic Act, s. 26000 et seq., Health and Safety Code.
17. Health and Safety Code s. 26670.
18. Health and Safety Code s. 26680 (d).
19. Health and Safety Code s. 26801.
20. Luminex, Inc., and McGhan Medical.
21. See letter of Victor Asch to Richard Hawkins, October 3, 1975.
22. Government Code s. 11503; Health and Safety Code ss. 26212, 26691.
23. Government Code ss. 11503, 11512.
24. CCP s. 1094.5.
25. CCP s. 1060; Government Code s. 11440; *Charles L. Harvey, Inc.,* v. *Contractors' State License Board* (1952) 39 C. 2d 561, 564.
26. CCP ss. 526 (2), 527; *Conover* v. *Hall* (1974) 11 C. 3d 842, 849.50.
27. Order of Honorable Norman R. Dowds, December 8, 1975, Case # C 133877, Superior Court of California, County of Los Angeles.
28. Public Law 94-295, 90 Stat. 539.
29. Public Law 94-295, 90 Stat. 575 s. 201 (h) F.
30. *Federal Register,* vol. 41, no. 67.
31. 90 Stat 573, s. 520 (1).
32. 90 Stat 577, s. 501.
33. 90 Stat 574, s. 520 (1).
34. 90 Stat 574, s. 520 (1).
35. 90 Stat 569, s. 520 (g).
36. 90 Stat 574, s. 521 (b).

CHAPTER 16

Future of pseudophakos surgery

Ophthalmology is a dynamic specialty in which innovations in surgical techniques occur rapidly. It is therefore difficult to predict with confidence the future of intraocular implant surgery. Before considering the future prospects, it is important to establish the current position of the intraocular implant lens as seen by most observers.

ADVANTAGES

1. In uncomplicated cases the quality of vision far exceeds that of a routine cataract extraction corrected with spectacles.
2. For those unable to manage a contact lens (elderly, arthritics, Parkinsonians, hemiplegics, mentally retarded, and so on), intraocular implant lens surgery is often the procedure of choice.
3. In a patient with bilateral cataracts, unilateral intraocular implant lens surgery may be adequate for the patient's needs.
4. The patient with a successfully implanted intraocular lens in one eye usually is more mobile than a patient who is bilaterally aphakic and wearing spectacles.
5. Long-wear contact lenses are still unproven.

DISADVANTAGES

1. The surgery is technically more difficult than a routine cataract extraction.
2. The rate of complications is greater, although only slightly greater, according to present knowledge. This varies with the skill of the surgeon.
3. Some complications associated with both intraocular implant lens surgery and routine cataract extraction are more serious with the former, for example, flat or shallow anterior chamber and retinal detachment.
4. Closer follow-up care, both short- and long-term, is required, especially if we are to assess the risks and advantages of intraocular lenses.
5. Colleague resistance. Complications are more severely criticized and more likely to lead to litigation, even though this may be unjustified.
6. Dependence on quality manufacturing.

CURRENT POSITION

1. Intraocular implant lens surgery should be performed only after adequate training.
2. For less experienced surgeons, the initial indications should be extremely conservative.
3. Surgery should be restricted to those not likely to manage a contact lens, in the judgment of the surgeon.
4. Surgery on two eyes within a short time span is unacceptable.
5. The patient's decision to undergo intraocular lens surgery should be based on a reasonable informed consent, which includes the advantages and disadvantages of the procedure as well as alternatives.
6. A surgeon who performs an adequate cataract extraction but feels insecure with the demands of intraocular im-

plant lens surgery or is unconvinced of its benefits is not remiss in not performing intraocular implant lens surgery.

7. There are still breakdowns in good manufacturing processes.

8. The long-range results are still uncertain. There is a need for well-documented retrospective studies.

9. The short-term safety is still controversial. There is a need for well-controlled prospective studies.

10. It is inevitable that the current position will change in the future.

FUTURE

The future of intraocular implant lens surgery will be determined by many factors. Some of these are now considered.

Safety and efficacy of intraocular lenses. Efficacy has been accepted by most ophthalmologists, but there remains considerable controversy over the safety of the intraocular implant lens. There have occurred several instances of intraocular infection and severe intraocular inflammation as a result of poor quality control by manufacturers. Hopefully, this will be remedied by the new federal devices legislation. The long-range safety of intraocular lenses has not yet been firmly established. Although intraocular lenses have enjoyed increased success over the past 20 years, there have occurred many important modifications in implant design and in the techniques of their implantation so that long-range studies of a single implant and its technique of implantation are virtually nonexistent.

Reasonable guidelines for indications and contraindications for intraocular implant lens surgery. This is a formidable task. It is very difficult to get surgeons to agree on who should undergo what is still considered by some to be a controversial procedure. As a result of experience, there have emerged several well-defined indications and contraindications for this surgery. Some surgeons tend to be more aggressive and some more conservative. Obviously they will differ in their guidelines. However, surgeons of good conscience consider the needs and welfare of their patients to be the overriding factor in their approach to implant surgery. They will carefully analyze the data presented by investigators of good reputation. There have been comprehensive reports presented in the past, and it is certain there will be a much greater number presented in the future. Out of these will emerge a reasonable set of guidelines for indications and contraindications acceptable to the profession.

Surgical training. The success of intraocular implant lens surgery depends greatly on the skill of the surgeon. Therefore it is mandatory that surgical training be given a high priority. Surgeons experienced in this technique must accept the responsibility for teaching their colleagues. Surgical instruction courses must be updated. A minimum requirement is the inclusion of practice surgery using the surgical microscope. Surgical education must be designed to meet the needs of the resident ophthalmologist and the ophthalmologist beyond the residency level. The former has the advantage of incorporating intraocular implant lens surgery into the overall structure of surgical education available in any accredited program. Many residency programs include implant surgery, and many more will surely do so in the future. The graduate ophthalmologist must seek his own instruction course. In the future more courses must be available and their content continually upgraded.

Community study groups. An excellent format for data collection exists in community study groups. Ophthalmologists in each community should be encouraged to register their implant patients with a central registry and have all patients examined annually by an assigned third party. The results may be reported at an annual professional meeting. This encourages community surgeons to adhere to reasonable guidelines and promotes a healthy atmosphere for mutual assistance at surgery and exchange of information. This approach has proved invaluable in the Miami community (Chapter 14).

Manufacturers' quality control. The ophthalmologist should remain the watchdog over the industry. He should not fall prey to the "buyer beware" philosophy. There is a wide variance in quality implants among the present manufacturers. Defects should be quickly reported. In the future the manufacturer will be closely supervised by the Food and Drug Administration of the U.S. Department of Health, Education, and Welfare. Provisions for this have been included in the new devices legislation that became law in 1976. Uniform methods of sterilization for all implants will become a reality. The trend is toward gas sterilization and away from the Frederick Ridley caustic soda method (Chapter 7).

Role of national implant organizations. Every surgeon who performs intraocular implant lens surgery should join the American Intra-Ocular Implant Society. This organization, currently consisting of well over 1000 members, plays an important role in disseminating the latest trends in implant surgery and provides a warning system for its members in the event of faulty design or contamination of implants. It has proven its worth in the past and should be invaluable in the future. The International Intraocular Implant Club is a smaller group with a limited membership. Therefore it cannot maintain a direct relationship with all implant surgeons. It has educational and advisory functions. Membership in a national society is particularly useful for implant surgeons in rural areas. In addition to being apprised of programs in lens implant surgery, they are placed in contact with experienced surgeons in the event of surgical complications.

Improvement in contact lens technology. Increasing sophistication in contact lens technology is likely to occur in the future. If long-wear contact lenses become successful, the surgeon will be faced with the dilemma of choosing between intraocular lens implant surgery or routine cataract surgery with long-wear contact lens correction. To date, long-wear contact lenses are still unproven.

Type of cataract extraction. The current controversy between proponents of the intracapsular and extracapsular cataract extractions promises to continue in the future. Hopefully, data will become available that will determine whether the incidence of postoperative retinal detachment and cystoid macular edema is favorably influenced by an extracapsular extraction. At the same time, data will accumulate as to the frequency of failure to localize small retinal breaks because of the retained capsular membrane and whether postoperative discission to improve visual acuity negates the value of the extracapsular extraction.

Secondary implantation. An equally heated exchange promises to highlight the future concerning the safety of the Choyce Mark VIII anterior chamber angle-supported implant in secondary implantations. The popularity of this concept is directly attributable to the frequent failure of patient acceptance of the spectacle-corrected aphakic situation. The safety of this concept will be determined in the future.

Federal activity. Ophthalmologists will be involved with intraocular lens manufacturers during a period of clinical evaluation of intraocular lenses by the Food and Drug Administration. At this time the scope and duration of the study are uncertain. In addition, the National Eye Institute will be involved in a retrospective and controlled prospective study of intraocular lenses.

SUMMARY

It appears incredible that nearly 30 years have passed since Ridley implanted his first posterior chamber lens. The past has been marked by heated controversy and numerous crises. The future promises more of the same.

Index

R